The Comprehensive Handbook of
BEHAVIORAL MEDICINE

Volume 3:
Extended Applications & Issues

The Comprehensive Handbook of
BEHAVIORAL MEDICINE

Volume 3:
Extended Applications & Issues

Edited by

James M. Ferguson, M.D.
Medical Director, Gifford Mental Health Center
Assistant Professor of Psychiatry
University of California, San Diego School of Medicine
and Department of Psychiatry, VA Hospital, La Jolla

and

C. Barr Taylor, M.D.
Assistant Professor of Psychiatry
Stanford University Medical Center
Stanford, California

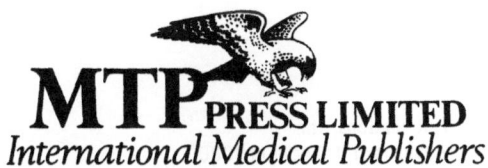

MTP PRESS LIMITED
International Medical Publishers

Published in the UK and Europe by
MTP Press Limited
Falcon House
Lancaster, England

Published in the US by
SPECTRUM PUBLICATIONS, INC.
175-20 Wexford Terrace
Jamaica, N.Y. 11432

ISBN-13: 978-94-011-6292-0   e-ISBN- 13:978-94-011-6290-6
DOI: 10.1007/978-94-011-6292-0

Contributors

W. STEWART AGRAS, M.D.
Laboratory for the Study of
  Behavioral Medicine
Department of Psychiatry and
  Behavioral Sciences
Stanford University School
  of Medicine
Stanford, California

BRUCE L. BIRD, Ph.D.
Department of Psychology
University of New Orleans
and
Hope Haven Institution
Marrero, Louisiana

DALE A. CALLNER, Ph.D.
The Children's Center
Kearns, Utah

EDWARD G. CARR, Ph.D.
Department of Psychology
State University of New York
  at Stony Brook
Stony Brook, New York

MICHAEL F. CATALDO, Ph.D.
Behavioral Psychology
John F. Kennedy Institute
  for Handicapped Children
Johns Hopkins University
  School of Medicine
Baltimore, Maryland

**EDWARD R.
  CHRISTOPHERSEN, Ph.D.**
Department of Pediatrics
The University of
  Kansas Medical Center
College of Health Sciences
  and Hospital
Kansas City, Kansas

**JACQUELINE M.
  DUNBAR Ph.D., R.N.**
Laboratory for the Study
  of Behavioral Medicine
Department of Psychiatry
  and Behavioral Sciences
Stanford University School
  of Medicine
Stanford, California

K. ANTHONY EDWARDS, Ph.D.
Human Services Program
North Kentucky University
Highlands Height, Kentucky

LEONARD H. EPSTEIN, Ph.D.
Department of Psychiatry
University of Pittsburgh School of
Medicine
Pittsburgh, Pennsylvania

JOHN W. FARQUHAR, M.D.
Stanford Heart Disease
Prevention Program
Stanford University
School of Medicine
Stanford, California

JAMES FERGUSON, M.D.
Department of Psychiatry
School of Medicine
University of California, San Diego
San Diego, California

ROBERT G. HALL, Ph.D.
Veterans Administration Hospital
Palo Alto, California

SHARON M. HALL, Ph.D.
Department of Psychology
California State University
San Francisco, California

FREDERICK J. HEIDE, Ph.D.
Department of Psychiatry
University of California,
Davis, Medical Center
Sacramento, California

O. IVAR LOVASS, Ph.D.
Department of Psychology
University of California,
Los Angeles
Los Angeles, California

ALFRED L. McALISTER, Ph.D.
School of Public Health
Harvard University
Cambridge, Massachusetts

MICHAEL J. MAHONEY, Ph.D.
Department of Psychology
Pennsylvania State University
University Park, Pennsylvania

JO A. MURRAY, Ph.D.
Department of Psychology
Ohio State University
Columbus, Ohio

JOYCE D. NASH, Ph.D.
Weight Watchers of
Northern California, Inc.
San Francisco, California

TERRY F. PECHACEK, Ph.D.
Laboratory of Physiological Hygiene
Department of Psychology
University of Minnesota
Minneapolis, Minnesota

MICHAEL A. RAPOFF, M.S., ED.
Department of Psychology
University of Kansas
Lawrence, Kansas

STEVEN M. ROSS, Ph.D.
Department of Psychiatry
Veterans Administration Hospital
Salt Lake City, Utah

DENNIS C. RUSSO, Ph.D.
Department of Behavioral Psychology
Children's Hospital Medical Center
Harvard Medical School
Boston, Massachusetts

LINDA C. SOBELL, Ph.D.
Behavioral Intervention
  Research Addiction
  Research Foundation
Toronto, Ontario
Canada

MARK B. SOBELL, Ph.D.
Sociobehavioral Treatment
  Research Addiction
  Research Foundation
Toronto, Ontario
  Canada

JAMES W. SMITH, M.D.
Schick's Shadel Hospital
Seattle, Washington

CRAIG BARR TAYLOR, M.D.
Laboratory for the Study
  of Behavioral Medicine
Department of Psychiatry
  and Behavioral Sciences
Stanford University School
  of Medicine
Stanford, California

JAMES W. VARNI, Ph.D.
Division of Hematology-Oncology
Children's Hospital of Los Angeles
Los Angeles, California

BRIAN T. YATES, Ph.D.
Department of Psychology
The American University
Washington, D. C.

Preface

Many of the greatest strides in medical care have neither been glamorous nor made the front page of *The New York Times*. They have been simple measures such as sanitation, immunization, and provision of clean, wholesome food. And even more glamorous medical breakthroughs and techniques like heart transplants are often last-ditch responses to largely preventable medical problems that required a lifetime to develop. Changing those life styles which may cause, worsen, or exacerbate disease and utilizing current medical knowledge may be the most important strides medicine will make in the next few decades. To meet this challenge, techniques have already been developed to change eating and nutritional patterns that may lead to obesity and heart disease. In addition, interventions are being developed for a wide variety of medical problems. Many of these techniques are based on behavioral principles.

Several years ago, one of the editors of this book gave a behavioral medicine seminar for psychiatry residents concerning behavioral principles and their application to medicine. As the seminar developed, it became evident that many of the important articles on the subject were scattered throughout a wide body of literature, which encompassed a variety of disciplines and journals. No single source was available to provide the state of the art of this emerging field. This book was spawned, in part, as an attempt to overcome this deficit. We wanted to provide a handbook to help health-care practitioners understand and use behavioral techniques appropriate to their areas of interest. However, we also wanted to develop a handbook that would be useful to researchers. To reach both audiences we decided to include a wide range of chapters, some focusing on practical and clinical issues, others focusing on theoretical or technical issues. We encouraged the contributors to speculate about future directions in their areas of specialty. We also decided to include several sections on basic physiology, to illustrate the potential for change in several systems.

Our contributors have been patient and supportive. They have watched as pages of "golden prose" disappeared under the hand of heavy editing. Many made last-minute additions to make their material as up-to-date as possible. And, we have been impressed with the many changes our contributors have undergone in their lives. Some have moved or received promotions, new degrees, and a variety of honors. They have married and divorced, had children, suffered the deaths of loved ones, and died themselves. Especially in light of these many personal changes, we thank them for their help.

We have also been impressed with the tremendous changes in the field of behavioral medicine. Since the field will undoubtedly continue to change, we intend to add volumes to the Comprehensive Handbook to keep it as up-to-date as possible.

In this work, we would like to acknowledge the help of many individuals. We received editorial assistance from Patricia Benefiel, Ph.D., and Francis Filloux, and many suggestions about content from our colleagues. The manuscript has been typed, retyped, and re-retyped tirelessly by Dottie Pakus. Tome Tomisawa has also helped enormously with preparation of the book. The project has been generously supported by a grant from the Janss Foundation, which helped with the multiple and miscellaneous expenses associated with manuscript preparation, and psychologically supported by the enthusiasm of the Foundation's President, Mr. Joseph Legett.

Introduction

The third volume of the *Comprehensive Handbook of Behavioral Medicine* addresses important issues and techniques in behavioral medicine related to prevention, compliance, addiction, rehabilitation, cost-effectiveness, pediatrics, geriatrics, chronic disease, maintenance, and mass media intervention. As such, it completes our comprehensive description of the state of the art in this field.

In the first volume, behavioral medicine is defined as the systematic application of behavioral analysis and behavior therapy techniques to medical problems. In the introduction to Volume 1, the process of behavioral analysis is described and basic behavioral principles are defined. These include respondent and operant conditioning; discriminative stimuli; positive and negative reinforcement; extinction and shaping; aversion, avoidance, and escape learning; and a variety of cognitive behavioral procedures. The behavioral therapy techniques which derive from these principles are also described: relaxation, systematic desensitization, environmental structuring with and without token economies, assertion training, modeling, feedback techniques, contingency contracting, stimulus control, and procedures for enhancing the effectiveness of information.

The first volume contains sections on the cardiovascular, central nervous, psycho-endocrine, genitourinary, and musculoskeletal systems. Each of these sections contains a group of chapters which summarize the relevant behavioral medicine literature.

In the second volume the application of behavioral principles to syndromes and symptom complexes is discussed. These include the eating disorders and a variety of gastrointestinal symptoms, pain, asthma, skin disorders, and habits.

Among these topics are the most thoroughly researched, and most completely developed clinical applications of behavioral medicine.

In the third volume of the *Handbook,* a series of chapters which do not fit into either the organ system, symptom, or syndrome outline used for Volumes 1 or 2 are grouped together. This volume presents a discussion of extended issues and other applications of behavioral technology to medical care. For many of these chapters, authors discuss relatively narrow topics, belonging to larger areas. For example, Edwards has limited his discussion of the elderly to behavioral approaches to nursing home care, rather than the general plight and treatment of problems in a geriatric population. A complete review of geriatric problems and their treatment would be premature; his work with nursing homes is widely applicable at this stage of development. For other topic areas, for example, the behavioral and treatment of addictions, several volumes could be devoted to lengthy descriptions and discussions. In this case, chapters are limited to relatively narrow topics.

Pediatrics: Although much of the basic human research in applied psychology has used a grade school population, behavioral research in pediatric medicine is sparse. For this text, two examples were chosen. Christophersen and Rapoff point out that much of normal pediatric medical practice involves giving advice, counsel, and simple instruction about psychological and developmental problems, a process which requires a large amount of practitioner time. If primary prevention can be enhanced by the use of clear, written guidelines for handling simple, common behavioral problems, fewer secondary treatment programs for disturbed children may be needed.

To discuss the behavioral analysis and treatment of well-defined maladaptive behaviors, this volume includes one of the initial behavioral problems to receive systematic behavioral analysis, with a complete description of discriminative stimuli and operant factors which maintained the behavioral pattern. Although the disorders discussed by Russo, Lovaas, et al., are unusual, future research can look to the basic findings with these children and apply the technology to similar disorders in children and adults. When the application of behavioral medicine principles to developmental and pediatric problems is viewed in its entirety, and the possibility of generalizing programs developed for other populations, for example weight control, are applied to children, the greatest potential impact of behavioral medicine may be found. Prevention of many chronic disorders, such as obesity, hypertension, drug addiction, and possibly heart disease should begin with this age group.

Aging: Current demographic surveys indicate that the percentage of elderly people in our society is increasing rapidly. At the present time, the medical profession has little to offer the "senile," the chronically infirm, and the socially isolated elderly. Often, these individuals are "warehoused" until they die. Edwards describes the use of behavioral analysis and treatment with this population. Operant techniques have been shown to be useful in training the senile to take care of themselves and to engage in social behaviors. He points out, "nursing homes, developed as cheap alternatives to hospitals, have become poor alternatives to living." This trend can be reversed by changing the basic structure of nursing homes by providing opportunities for the staff to interact with the patients, restructuring staff duties and by changing reinforcement patterns for staff and patient behaviors. Systematic environmental changes, for example, provision of a roommate, social activity programs with cues or reminders to take part in them, and reality orientation can markedly alleviate some of the symptoms of senility. In this population, outcome is not assessed by "cure," but in terms of quality of remaining lifetime. The return to sociability after seclusion to a back room because of sloppy eating habits or lack of toilet training can be considered a major achievement in most nursing home situations.

Chronic Disorders: The chapter on chronic disorders by Cataldo, et al., emphasizes that large numbers of individuals currently suffer from chronic disorders and that in the future, as our population ages, more people with a variety of age-related chronic disorders will need care. The cost of care for these disorders to society and to the individual patient is large. Treatment strategies for the prevention and remediation of these conditions are urgently needed. Currently, a combination of medical and behavioral treatment appears to be most appropriate. These approaches are similar in many ways; both require a detailed history with specific reference to exacerbations, remissions, antecedent events, and apparent reinforcing environmental events with clearly specified treatment goals and outcome possibilities. The authors present three chronic disorders in some detail, in order to illustrate the application of behavioral technology to chronic medical disorders. In each of these disorders, health "skills" can be taught to patients to allow them to reduce their consequences of the disorders.

Cognitive Strategies: In the last few years, operant psychologists have begun looking at the world of cognitions. Heide and Mahoney discuss the application of cognitive strategies to medical disorders. They describe several therapies, including those based on cognitive learning theories and covert conditioning techniques. To date, the application of covert or cognitive techniques have been limited to headaches, Type A behaviors, alcoholism, and obesity. In each case, there has been significant influence by these techniques. Although these procedures are relatively weak, research into cognitive therapy with depressed populations indicates that there may be ways to increase the effectiveness of such procedures.

Compliance: Dunbar and Agras provide an extensive review of the problem of compliance with medical instructions. The problem of poor adherence to medical regimens has been well documented and, in some cases, the percentage of noncompliant patients is extemely high. For individual patients, the results of the failure to receive benefit from health programs and medications are obvious. From a larger viewpoint, it is impossible to monitor treatment efficacy, safety, and side effects without knowing the rate of compliance to drug prescription or other therapeutic instructions. Studies in this area are too recent to know long-term outcome for various intervention strategies. The technology which has been developed, stresses factors such as clinic organization, methods and schedule of medication administration, the quality of patient/physician interaction, inter-actions with other staff members, and patient health care benefits. Although it is still not clear why patients fail to follow treatment advice, answers are beginning to emerge, and the technology is beginning to be developed to change the course of poor adherence.

Maintenance: Hall and Hall discuss one of the more difficult areas in behavioral medicine, maintaining change. The technology has been developed to change habits in the area of addictive behaviors, to change health-seeking behaviors, and to intervene in parent-child and parent-parent interactions. Follow-up indicates that, in many cases, these behavior changes are not maintained over time. Relapse, for example, in the case of an alcoholic, can be precipitated by stimulus conditions, for example, having alcoholic friends that continue to drink and no *non-alcoholic* friends. Relapse can also be caused by biological pressures, for example, a childhood-onset obese individual who manages to lose weight, or from external reinforcement, for example, a child who finds the only way to gain attention with her family is to starve herself. The authors review the literature of maintenance and point out that some technology is currently available which appears to increase the probability of maintaining change. This includes booster sessions, which need not be either frequent or extensive, making follow-up visits as much like treatment as possible, and continued concern on the part of the therapist. The simplicity of these recommendations, they point out, reflects the state of the art.

Cost Effectiveness: In an era of increased accountability and mounting pressure to spend health care dollars in an efficient, effective way, it is necessary to look at the technology for determining cost effectiveness. Yates explores this seldom talked about, and less often understood, area in some detail. Behavioral medicine offers one way to institute preventive measures that may reduce health care costs. Cost effectiveness, cost benefit, and cost utility analysis provide the methodology for comparing new programs with traditional ones.

Addictions: If Americans would stop overeating, smoking, and abusing ad-dicting substances, the resulting changes in mortality and morbidity from disease, and consequent decreases in the cost of health care would be significant. The area of addictions is a broad one in which definition is not clear. The use of harmful substances are more common in our society now than at any time. More than nine million people are considered to be alcoholics; six percent of high school seniors consume alcohol each day. Despite massive media campaigns designed to educate the public about the dangers of smoking, the absolute number of smokers remains constant as younger individuals replace the older ones who quit. The use of narcotics and related substances has leveled off at a very high rate, especially among the younger age group. This high rate of substance abuse would be further increased if iatrogenic addiction to minor tranquilizers, pain killers, and hypnotics were included.

The treatment of alcoholics is difficult, frustrating, and often unrewarding. Perhaps nowhere in the behavioral literature do treatment philosophies collide head on more resoundingly than in the area of alcohol studies. This section begins with a discussion by Sobell and Sobell of their treatment approach, "nonproblem" drinking; their data show that some alcoholics can learn to control their drinking and maintain this control for a considerable time. Although success is not universal, the results, appear promising. At the other extreme, many clinicians and researchers feel that abstinence is the mainstay of alcohol treatment. Most traditional clinical programs and Alcoholics Anonymous with its related programs, have proven their worth. The chapter by Smith discusses two traditional programs, the Schick program which uses aversive conditioning and Alcoholics Anonymous.

Although it would appear to be a relatively simple, easily defined behavior, drug abuse involves a complex series of activities that extend beyond the use of narcotics. It includes drug seeking, environmental interactions of the addict with others, and the development of coping skills in a usually hostile drug oriented world, in addition to the drug use and consequent pleasurable state. Callner and Ross discuss the problem of addiction in terms of respondent and operant conditioning, with positive and negative reinforcement under a variety of schedules, multiple environmental discriminative stimuli all combined with peer pressure, biological responses to a drug, modeling, threatened exclusion and punishment—all of which in addition play an important role in determining the narcotic habit. Although, as with alcoholism, many types of treatment have been used in an attempt to free people of drug abuse habits, it appears that a combination of techniques devoted to eliminating each link in the behavioral chain leading to drug taking is most effective. Despite extended behavioral analyses, and many interventions, these programs unfortunately have not matched up to the enthusiasm of their designers.

A final area of addiction research describes the habit of smoking and its effective control. Although the inclusion of smoking among the addictions may be controversial, the outcome is hardly different from the others. Pechacek and McAlister present a comprehensive review of the currently available behavioral technologies which have proven useful in the short run for helping individuals stop smoking. Unfortunately, for the majority, these techniques have a high recidivism rate at one year of follow-up. Their own work in the areas of prevention, community-wide programs, and media programs are most exciting.

A detailed behavioral analysis of the behaviors which initiate the smoking habit may be most fruitful in defining an optimal time when a behavioral intervention will be maximally effective, instead of concentrating on the habit once it is firmly established.

Dentistry: Dental problems have received scant attention in the area of preventive medicine. Murray and Epstein discuss the acquisition of oral hygiene skills. They summarize the literature which describes basic research in compliance with dental instructions, and the unique technology that has been developed to monitor dental habits. Toothbrushing represents a habit pattern that responds to instruction, cueing, and operant techniques, and as such can serve as a model for behavioral interventions in other disease processes where health care habits need to be developed to prevent pathological processes from occurring.

Preventive Medicine Programs: The final chapter in this volume describes the application of behavioral medicine technology to a total community. Nash and Farquhar describe their experiment using three communities, each of which had 15,000 inhabitants. They systematically provided behavioral techniques to reduce cardiac risk, using the mass media and face-to-face intervention for high risk individuals. With exquisite attention to a variety of dependent variables, statistical analysis, and follow-up technology, they were able to demonstrate a significant reduction in cardiovascular risk in the city where intensive instruction in addition to mass media interventions were provided. This type of behavioral intervention for establishing a preventive medicine program may be one of the major advances of the behavioral medicine movement. Through the use of preventive techniques, the need for secondary and tertiary treatment facilities may be reduced, the quality of life increased, and the cost of care markedly minimized. Since the initial publication of their studies, a replication in Finland has been carried out, and the authors are in the process or replicating their own work in larger population groups in the United States.

Contents

The Comprehensive Handbook of
BEHAVIORAL MEDICINE

Volume 3:
Extended Applications & Issues

Introduction To
Pediatric Strategies

Much of the basic human research in the applied behavioral sciences has been devoted to the study and treatment of children. Unfortunately, in the field of behavioral medicine, the behavioral research on pediatric problems is sparse with the exceptions of enuresis and self-injury.

The chapter on biosocial pediatrics discusses the interface between pediatric practice and psychological issues that arise in normal development. The authors point out that perhaps as much as 85% of a normal pediatric practice is spent giving advice, guidance, and counseling about psychological and developmental problems. To minimize the time needed by health givers to provide this service, the authors have developed a series of guides and associated materials to be given to parents. For instance, they offer written guidelines for handling common behavioral problems such as bedtime crying, temper tantrums, dressing oneself, inappropriate use of automobile car seats, and toilet training. The area of biosocial pediatrics goes beyond the specific treatment of pathology by a pediatrician and helps in the area of prevention. For example, each of the behavioral problems mentioned above is a potential point of conflict between parent and child which can be avoided by preparing the parents in advance and teaching them how to train their children in a nontraumatic, nonthreatening way.

The second chapter in this section, Self-Injury in Pediatric Populations, is an extension of earlier work by Lovaas et al. which describes behavioral treatment for this group of unfortunate children. Self-injurious activity is one of the most striking behavioral aberrations. Children who self-injure may bite their fingers off, gouge their eyes out, or repeatedly bang their heads against the wall until losing consciousness or creating severe brain damage. A wealth of basic research has shown that many of these behaviors are under operant control, and that appropriate treatment strategies to end the reinforcement for the behavior and to substitute alternative behaviors provide an effective treatment. In other cases, such as Lesch-Nyhan Syndrome, the behavior appears to be superimposed on a genetic component but is still modifiable by behavioral techniques. Although the disorders discussed by Russo et al. are unusual, they can be specified and quantified precisely, which makes them excellent "model" disorders to test behavioral hypotheses and behavioral control techniques. Future research can apply basic findings in these children to other pediatric disorders, and possibly to disorders in adults.

Other pediatric problems are discussed in detail elsewhere in this volume. Drabman presents data about obesity in children and suggests treatment strategies. Thoreson and Coates discuss the problem of obesity in adolescents and indicate several encouraging interventions in an otherwise discouraging field. Cataldo et al. discuss chronic disorders in children, including pain, neuromuscular disturbances, and seizure disorders. They provide guidelines for evaluation and treatment strategies that are based on firm experimental evidence. The problems of enuresis and encopresis are discussed in detail by Doleys in the first volume of this text.

It may be in the area of pediatrics that behavioral medicine will eventually have its greatest impact. Prevention of many chronic disorders such as obesity, hypertension, and possibly heart disease should begin in this age group. The chapters in this section are a beginning to developing a literature which hopefully will continue to expand.

CHAPTER 1

Biosocial Pediatrics

Edward R. Christophersen
Michael A. Rapoff

A Task Force on Pediatric Education was established in 1976 by the American Academy of Pediatrics, with the support of ten other clinical and research societies. Released in 1978, the Task Force Report identifed several priorities for pediatric education programs. One of the top priorities was the area of "biosocial pediatrics." This term was chosen to reflect the emphasis that the Task Force felt should be placed on socially influenced pediatric problems. This shift in emphasis in pediatric training programs was long overdue. Anderson (2), in an address to the American Medical Association in 1930, had discussed the relation of pediatrics to child psychology, stating that he was prompted to do so by the "increasing emphasis being placed on methods of child training and problems of adjustment in this age and the many demands that are made on the physician, educator and scientist for information and assistance."

Considerably later, Kagan (35) proposed a cooperative effort by pediatrics and child psychology to aid both in accomplishing their mutual goals. From 1967 on, increasingly more emphasis has been placed on the symbiotic relationship between pediatrics and child psychology. Wright (62, 63) chronicled the changes that had taken place since Anderson's "prophesy" of the impact that psychology could have and was having on pediatrics. In 1969 he wrote of the establishment of the Society of Pediatric Psychologists, which at this writing has over one thousand members, to represent psychologists working with children in "non-psychiatric medical settings."

Salk (52) suggested that the psychologist could assist the pediatrician in the early diagnosis of behavioral and developmental problems, in staying abreast of new developments in the behavioral sciences, and with their knowledge of child-rearing practices. What follows is a relatively brief overview of some of the developments that have taken place between the psychologists' recognition of the need for the kinds of information arising from "biosocial pediatrics" and the formal recognition of such a need by pediatrics. For a much more detailed discussion of the accomplishments of pediatric psychology the reader is referred to the book, *Encyclopedia of Pediatric Psychology,* by Dr. Logan Wright et al. These accomplisments can be, and probably will be, extensively utilized by training programs for biosocial pediatrics.

This chapter presents material in the order of its importance to pediatric health care providers. The topics—prevention, early detection, and common behavior problems—are well within the province of the average pediatrician or family practitioner.

PREVENTION

Brazelton (15) estimates that he spends 85% of a 60- to 70-hour week in a general pediatric practice giving advice, guidance, and counseling about psychological or developmental problems and preventive anticipatory guidance. Under the general consideration of prevention of behavior problems, Christophersen (23) describes a number of points that the pediatrician might cover prenatally as well as during well-child visits in the first few years of life. The notion that behavior problems can be prevented or at least minimized is expressed by both Brazelton and Christophersen, but is as yet unproven. Although there is minimal empirical proof that preventive counseling is of value, the likelihood that this type of counseling is detrimental is remote. The following outline has been used successfully in prenatal classes on parenting. A much more comprehensive description of prevention programs for common childhood behavior problems is included in Becker and Becker (11) and Christophersen (21).

"Preparing For Parenthood"

1. *Select the doctor you want to care for your child before your expected delivery date and schedule at least one appointment with him to discuss any part of health care about which you have questions or concerns.
2. After delivery, make sure that someone teaches both the mother and the father basic caregiving skills such as bathing, diapering, feeding, and dressing the infant. Both parents should experience holding, diapering, feeding, and

---

*© Edward R. Christophersen, 1978.

dressing their infant before discharge from the hospital.

3. If you have help coming to your home after you deliver, ask them to *please* help with household tasks and let you adjust to caring for the new baby.

4. Talk to your baby while you are taking care of him. Use normal speech, not baby talk, and look at his face while talking.

5. Spend time playing with and examining your new baby. Make sure both parents have ample practice with the baby! Be sure to *make time* for this while your baby is rested, fed, and happy.

6. Try to develop standard caregiving routines and, within reason, stick with them. For example, it's a good idea to use the same place and the same procedures each time you diaper or bathe your baby.

7. Try very hard to hold and play with your child when he is quiet and happy instead of waiting for him to cry. Babies learn very quickly which behaviors gain them attention.

8. You will teach your infant something each time that you interact with him, so begin giving attention very early to those things that you want your baby to do.

9. Purchase an infant car seat before your baby is discharged from the hospital and use it on every trip you make in an automobile.

EARLY DETECTION

Christophersen, Rainey, and Leake (24) described a procedure whereby the pediatrician and the pediatric psychologist conduct their interviews simultaneously. They suggested that this procedure helps both professionals to arrive at a diagnosis more effectively than traditional independent evaluations. One part of the procedure has parents describe portions of a typical day. For example, the parents were asked what time the child got up, when he had breakfast, and who selected breakfast. In addition, Christophersen (23) had the clinician ask specific questions about various parent-child interactions during an average day. This type of interview is analogous to a pediatrician's interaction with a parent when examining a child with somatic complaints. For example, if otitis media is suspected, the pediatrician asks about fever, crying, rubbing the suspected ear, sleeplessness, etc., to arrive at a diagnosis of otitis media. For behavior problems, the procedure is similar. The clinician asks specific questions relevant to common problem areas such as bedtime, mealtime, dressing, and compliance. In each case the therapist uses the parent's answers to specific questions to determine whether or not a problem exists. The major difference between the pediatrician conducting an examination for a somatic complaint and a therapist asking questions regarding behavior problems is that the therapist can explore one or several high-probability problem areas during routine well-child visits *before* the parents indicate concern about the child's behavior. The following guideline gives an example of the type of questions used to probe for bedtime problems.

"Early Detection of Behavior Problems"

Guidelines for Health Care Providers

Bedtime Problems. Many parents experience minor behavior problems with their children that they do not tell to their health-care provider. This may be due to a lack of understanding of "normal" behavior, or it may be because they are embarrassed to admit that they might be having "problems." Usually, asking parents if their children have behavioral problems is inadequate, since many parents will give a negative answer.

The following guidelines are designed to assist the health-care provider in determining what problems exist.

1. *Ask specific data-based questions: For example, for bedtime problems you might ask:
   a. What time do you start putting him to bed?
   b. What time is he in bed?
   c. What time is he asleep?
   d. How many times does he awaken during the night?
   e. Where does he sleep?
2. Pursue any of these questions if the parent's answers suggest that a problem exists. For example, if the parents report two and one-half hours for a bedtime routine, ask them how they spend that time and what else they could do during that time.
3. Observe the child during your interview and the physical exam for general compliance.
4. If you think that the parents are having problems with their child, direct your suggestions toward specific information received in response to your questions. For example, tell the parents that there is no need for the bedtime routine to take two and one-half hours, that this is a very common area where parents run into problems, and that you have a set of procedures that the parents can use to make bedtime more pleasant.
5. Request that the parents call your office frequently to leave "progress reports" with your nurse or receptionist. If you are not getting these "progress reports" or if the reports don't seem to indicate much progress, call the parents for more information. If the reports indicate progress, call the parents to encourage them to continue following the procedures.

---

*© Edward R. Christophersen, 1978.

Whether the parent comes to the clinician because of a specific behavior problem or the clinician detects the problem prior to the parent's identification of the problem area, the management is the same. The following section on Common Behavior Problems discusses some problem areas that are commonly encountered by pediatric health services and presents examples of written guidelines for parents suggesting ways in which these problems can be managed.

COMMON BEHAVIOR PROBLEMS

Little systematic research has evaluated the minor behavior problems that are frequently brought to the attention of pediatricians by parents. If untreated, problems such as tantrums, refusal to eat, minor sleep disturbances, etc., can probably cause parent-child conflicts. Several behavioral problems will be briefly discussed and specific guidelines for treating them suggested. These guidelines have evolved over the last few years and are based on experience with over three hundred families seen in a pediatric outpatient clinic. These are the kinds of problems that can be detected early and successfully treated in families where there is no psychopathology.

Bedtime Problems

In a review of sleep disturbances in childhood, Anthony (3) presented a description of these disorders and an estimate of their incidence in child populations. He found that minor disturbances, including restlessness, mumbling, talking, teeth grinding, early or frequent waking, and difficulty in falling asleep, account for 46% of all sleep disturbances in children. Nocturnal enuresis accounted for an additional 26%, while nightmares, night terrors, and sleepwalking accounted for 7%, 2%, and 1% respectively. The most frequent sleep-related problems are those which are "minor." (The more severe sleep disturbances of childhood are reviewed in references 1, 32, 36, 37.) The following section specifically addresses the problem of resistance to going to bed, getting out of bed, getting into bed with the parents, and crying at bedtime. This final problem will be discussed in some detail to provide a model for dealing with this type of minor behavior problem at bedtime. Because very little systematic research has investigated these problems, most of the treatment procedures described are based on clinical experience.

In a classic case study, Williams (61) reported the elimination of crying and tantrum behavior in a 21-month-old child by extinction procedures. The child cried when the parents left his room, whereupon they would return and wait an average of one-half to two hours until he fell asleep. The parents were advised to change the bedtime routine so that after putting the child to bed and exchanging pleasantries they left the room and did not reenter. By the tenth occasion, the child no longer cried when the parents left the room. A week later the child cried and an aunt reentered the room, thus reestablishing the crying behavior and necessitating a second extinction trial. The behavior was no longer evident on the ninth occasion of the second trial. During the next two years no further tantrums at bedtime were reported. One and one-half years later, the child showed no negative side effects. This straightforward strategy has been suggested by others (24, 27, 56). Wright, Woodcock, and Scott (64) reported on a similar problem with a three-year-old adopted child who would tantrum and indicate that there were spiders in his bedroom. These tantrums and "phobic displays" typically lasted 90 minutes, and parents reported that the child had not slept more than five consecutive hours on any night for two years. Treatment consisted of giving the child undivided attention one hour before bedtime, putting the child to bed at a specific time each night, saying goodnight, leaving the room, locking the door, and not reentering until 7 o'clock the next morning. The investigators were present in the home for the first three nights and maintained weekly contact for ten weeks. Within 35 days the duration of nightly crying decreased from 90 to 0 minutes. At a follow-up conducted after 30 weeks the parents reported that the child was sleeping 10 to 11 hours per night.

Resistance to going to bed is a problem that generally takes two forms: passive and active. In passive resistance the child effectively stalls for more time by requesting drinks, talking, and ignoring parental commands. In active resistance the child may tantrum, run off to other parts of the house, slump on the floor, or get out of bed frequently. If a child is stalling bedtime by 45 minutes or more, it should be considered to be a problem. Christophersen (21) recommends that parents should precede bedtime with 30 minutes of quiet activity, including bedtime rituals (story, kiss, prayers, etc.) after which the parents should leave the room and should not reenter. If the child leaves the bedroom, one swat on the bottom should be administered and the child placed back in his own bed. Patterson (47) outlined a simple contingency program consisting of informing the child that if he stays in bed, the next evening a bedtime story will be read. If he gets out of bed, the story will be omitted and the child will be placed in time-out each time he gets out of bed. He suggested a similar program for children who get in bed with their parents during the night. The child is told if he remains in his own bed one of the parents will climb in with him in the morning and read a story. If the child does get in bed with the parents he is returned to his own bed and loses the opportunity to hear the morning story. Spock (56) indicated that the child who climbs into bed with his parents should promptly and firmly, though not angrily, be returned to his own bed as many times as necessary. To shorten the temporal gap between the time the child leaves his own bed and is found in the parents' bed a cowbell or similar device on the top of the child's door will signal his exit from his room.

As suggested in the above examples, common bedtime problems can be effectively diminished or eliminated within one to two weeks if parents consistently apply the recommended procedures. Clinical experience suggests that close supervision by a clinician (usually by phone) is essential to the success of any change strategy. This supervision is especially important during the first week of treatment. Clearly, these problems seem to be amenable to environmental manipulation, although systematic research is needed to confirm the efficacy of recommended procedures.

The following guidelines, based on the literature and referenced above, have been given to parents attending a pediatric outpatient clinic.

"Bedtime Problem—Crying"

Guidelines for Parents

1. *Establish a reasonable time for bedtime or naptime, and under normal day-to-day circumstances put your child to bed at that time.
2. About 30 minutes prior to bedtime, start "quiet time," during which your child should engage in quiet activities rather than roughhousing, etc.
3. Go through your regular bedtime routine (bedtime story, drinks, kisses, etc.).
4. At the established bedtime have your child in bed. Tell him goodnight and that you will see him in the morning, turn off the light, leave the room, and close the door (optional).
5. Do *not* go back into the room. Your child may cry for a very long time, but if after one or two hours you go in and pick him up, you will teach him that all he has to do is cry for a long time and then Mommy will come back in. Your child may also try a variety of different noises, calls, etc., in an effort to get you to give in but don't fall for these. Stay out of the room.
6. Don't get discouraged. It only takes a few nights.
7. After your child is regularly going to bed without crying for more than a minute or two, it is all right to check on him if he continues to cry to make sure he is all right.

Follow these suggestions for any bedtime crying to avoid having the bedtime problem recur:
a. Do not talk to your child after he is down for the night.
b. Check diapers, etc., as quickly as possible.
c. If everything is okay, leave the room without saying a word or holding your child.

---

*© Susan K. Rainey, Edward R. Christophersen, and Hunter C. Leake, 1976, Department of Pediatrics, University of Kansas Medical Center.

Similar Guidelines are available for the child who gets out of bed. These and other guidelines mentioned in this chapter can be obtained from the first author upon request.

Mealtime Problems

Most of the literature on mealtime problems involves teaching appropriate social and self-feeding skills to retardates. Leibowitz and Holcer (40) reported a shaping program which successfully increased the variety of foods accepted by a retarded child while concurrently developing self-feeding skills. Barton et al. (8) successfully decreased undesirable mealtime behaviors (such as stealing food and using fingers) in institutionalized retarded persons by applying time-out procedures. O'Brien and Azrin (45) demonstrated that institutionalized retarded subjects could acquire proper "table manners" and maintain these manners in a public restaurant and group dining setting. Their training program involved the combined use of verbal instruction, imitation, and manual guidance and could be easily carried out by regular staff. There are other studies reporting successful interventions at mealtime with retarded persons (4, 12).

Although the literature in the area of mealtime problems with retardates is fairly well developed, there are few papers describing mealtime problems and their treatment in normal children. In one of the few published adaptations of procedures developed for retardates to the mealtime problems of normal children, Palmer et al. (46) describe a normal-IQ six-year-old who refused solid foods. They suggested that feeding problems frequently involve "behavioral mismanagement," and that parents can be taught behavioral techniques to manage problems such as mealtime tantrums, multiple food dislikes, and prolonged subsistence on puréed foods. Spock (56) offers parents some specific guidelines for feeding problems with infants and young children. These guidelines are quite extensive and continue to be a major source of information. Christophersen (21) discusses eating problems such as food dislikes, poor eating habits, and slow eating and offers specific remedies for parents.

Dressing Problems

The authors know of no systematic research with normal children that investigates teaching dressing skills or managing behavior problems associated with dressing. Child management books (21, 38) remain the major sources of information in this area. Written guidelines have been developed for teaching dressing skills and dealing with stalling when dressing. These are available from the authors.

Minor Tantrums

The literature clearly shows that parents can be taught to effectively manage temper tantrums as well as noncompliant or aggressive behaviors displayed by their children (13, 33, 34). Most books on child rearing discuss procedures to control tantruming in children (10, 48). Time-out has been particularly effective in controlling tantrums and other objectionable behaviors (28, 43, 59). Guidelines to help parents whose children display mild tantrum behavior or objectionable behaviors in public are available from the authors.

Automobile Travel

Auto-related accidents are the leading cause of death and disability in young children in the United States (44). Although parents may report using child-restraint devices, roadside observations have generally shown that less that 15% of children under ten years of age are actually restrained (49, 60). Several thorough discussions of child-restraint devices are available offering comparisons of devices on the market and specifying guidelines for ensuring the safety of children (17, 19, 26, 54). The task of effectively influencing parents to routinely use car seats has been conceptualized as an educational problem. Several authors have recommended that pediatricians take a major role in shaping parental attitudes by offering literature and "face-to-face" guidance to parents as part of "preventive medicine" (9, 22, 25, 39, 53).

Parents are usually told that the reason they should use restraint devices is to avoid the possibility of the death or disfigurement of an unrestrained child in the event of a collision (51). However, in the only well-controlled study of its kind, Christophersen (22) demonstrated that the introduction of car-seat use significantly reduced levels of disruptive behavior—e.g., standing, climbing, kicking, screaming, etc.—displayed by young children with concomitant increases in appropriate behaviors which were maintained at a follow-up three months later. Christophersen suggested that pediatricians can use potential behavioral improvements brought about by car-seat use as a "selling point" in discussions with parents; in.addition to the safety benefits, car seats can make automobile travel more pleasant for parents and children. Parents can make travel more enjoyable for their children by involving them in conversation and attending to them when they are behaving appropriately (22). The following guidelines can be given to parents to help them induce children to use seat belts and car seats during travel. An evaluation of the use of this handout has recently been completed, and showed a dramatic increase in the use of car seats.

Using Automobile Car Seat

Guidelines for Parents

Car riding can and should be a pleasant time for you and your child. This is an excellent time for pleasant conversation and for teaching your child acceptable and appropriate behavior in the car. It is also the safest mode of travel, even for short trips, for your child.

1. *Introduce the car seat to your child in a calm, matter-of-fact manner as a learning experience. Allow him to touch it and to check it out.

2. Remind the child about the rules of behavior *nicely* before the first ride and in between rides.

3. Your first rides with the seat should be short practice rides to teach him the expected and acceptable behaviors; *perhaps once around the block.* Point out interesting things that he can see. Make it a positive experience for both of you.

4. Praise him *often* for appropriate behaviors (Example: "Mike, you are sitting so quietly in your seat. Mommy is proud of you. You are a good boy...."). This explanation teaches him the expected and appropriate behavior. Young children need specific directions. They cannot make the opposite connection of what is meant by "Quit that!" Catch him being good! You cannot praise him too often.

5. Include the child in pleasant conversation. (Example: "That was sure a good lunch... You really like hot dogs... You were a big help to me in the store... It'll be fun visiting grandma...").

6. This is also a good time to teach your child about his world. (Example: "Jon, see that *big, red* fire truck. Look at how *fast* it is going. What *do* firemen do? The light on the *top* is *red*... What else is red?...") This needs to be geared to the age of the child.

7. By your frequent praise, teaching, and pleasant conversation, your child will remain interested and busy and will not spend his time trying to get out of the seat. You will have his frequent attention.

8. Ignore yelling, screaming, and begging. The instant he is quiet praise him for being quiet. You, too, should not yell, scream, or beg. Remember, remain calm and matter-of-fact. Keep your child busy in conversation and observations of his world. Do not give in and let him out. This only teaches him that yelling, screaming, and begging will finally get Mom or Dad to let him do what he wants. Who's the boss!

9. Older siblings should also be expected to behave appropriately. If the young child sees an older sibling climbing and hanging out the window, he will

---

*© Jo-Eileen Gyulay and Edward R. Christophersen, 1978.

want to become a participant. The older siblings should also be included in the conversation, praise, and teaching.

10. Provide one or two safe toys that your child associates with quiet play, such as books, stuffed animals, dolls, etc. It may help to have special quiet riding toys that are played with only in the car. This decreases boredom. Remember, the young child's attention span is *very* short. Do not expect him to keep occupied for more than a couple of minutes, particularly at the beginning, depending upon his age. *Anticipating* this will *prevent* throwing of toys, temper tantrums, crying, or fussing.

11. Immediately after the ride, reward him with five to ten minutes of your time participating in an activity that he likes, such as reading a story, playing a game, helping prepare lunch, helping put away the groceries, etc. Do not get into the habit of buying your child favors or presents for his good behavior. He enjoys time *with you* and it's less expensive and more rewarding for both of you. Remember, CATCH HIM BEING GOOD—AND PRAISE HIM OFTEN!

12. If your child even begins to try to release his seat belt or to climb out of the car seat, immediately tell him, NO! in a firm voice. On your first few trips, which should just be around the block, stop the car if you think that is necessary. Also, consider stating the rule once, clearly, "Do *not* take off your seat belt!" and administer one firm slap on his hands.

13. Remember, without the praise and attention for good behavior in the car, your child will learn nothing from the training trips. The combination of praise and attention, with an occasional hand slap, will teach the behavior you want in the car.

Toilet Training

Bowel and bladder control is considered to be a major milestone in the physical and social development of children. By the age of 36 months most children have achieved diurnal control, although occasional accidents may occur until the age of five years (55). Although much importance has been attached to this developmental task, little evaluative research has been done to date. Several reasons for the paucity of research have been suggested: This area has often been viewed as taboo; data collection on children of this age is difficult because they are at home and are not as accessible as children in structured school settings; and the amount of time necessary to study the toilet-training process can be prohibitive (50). Another possible deterrent to research has been the lack of established procedures.

Central to the task of toilet training is the concept of "readiness." Brazelton (14) suggested several physiological and psychological readiness criteria. According to him, physiological readiness includes reflex sphincter control, which can be elicited as early as nine months, and myelinization of the pyramidal tracts, which is completed between 12 and 18 months. Psychological and developmental readiness includes established sitting and walking, some verbal understanding, positive relationships with parental figures which are evident in the desire to please, identification with and imitation of parents and significant others, and the desire to be autonomous and master of "primitive impulses." He suggests that readiness begins to peak at 18 months and increases to 30 months with most children.

Azrin and Foxx (6), in their popular book on toilet training, have suggested several specific readiness criteria that parents can use to decide when to begin training.

1. *Bladder Control.* The child should empty his bladder completely when voiding, stay dry for several hours, and indicate when he is about to urinate by facial expression or posturing. Control is evident when the child consistently exhibits the first two behaviors.

2. *Physical Readiness.* The child should exhibit fine and gross motor coordination sufficiently to be able to pick up objects easily and to walk well without assistance.

3. *Instructional Readiness.* The child should have enough receptive language to enable him to follow one- and two-stage directions (e.g., "Show me your nose." "Put the dolly in the wagon.").

They suggest that most children over 20 months can usually pass these criteria. Initial bladder control and physical coordination are considered by Azrin and Foxx to be maturational in nature, while instructional readiness can be taught by the parent before actual training is begun. They caution parents not to count on "advancing age" as a remedy for negativism. When children attain these readiness criteria, Christophersen (21) suggests that parents wait an additional three months before actually beginning to train, which means that training with most children will begin between 24 and 30 months of age.

Until recently, a major source of information about toilet training has been child-rearing books, e.g., Spock's *Baby and Child Care.* Several direct attempts to expedite the toilet-training process have been reported in the literature based on operant conditioning principles with both normal (16, 42, 50) and retarded (31, 42, 58) subjects. A major criticism of this research is that few subjects were involved, and this fact severely limits the generality of the findings.

Madsen et al. (41) reported on the only group study which compared training procedures with a no-treatment control group. Their study involved 70 children who were randomly assigned, with a few exceptions, to one of the following groups: No-contact control group; parents' method group; reinforcement schedule group where contingent rewards were used to shape training; buzzer-pants group where a urine-sensing device was sewn into the child's underpants; and reinforcement plus buzzer-pants group. The study was designed to compare the effectiveness of different techniques over a six-week period (one week of baseline, four weeks of training, and one week of posttraining data collection). It was expected that the children would not be completely trained. They found significant treatment effects for the reinforcement and reinforcement plus buzzer-pants groups over the parent, control, and buzzer-pants only groups. Although the reinforcement and reinforcement plus buzzer-pants groups did not differ significantly, they suggested that the addition of the buzzer did decrease the number of accidents. They concluded that reinforcement procedures can enhance toilet training in normal children.

Brazelton (14) has outlined a more indirect method of toilet training which has been quoted frequently in the pediatric literature. This "child-oriented" approach consists of several phases through which the child proceeds at his own pace. During the first phase, sometime after 18 months of age, the child is introduced to the potty chair and invited to sit on it while fully clothed. After a week or two of this introductory phase, the child is taken to the potty chair to sit with diapers off, although no results are expected. Next, the child is taken to the chair once daily to empty soiled diapers with the intent of establishing the chair as a convenient receptacle for waste. The next phase involves placing the potty in the child's room or play area periodically throughout the day. The child does not wear diapers and the parent explains that he may use the potty if he wishes. After cooperation has been achieved through these preceding phases, the child is dressed in training pants and encouraged to use the potty. Brazelton emphasizes the voluntary cooperation of the child and limited guidance by the parent. Of the 1170 primarily upper-middle-class children for whom this protocol was suggested over ten years of pediatric practice, 80.3% were completely trained (diurnal and nocturnal) by three years of age. The average age for day training was 28.5 months and for day and night training was 33.3 months. Among this group of children he reports a lower incidence of residual symptoms such as enuresis and encopresis. Although there is much surface appeal for this approach, he does not specify how the data he reports were obtained. As is the case generally in this area, systematic investigations are needed to validate and extend these findings to children of differing socioeconomic backgrounds.

Foxx and Azrin (29) reported a rapid and effective procedure for toilet training normal children which has been popularized in book form for parents (6). This method was first tested with retarded subjects (5, 30) and later extended to normal subjects. There are at least 16 major characteristics of this training program, which includes practice and reinforcement of dressing skills, immediacy of reinforcement for correct toileting, and learning by imitation. The original study with normal children involved a sample of 34 children with a mean age of 25 months. The training was conducted in the child's home or in the home of the trainer with family members absent. All 34 children were trained in an average of 3.9 hours (with a range of one-half to 14 hours). Accidents within the first posttraining week had decreased by 97% to 0.2 accidents per day per child, about one per week. Accidents remained at a near-zero level during four months of follow-up study. Foxx and Azrin suggest that the results of their study indicate "virtually all" healthy children 20 months and older can be trained within a few hours. However, they caution that because this method relies heavily on verbal, instructional, and symbolic procedures, rapid training may not be possible with a less verbal child. Although these results are quite impressive, the authors know of only one unpublished study (7) that has attempted to replicate these procedures using an adequate experimental design. This study differed from the Foxx and Azrin study in that parents conducted the training. The efficacy of this method needs to be established by a large number of successful replications by parents.

Questionnaire surveys indicate that parents may have unrealistic expectations about when toilet training should be begun and when it should be completed (20, 57). Discussions with parents about toilet training should begin when the child is about nine months of age (14). The primary health-care provider is in a unique position to initiate such discussions. Actual training should not be attempted until the child is at least 20 months of age, when training can be more rapidly achieved with less difficulty for the parent and child (21, 29).

For toilet training, the clinician has few options. The Foxx and Azrin study is the most impressive empirical demonstration to date, but in our experience, training is rarely achieved in one day. Although the procedure has been popularized in book form for parents, many parents may not be able to successfully carry out the program (18). If parents consistently adhere to the procedures, complete training can be realistically achieved within two to three months. The dry-pants procedure is quite intensive and may be too demanding for some parents. Brazelton's approach is appealing in that the response cost to the parent is low; however, components of the training are not as clearly specified and sequenced as with the Foxx and Azrin method. In addition, some children may not possess sufficient motivation to enable them to progress at an adequate pace. This may elicit impatience and coercive behaviors from parents. Further research is needed to determine which approach is likely to be efficient and palatable for particular parent-child dyads. There are several recommendations which can be suggested, irrespective of the approach taken to training.

Toilet Training

Guidelines for Parents

1. *Long before training is begun, parents can begin to teach their children dressing skills. These must be shaped in small steps (18).

---

*© Michael A. Rapoff and Edward R. Christophersen, 1978.

2. Children learn much by observing and imitating their parents. The child can occasionally accompany his parent to the bathroom. The parent can then use his own preferred vocabulary to describe the elimination process.
3. Children can be taught to follow one- and two-stage directions. The understanding and expression of language greatly facilitates the training process.
4. Training should not begin before 20 months. The efforts necessary to train a child much younger cancel out any potential benefits.
5. Children should not be required to sit on the potty for extended periods of time. Five to ten minutes is sufficient. Adults do not eliminate on command and this should not be required of children.
6. As much as possible, the training process needs to be pleasant for both children and parents. Physical punishment definitely has no place in training. Punishment does not teach, and the resulting negative side effects disrupt the parent-child relationship.

Whichever approach is suggested, the clinician can give parents specific guidelines that can help to prevent unnecessary complications.

DISCUSSION

From this review, it is evident that there is a developing literature to support the growing emphasis that pediatric education is beginning to place on socially influenced pediatric problems, or "biosocial pediatrics." This shift in focus, mandated by the 1978 Task Force Report on Pediatric Education, presents a substantial challenge to pediatric educators. Ideally, this challenge would be met by training new health-care providers in all of the well-documented prevention and treatment techniques that currently exist. Unfortunately, as the present review indicates, much of behavioral pediatrics is still in a state of development. Much of the literature is case-study material. Although frequently of enormous interest to the practicing clinician, case studies do not take the place of good experimental designs with adequate controls which *demonstrate* the efficacy or lack of efficacy of specific procedures. It is to be hoped that this new emphasis on biosocial pediatrics will stimulate research studies in addition to the case reports that will undoubtedly continue to be published, and that the controlled investigations currently being carried out by psychologists, educators, and physicians will begin to appear in a form that is useful to the pediatrician.

Beyond the concern for documenting treatment efficiency, substantial effort needs to go into developing and packaging treatment strategies that can be easily implemented by the health-care provider. Rare is the pediatrician who does not recognize the influence of socioenvironmental variables on his patients; however, pediatricians often do not have the *time* to include behavioral pediatrics in their routine practice. This problem may not be due to the procedures themselves, but to the fact that the pediatrician does not have the technology to implement the procedures without substantially lengthening the average time of a well-child visit. The "Guidelines" presented in this chapter have provided information and treatment strategies for over 500 pediatricians and 250 nurses. This is an example of how the pediatrician or nurse can incorporate child-rearing counseling into their practice without disrupting their ongoing medical management of the child. With appropriate materials, the pediatrician has a way to implement behavioral counseling that is both comfortable and time efficient. When effective treatment procedures, packaged for efficient office distribution, are available to pediatricians, we expect to see an increase in the number of pediatricians incorporating behavioral pediatrics into their clinical practice.

ACKNOWLEDGMENTS

Preparation of this manuscript was supported by a grant (HD 03144) from NICHD to the Bureau of Child Research, University of Kansas, Lawrence, Kansas.

REFERENCES

1. Anders, T.F., and Weinstein, P. Sleep and its disorders in infants and children: A review. *Pediatrics* 50:312-324, 1972.
2. Anderson, J.E. Pediatrics and child psychology. *JAMA* 95:1015-1020, 1930.
3. Anthony, J. An experimental approach to the psychopathology of childhood: Sleep disturbances. *Br. J. Med. Psychol.* 32:19-37, 1959.
4. Azrin, N.H., and Armstrong, P.M. The "mini-meal"—A method for teaching eating skills to the profoundly retarded. *Ment. Retard.* 11:9-13, 1970.
5. Azrin, N.H., and Foxx, R.M. A rapid method of toilet training the institutionalized retarded. *J. Appl. Behav. Anal.* 4:89-99, 1971.
6. Azrin, N.H., and Foxx, R.M. *Toilet Training in Less Than a Day.* New York: Simon & Schuster, 1974.
7. Barnard, J.D., Christophersen, E.R., and Wolf, M.M. A replication and evaluation of "dry pants" toilet training procedures. Unpublished manuscript, 1977.
8. Barton, E.S., Guess, D., Garcia, E., and Baer, D.M. Improvement of retardates' mealtime behaviors by timeout procedures using multiple baseline techniques. *J. Appl. Behav. Anal.* 2:77-84, 1970.
9. Bass, L.W., and Wilson, T.R. The pediatrician's influence in private practice measured by a controlled seat belt study. *Pediatrics* 33:700-704, 1964.
10. Becker, W.C. *Parents Are Teachers.* Champaign, Ill.: Research Press, 1971.
11. Becker, W.C., and Becker, J.W. *Successful Parenthood: How to Teach Your Child Values, Competence and Responsibility.* Chicago, Ill.: Follett Publishing, 1974.
12. Berkowitz, S., Sherry, P.J., and Davis, B.A. Teaching self-feeding skills to profound retardates using reinforcement and fading procedures. *Behav. Ther.* 2:62-77, 1971.

13. Bernal, M.E. Behavioral feedback in the modification of brat behaviors. *J. Nerv. Ment. Dis.* 48:375-385, 1969.
14. Brazelton, T.B. A child-oriented approach to toilet training. *Pediatrics* 29:121-128, 1962.
15. Brazelton, T.B. Anticipatory guidance, in S. Friedman (ed.), *The Pediatric Clinics of North America.* Philadelphia: W.B. Saunders, 1975.
16. Brown, R.M., and Brown, N.L. The increase and control of verbal signals in the bladder training of a seventeen-month-old child: A case study. *J. Child Psychol. Psychiat.* 15:105-109, 1974.
17. Burg, F.D., Douglass, J.M., Diamond, E., and Siegel, A.W. Automotive restraint devices for the pediatric patient. *Pediatrics* 45:49, 1970.
18. Butler, J.F. The toilet training success of parents after reading "Toilet Training in Less Than A Day." *Behav. Ther.* 7:185-191, 1976.
19. Car safety restraints for children. *Consumer Reports* Feb.:108-112, 1974.
20. Carlson, S.S., and Asnes, R.S. Maternal expectations and attitudes toward toilet training: A comparison between clinic mothers and private practice mothers. *J. Pediatrics* 84:148-151, 1974.
21. Christophersen, E.R. *Little People: Guidelines for Common Sense Child Rearing.* Lawrence, Kan.: H & H Enterprises, 1977.
22. Christophersen, E.R. Children's behavior during automobile rides: Do car seats make a difference? *Pediatrics* 60:69-74, 1977.
23. Christophersen, E.R. Behavioral pediatrics for the pediatric clinician, in D.P. Hymovich and M.U. Barnard (eds.), *Family Health Care,* 2nd ed. New York: McGraw-Hill, 1979.
24. Christophersen, E.R., Rainey, S.K., and Leake, H.C. Simultaneous evaluation by the pediatrician and the pediatric psychologist. *Ambulatory Pediatrics Association Proceedings, 1975.*
25. The Committee on Accident Prevention of the American Academy of Pediatrics. Seatbelts in the prevention of automobile injuries. *Pediatrics* 30:841-843, 1962.
26. The Committee on Accident Prevention of the American Academy of Pediatrics. Auto safety for the infant and young child. *Clinical Pediatrics* 14:122-133, 1975.
27. Dreikurs, R. *Coping With Children's Misbehavior: A Parent's Guide.* New York: Hawthorn Books, 1972.
28. Forehand, R., and MacDonough, S. Response contingent time out: An examination of outcome data. *European J. Behav. Anal. Mod.* 1:109-115, 1975.
29. Foxx, R.M., and Azrin, N.H. Dry pants: A rapid method of toilet training children. *Behav. Res. and Ther.* 11:435-442, 1973.
30. Foxx, R.M., and Azrin, N.H. *Toilet Training the Retarded.* Champaign, Ill.: Research Press, 1973.
31. Giles, D.K., and Wolf, M.M. Toilet training institutionalized severe retardates: An application of operant behavior modification techniques. *Am. J. Ment. Deficiency* 70:766-780, 1966.
32. Guilleminault, C., and Anders, T.F. Sleep disorders in children, in I. Shulman (ed.), *Advances in Pediatrics.* Chicago: Year Book Medical Publishers, 1976, pp. 151-174.
33. Hall, R.V., Axelrod, S., Tyler, L., Grief, E., Jones, F.C., and Robertson, R. Modification of behavior problems in the home with a parent as observer and experimenter. *J. Appl. Behav. Anal.* 5:56-64, 1972.
34. Johnson, C.A., and Katz, R.C. Using parents as change agents for their children: A review. *J. Child Psychol. Psychiat.* 14:181-200, 1973.
35. Kagan, J. The new marriage: Pediatrics and Psychology. *Am. J. Dis. in Children* 110:272-278, 1965.

36. Kales, A., and Kales, J.D. Sleep disorders: Recent findings in the diagnosis and treatment of disturbed sleep. *New England J. Med.* 290:487-499, 1974.
37. Keith, P.R. Night terrors: A review of the psychology, neurophysiology, and therapy. *J. Am. Acad. Child Psychiatry* 14:477-489, 1975.
38. Krumboltz, J.D., and Krumboltz, H.B. *Changing Children's Behavior.* Englewood Cliffs, N.J.: Prentice-Hall, 1972.
39. Lieberman, H.M., Emmett, W.L., and Carlson, A.H. Pediatric automotive restraints, pediatricians, and the academy. *Pediatrics* 58:316-319, 1976.
40. Liebowitz, J.M., and Holcer, P. Building and maintaining self-feeding skills in a retarded child. *Am. J. Occupational Ther.* 28:545-548, 1974.
41. Madsen, C.H., Hoffman, M., Thomas, D.R., Koropsat, E., and Madsen, C.K. Comparisons of toilet training procedures, in Gelfand, D.M. (ed.), *Social Learning in Childhood.* Belmont, Cal.: Brooks/Cole, 1969.
42. Mahoney, K., Van Wagenen, R.K., and Meyerson, L. Toilet training of normal and retarded children. *J. Appl. Behav. Anal.* 4:178-181, 1971.
43. Murray, M.E. Modified time-out procedures for controlling tantrum behaviors in public places. *Behav. Ther.* 7:412-413, 1976.
44. Newmann, C.G., Newmann, A.K., Cockrell, M.E., and Banani, S. Factors associated with child use of automobile restraining devices. *Am. J. Dis. Child* 128:469-474, 1974.
45. O'Brien, F., and Azrin, N.H. Developing proper mealtime behaviors of the institutionalized retarded. *J. Appl. Behav. Anal.* 5: 389-399, 1972.
46. Palmer, S., Thompson, R.J., and Linsheid, T.R. Applied behavior analysis in the treatment of childhood feeding problems. *Developmental Med. Child Neurology* 17:333-339, 1975.
47. Patterson, G.R. *Families: Applications of Social Learning to Family Life,* (Rev.) Champaign, Ill.: Research Press, 1975.
48. Patterson, G.R., and Gullion, M.E. *Living With Children,* (Rev.) Champaign, Ill.: Research Press, 1968.
49. Pless, I.B., Roghmann, K., and Algranati, P. The prevention of injuries to children in automobiles. *Pediatrics* 49:420-427, 1972.
50. Pumroy, D.K., and Pumroy, S.S. Systematic observation and reinforcement technique in toilet training. *Psychol. Rep.* 16:467-471, 1965.
51. Robertson, L.S., O'Neill, B., and Wixom, C.W. Factors associated with observed safety belt use. *J. Health Soc. Behav.* 13:18-24, 1972.
52. Salk. L. Psychologist in a pediatric setting. *Professional Psychol.* 1:395-396, 1970.
53. Shelness, A., and Charles, S. Children as passengers in automobiles: The neglected minority on the nation's highways. *Pediatrics* 56:271-284, 1975.
54. Siegel, A.W., Nahum, A.M., and Appleby, M.R. Injuries to children in automobile collisions. Reprint from 12th Stapp Car Crash Conference. Society of Automotive Engineers, Inc., 1968.
55. Simonds, J.F. Enuresis: A brief survey of current thinking with respect to pathogenesis and management. *Clin. Pediatrics* 16:79-82, 1977.
56. Spock, B. *Baby and Child Care,* (Rev.) New York: Pocket Books, 1976.
57. Stehbens, J.A., and Silber, D.L. Parental expectations in toilet training. *Pediatrics* 48:451-454, 1971.
58. Van Wagenen, R.K., Meyerson, L., Kerr, N.J., and Mahoney, K. Field trials of a new procedure for toilet training. *J. Exper. Child Psychol.* 8:147-159, 1969.
59. Wahler, R.G. Oppositional children: A quest for parental reinforcement control. *J. Appl. Behav. Anal.* 2:159-170, 1969.
60. Williams, A.F. Observed child restraint use in automobiles. *Am. J. Dis. Child* 130:1311-1317, 1976.

61. Williams, C.D. The elimination of tantrum behavior by extinction procedures. *J. Abnorm. Soc. Psychol.* 59:269-270, 1959.
62. Wright, L. The pediatric psychologist: A role model. *American Psychologist* 22:323-325, 1967.
63. Wright, L. Pediatric psychology—Prospect and retrospect. *Pediatric Psychology Newsletter* 1:1-2, 1969.
64. Wright, L., Woodcock, J., and Scott, R. Treatment of sleep disturbance in a young child by conditioning. *Southern Med. J.* 63:174-176, 1970.

The Comprehensive Handbook of Behavioral Medicine, Volume 3

CHAPTER 2

Self-Injury In
Pediatric Populations

Dennis C. Russo
Edward G. Carr
O. Ivar Lovaas

A large number of children will, at some time during their development, exhibit self-injurious behavior. In all probability, the first health-care professional to be made aware of this behavior will be the child's pediatrician. In these cases, the initial assessment of the dangerous potential that the behavior represents for the child, the likelihood that the behavior will become chronic, the evaluation of causative or contributing factors, and the prescription of treatment are all critical issues that must be carefully considered.

The purpose of this chapter is to evaluate the demographics, etiological and motivational underpinnings, existing treatment technologies, and methods for behavioral diagnosis of self-injury in pediatric populations. The cooperative efforts of both the behavioral and the medical practitioner must be brought to bear in early intervention for children with self-injurious behaviors.

DEMOGRAPHICS

Self-injurious activity is perhaps the most striking of all behavioral aberrations. Children exhibiting self-injury may hit, bang, slap, gouge, or pinch parts of their body, especially the head and face, with other parts of their body or objects from their environment. The frequency of the behavior may vary from several times per day to several times per second. Trauma from this activity is usually minor with some skin discoloration or swelling. However, there are many cases where this type of behavior has posed a serious threat to the child's life, either directly from the activity itself, e.g., subdural hematomas and concussions resulting from head banging, or secondarily due to recurrent infection caused by repeated self-injury. Permanent impairment may result from chronic or very intense bursts of self-injurious activity—for example, the loss of body members such as fingers from biting; removal of tissues overlying bone as the result of biting or gouging; and permanent blindness due to self-ennucleation, or retinal detachment produced by the repeated impact of the head against walls or other objects. In addition to physically abusive behavior, self-injury may also take the form of recurrent vomiting, rumination, or the self-induction of organic pathological processes like epileptic seizures. Self-injury may best be defined as any behavior that produces physical trauma or abnormal physical symptoms, such as severe weight loss. The diagnosis is based on the outcome rather than the intent of these behaviors.

Self-injurious behavior occurs in a variety of populations. It is seen in 9% to 17% of children between nine months and two years of age (77) and, as such, may be viewed as a normal developmental phenomenon (42). Behavior like periodic head banging against the sides and floor of the crib usually decreases and finally disappears without treatment in the course of normal development. However, in some young children self-injurious behaviors will be of sufficient intensity and frequency to pose a significant threat to their life.

The risk of severe, chronic self-injury appears to be increased in psychiatric and developmentally disabled pediatric populations (5). Prevalence rates of 4% to 5% have been reported in children diagnosed retarded, organically brain damaged, autistic, or schizophrenic (29, 64). Among institutionalized children, self-injurious behavior is most common among the female patients, but most severe among the males (33).

Although in chronic, severe cases, permanent physical damage may occur, no instances of death due directly to physical self-injury, such as biting or head banging, have been reported (68). The absence of fatalities from physical self-injury is probably due to the widespread use of complete physical restraint and sedation, which can be applied on an emergency basis. Under even the most optimal circumstances, self-injury presents a continued danger to the child, and its presence may minimize the impact of rehabilitative procedures and in general worsen the prognosis for the child exhibiting the behavior (10).

In this chapter we will describe a therapeutic approach to self-injury within the context of the practice of behavioral medicine. We will discuss some of the hypotheses of etiology and treatment of self-injury. A more detailed discussion of this topic can be found in references 1, 4, 10, 29, and 79.

ETIOLOGICAL AND MOTIVATIONAL ASPECTS OF SELF-INJURY

Self-injury has received a great deal of attention from theorists and therapists. Many hypotheses describe the cause and maintenance of these behaviors. Organically based theories have attempted to relate self-injury to the presence of pathology resulting from genetic defects, sensory deficits, or infectious agents. These theories explain the deviant behavior as a symptom of an underlying organic pathological state. Other hypotheses emphasize factors responsible for the maintenance or motivation to continue this type of behavior; the *function* rather than the *cause* of the behaviors. Carr (10) suggests that self-injury is a learned response which provides a type of environmental control to otherwise behaviorally deficient children. The behaviors are maintained by providing social attention (Positive Reinforcement hypothesis), terminating or avoiding environmental demands (Negative Reinforcement hypothesis), and/or providing kinesthetic, vestibular, and tactile sensory input (Self-Stimulation hypothesis).

Organic Conditions as a Cause of Self-Injury

For some children with self-injurious behavior, it has been suggested that an aberrant physiological process exists, originating in a genetic defect, sensory deficit, or disease process. Several organic conditions are often accompanied by self-injurious behavior. In these cases, the functional relationship between the organic pathology and the behavior disorder is unclear.

Lesch-Nyhan Syndrome

This is an X-linked genetic disorder occurring exclusively in males (60, 62, 74). Its symptoms include mental retardation, athetoid cerebral palsy, hyperuricemia, and a lack of the enzyme hypoxanthine guanine phosphoribosyl transferase (HGPRT) which results in the failure of purine metabolism (47). Self-injurious, rejective biting of the lips, tongue, and fingers accompanies the disorder and results in tissue loss and damage in the majority of cases (40, 47).

Some investigators have speculated that the self-injurious behavior of these children is produced directly by the underlying organic pathology (74, 75). Hoefnagel (39) suggested that the self-injury might be the result of elevated uric acid levels in the saliva, which might account for the observation that the self-injury is commonly directed to the tongue and lips. Unfortunately, early treatment with allopurinol to prevent high uric acid levels did not block the eventual appearance of self-injury in these children (54).

Other pharmacological treatments have produced conflicting results. For example, although some investigators have found L-5-hydroxytryptophan (L-5-HTP), a serotonin precursor, successful in reducing self-injury (56), Nyhan reported no success with the use of this drug, but did report that L-5-HTP in combination with carbidopa (a drug used to facilitate central uptake of L-5-HTP) produced promising results (61). Systematic evaluation of the effects of various pharmacological agents on self-injurious behavior in Lesch-Nyhan disease is only beginning.

Nonpharmacological studies raise questions about a purely organic basis for self-destructive behaviors in this disorder. Although most children with Lesch-Nyhan Syndrome exhibit the characteristic symptomatology of self-injury to the tongue, lips, and fingers, a number of children exhibit discrepant forms of self-mutilation such as eye gouging or head banging (18, 19, 40). Even more puzzling, some children show no self-injury (73, 74). These anomalies become somewhat more comprehensible in the light of recent reports suggesting that the self-injurious behavior in these children is susceptible to social reinforcement and may therefore have a learned component to it (1, 19).

Further research is required to assess roles of organic factors and learning, in the form of operant conditioning, in the initiation and maintenance of self-destructive behaviors in children with Lesch-Nyhan Syndrome. Beyond questions of causality, recent research suggests that operant interventions may constitute an appropriate treatment for the behavior problems that arise from the organic pathology (13).

Cornelia de Lange Syndrome

Cornelia de Lange Syndrome (16) is diagnosed by identifying a constellation of physical characteristics including low birth weight, mental and growth retardation, hirsutism, and an unusual appearance distinguished by prominent synophrys, long eyelashes, a small nose, micrognathia, thin turned-down lips, and relative diminutiveness of the face and hands (8). While karyotypic examinations have shown the presence of chromosomal fragments in the cells of some of these children, no clear-cut etiology has been found (43).

Self-injury in this population occurs with a much greater frequency than in the institutional population at large; for example, Bryson et al. (8) reported the presence of self-injury in four of seven children in one institution. The topography of injury in children with Cornelia de Lange Syndrome includes hitting their face, picking at their eyelids, and biting their lips (76), with no definite pattern of self-injury seen across children. No phenotypic differences have been found between those children who exhibit self-injury and those who do not (8). The lack of an identifiable genetic basis for the disorder, the variability in the topography of self-injury, and the successful treatment of the behavior by operant conditioning (76) all suggest that self-injury in Cornelia de Lange Syndrome may not simply be the product of organic abnormalities, and that it is influenced by environmental factors.

Other Conditions

A number of additional conditions with a high incidence of self-injury have been reported in the medical treatment literature. These conditions fall into three general categories: 1) self-injury associated with medical disorders; 2) self-injury as a result of abnormal pain thresholds; and 3) self-injury associated with developmental or psychiatric disorders.

Nongenetic syndromes and medical disorders

Infants and young children may have episodes of serious chronic vomiting at some time during their development. This type of chronic vomiting is usually the result of a brain-stem lesion, structural defect or infection of the esophageal or gastrointestinal tract, or a reaction to ingested substances. Some children, usually between 2½ and 12 months of age (45, 49), exhibit chronic vomiting or rumination for which no structural defect of other physical cause can be found. This "infant rumination syndrome" is discussed at length in Chapter 4.

Self-injury may also accompany otitis media, a painful middle ear infection frequently found in pediatric populations. De Lissovoy (17) found otitis media in 6 of 15 children who were head-bangers, and Harkness and Wagner (35) suggested that this type of self-injury may occur as a form of pain relief, especially when the ear infection becomes severe enough to inflame sensory nerves. It is possible that an increase in the rate of self-injury in an already self-injurious child or an unexplained onset of this behavior might indicate the presence of physical illness. A complete medical evaluation should always be included in the evaluation of these children.

Self-injury may also take the form of the self-induction of symptoms of underlying organic pathological conditions. For example, Fabish and Darbyshire (21) described self-induced seizures in epileptic patients by hyperventilation. Other authors have reported self-induced seizures from moving the hands rapidly in front of the eyes or blinking (88). The evaluating physician should show a special concern for the function of the symptoms in these cases.

Abnormal Pain Reactions

The absence of an appropriate pain reaction commonly accompanies severe self-injury. Bursts of self-injury may produce severe tissue damage with little or no behavioral indication of pain by the child. For example, Goldfarb (32) found that 23 of 31 schizophrenic children had aberrant pain reactions, such as failing to show pain when catching their finger in a door. None of the seven self-injurious children in the group showed pain reactions to self-injury. Pain is a subjective phenomenon which is capable of modification through learning (25), and endurance of pain to elicit social reinforcement (78) and habituation to painful stimuli (83) are well-known phenomena which might partially explain this insensitivity. Finally, one cannot rule out the possibility that the abnormal pain reaction is the result, rather than the cause, of the self-injurious behavior.

Associated Developmental and Psychiatric Disorders

The risk of self-injurious behavior appears to be higher in children with developmental disorders such as mental retardation, autism, brain damage (10), sensory neuropathy, dysautonomia (46), and psychiatric disorders such as childhood schizophrenia (29). Self-injury in these behaviorally deficient populations must be looked at in terms of organic pathology and environmental factors that predispose these populations to an increased risk for the behavior disorder.

Motivational Aspects of Self-Injury

Although the original causes of self-injurious behavior are generally not known, a number of studies in the past 15 years have helped to isolate some of the variables that *maintain* self-injury (10). We can describe some of the factors controlling the frequency of self-injury as well as delineate some of the situations in which the behavior is likely to occur. One major conclusion that can be drawn from these studies is that self-injury is usually a *learned response;* that is, it is controlled by the effects it has on the behavior of those who interact with the child. This conclusion forms the basis of two theories of self-injurious behavior: the positive reinforcement hypothesis and the negative reinforcement hypothesis. A third formulation, the self-stimulation hypothesis, states that some forms of self-injury are maintained by the sensory stimulation caused by the performance of the behavior.

Positive Reinforcement Hypothesis

Self-injury often appears to function as a means for obtaining adult attention. Our earliest understanding of this type of behavior comes from a study by Lovaas, Freitag, Gold, and Kassorla (50). These investigators worked with a nine-year-old schizophrenic girl who had severe self-injury, particularly head-banging. As part of an educational treatment intervention, the child had been taught to sing and dance, reinforced by adult attention and approval. Significantly, Lovaas et al. found that on those occasions when adult attention was withdrawn from music behaviors, the child increased her rate of self-injury. Based on these observations, they speculated that some children may learn to exhibit self-injury as a means of reinstating adult attention. Other studies (14, 63) have suggested that some psychotic children may display self-injury to motivate adults to return favorite objects which have been removed temporarily. The studies in the experimental literature strongly suggest that the withdrawal of positive reinforcement, such as adult attention or preferred objects, is an important condition for the occurrence of self-injury.

Several studies have demonstrated that the most common reactions of adults to self-injury, though well intentioned, usually make the behavior worse. For example, one reaction to seeing a child hurt himself is to comfort him, a typical response of parents and institutional staff members. This response to self-injury dramatically increases the rate of self-injury (50). A second adult reaction is to "distract" the child when he begins to engage in self-injury in the hope that he will become interested in the distraction and stop mutilating himself. Lovaas and Simmons (53) systematically explored this strategy with one retarded child. They permitted the child to play briefly with a favorite toy whenever he began to engage in self-injurious behavior. The effect of this "distraction" therapy was to produce a precipitous increase in the rate of self-injury. A third method of dealing with self-injury is to try to persuade the child not to engage in the behavior because of its unpleasant consequences. For example, Carr and McDowell (11) described a normal child who had begun scratching himself in response to contact with poison oak. His continued scratching produced new lesions and these persisted long after the contact allergy had resolved. They found that whenever the child's parents attempted to verbally persuade him not to scratch, the rate of scratching sharply increased. These studies demonstrated that positive reinforcement, in the form of comfort, distraction, or verbal persuasion, presented contingently on the performance of self-injury, worsens self-destructive behaviors.

It appears that self-injury is often highly correlated with positive reinforcement from adults, and that this type of behavior has clear functional utility for the child. This relationship between reinforcement and self-injury is supported by a number of studies showing that animals can be taught to severely injure themselves using food as a reinforcement (41, 72). The positive reinforcement hypothesis explains why self-injury often is under strong stimulus control, occurring at a high rate when adults are present but at a low rate when the child is alone (9, 70). The children appear to gradually learn that attention for self-injury only occurs when an appropriate, rewarding adult is present. Over time, self-injury tends to occur only in the presence of these adults.

Negative Reinforcement Hypothesis

Some self-injurious behaviors are apparently maintained by negative reinforcement contingencies. For example, in teaching situations, an adult will typically make demands of a child. To the extent that the child has difficulty with the demands, the teaching situation becomes aversive. Under these circumstances, some children show high rates of self-injury. This behavior frequently causes adults to terminate their demands and effectively teaches the child that escape is possible if self-injury is displayed (55, 86).

Carr, Newsom, and Binkoff (12) carried out a detailed analysis of this type of behavior in an eight-year-old schizophrenic boy. When the child was left alone, his rate of self-injury was negligible. However, when an adult made demands of him, his rate of punching and slapping himself immediately increased to a very high level. When he was told the session was over, his rate of self-injury returned to a low level; apparently an example of avoidance or escape learning. Self-injurious behavior often resulted in a cessation of demands, and stimuli which signaled the end of a teaching situation effectively stopped self-injury.

Adults frequently negatively reinforce self-injury by allowing a child to leave the demand situation because a cessation of demands makes the behavior less frequent. This strategy is only temporarily effective, and there is ample evidence to indicate that allowing the child to leave may actually *increase* the rate of self-injury over time (80).

Self-Stimulation Hypothesis

This hypothesis assumes that each individual requires an optimal level of stimulation in order to function adequately and that self-injury represents an effort to generate sensory stimulation under conditions of relative environmental deprivation. Two sets of data favor this hypothesis. First, animal studies (36, 37) have demonstrated that monkeys raised in environments that severely restrict social and sensory stimulation are more likely to exhibit stereotyped behaviors including self-injury, than monkeys raised under normal conditions. Second, a series of studies of retarded individuals (4, 6, 15) demonstrated that higher rates of stereotyped behaviors, including self-injury, occurred under impoverished environmental conditions than under conditions rich in opportunities for play and stimulation. These data are consistent with the hypothesis that individuals deprived of adequate external stimulation may stimulate themselves by self-injury and other stereotyped or repetitive behaviors. A test of this hypothesis is meaningful only if the level of environmental stimulation is measured *independently* of the occurrence or nonoccurrence of the self-injurious behavior. Such measurement is rarely reported in the literature. However, one study (58) demonstrated that high levels of environmental stimulation, defined in terms of the amount of vibratory stimulation, were inversely related to the rate of self-injury for one autistic child.

Summary and Evaluation

Self-injury may be maintained by three different factors, which in clinical work vary among individuals, and often the factors maintaining these behaviors vary from situation to situation *for the same individual.* To make effective treatment decisions, the clinician must consider the possibility of multiple maintaining factors both within and among individuals.

BEHAVIORAL TREATMENT OF SELF-INJURY

Since self-injurious behavior is controlled by a number of variables, it is not surprising that a variety of procedures have evolved for treating this behavioral disorder. Two points must be noted for treatment programs. First, the majority of children with self-injury are unteachable as long as they exhibit the behavior; it must be eliminated or markedly decreased prior to undertaking any educational or skill training (10, 65). Second, any treatment program that focuses solely on the elimination of self-injury is incomplete. The goal of treatment is to *replace* the self-injurious behavior with a variety of socially appropriate behaviors. These two points should be kept in mind when reading the material discussed below.

Background

The initial studies of this phenomenon were designed to evaluate the relationship between self-injury and the principles of learning. The primary focus of this work was to discover environmental events whose systematic manipulation would produce reliable and replicable changes in the frequency of self-injurious behavior. Early studies may be classified into two groups: those manipulating social reinforcement variables, such as attention; and those using punishment procedures, such as electric shock.

Early studies demonstrated the role of positive social reinforcement in the motivation and maintenance of self-injury (50, 53, 86). In these studies, changes in the rate of self-injury were correlated with the application (50) or removal (9) of adult social attention. The work of Lovaas et al. (50) demonstrated the disastrous effects that could be produced by the well-meaning concerned reactions of parents and other care-givers. Attention in the form of statements of concern contingent upon self-injury produced sharp increases in the rate of the behaviors. Withdrawing all attention for the behaviors produced dramatic decreases in the rate of the behaviors (9, 53).

Punishment procedures demonstrated the "lawfulness" of self-injurious behavior. A number of studies (14, 52, 53, 66, 82) documented the rapid elimination of self-injury following the contingent application of a small number of localized electric shocks and the highly specific nature of the control provided by this technique. In the case of one boy, Lovaas and Simmons (53) measured self-injurious behavior in two situations: When he was sitting on the therapist's lap and when he was in his bedroom. During baseline, he had a steady high rate of self-injurious behavior in both situations. A single electric shock reduced the behavior to zero in the situation in which it was administered (the therapist's lap). Little or no decrease was seen in the frequency of the behavior in his bedroom, and there was only a temporary suppression in the presence of other adults who had not shocked the child. These data suggest that the child quickly learned which situations would produce punishment for self-injury and which would not. The suppression of this behavior generalized only after several shocks were administered by different experimenters in several settings.

In recent years, self-injury has continued to provide a forum for the investigation of both motivational constructs (10, 12, 13, 71) and treatment procedures (4, 22, 29, 51, 68, 79, 80). Current treatment procedures for self-injury are perhaps best classified according to the locus of treatment application and may be divided into two groups: Those treatments directly manipulating the occurrence of self-injury through the placement of specific *contingencies* on the self-injurious responses; and those treatments seeking to reduce the self-injury either by focusing on *antecedents* to the behavior or by training the child to make *alternative responses*.

Contingency Management Interventions

Two paradigms are available to produce a direct reduction in the probability of self-injurious behavior. The first withholds or removes social reinforcement contingent upon the emission of self-injurious behavior. The second applies an aversive stimulus contingent upon the occurrence of the self-injury. The first paradigm uses extinction and time-out from positive reinforcement, while the second uses punishment. Each of these paradigms is response contingent—consequences are contingent upon the occurrence of the behavior.

Extinction procedures use the withdrawal of social reinforcement, e.g., attention, contingent on the occurrence of self-injurious behavior. This technique was one of the first applied clinically to control the behavior (9, 24, 31, 34) and is still widely used (44, 57, 70). The major advantage of extinction is that it is easy to apply; it involves ignoring the behavior when it occurs. Several factors need to be considered prior to using it as a treatment of choice. First, the initial effect of extinction is usually a transitory increase in the frequency and intensity of the behavior, often called an "extinction burst." Second, extinction may be a time-consuming treatment requiring that the child make and the therapist ignore thousands of self-injurious responses before the rate approaches zero. Because of these considerations, it is usually applied to mild cases of self-injury.

Time-out from positive reinforcement is a second procedure that has been used successfully to treat self-injury (31, 34, 87). During time-out, the child is isolated from all sources of positive reinforcement for a fixed period of time after he performs a self-injurious act. Typically, the child is placed in a "time-out room" which is empty of people or stimulating events. Time-out is often plagued by the same problems as extinction. Additionally, concern about the isolated self-injurious child often makes the procedure unpalatable to clinicians. The use of both extinction and time-out is predicated on the assumption that the self-injury is maintained by social reinforcement. To the extent that this assumption is unwarranted, application of these procedures is inappropriate (10, 71).

Punishment Procedures

Punishment is the most widely used procedure for the control of self-injury. Typically, a localized electrical shock is administered by an "inductorium" or "training wand," or other less frequently used devices such as a special belt (30) and helmet (89). Studies using electric shock have consistently demonstrated rapid suppression of self-injurious behavior (14, 48, 52, 53, 82). However, problems in producing generalization of treatment effects across therapists and in different environments, together with the potential for abuse of the procedure, have made some clinicians wary of applying this technique. Lovaas and Newsom (51) review these and other issues pertaining to the use of electric shock.

Overcorrection procedures (2, 26, 27) are a punishment technique (20) which can be used as an alternative to electric shock. With this technique the child repeatedly practices a response that is incompatible with the self-injurious behavior. For example, a child who usually bangs his head with his fist would be made to practice holding his hands by his sides for a period of time after every occurrence of self injurious behavior. The experimental support for this technique (3, 37) and its relatively noncontroversial nature make it a promising one for the control of self-injury.

Some Further Considerations

Recent reviews of the multiple motivational factors controlling self-injury (10) make treatment on the basis of response topography alone no longer appropriate (71, 84). Treatments now should be selected on the basis of probable maintaining variables, and the clinician must consider other dimensions such as potential abuse (13, 71), possible side effects (9, 66, 85), and use of the least restrictive appropriate procedure (13); the generalizability of treatment (81); and the likely public reaction to a given treatment (67). All behavioral medicine efforts, including the treatment of self-injury, must be governed by procedural outcome and by the current ethical standards of medicine and behavioral psychology (13). It is partly in reaction to the above issues that researchers have continued to search for new ways of controlling self-injury.

Antecedent Stimulus and Alternative Response Interventions

Antecedent stimulus and alternative response procedures share a common treatment strategy: Each procedure involves an attempt to weaken self-injurious behavior *indirectly* by increasing the probability that a non-self-injurious behavior will occur. These methods contrast with treatment strategies that attempt to weaken self-injury by placing a contingency *directly* on the behavior itself.

Antecedent stimulus interventions are based on the observation that self-injury appears to occur more frequently in some settings than in others (7, 12, 13, 22, 69, 71). By introducing stimuli which normally control a low rate of self-injury, viz., a high rate of non-self-injurious behaviors, one should be able to decrease the rate of the unwanted behavior. Carr et al. (12) observed that self-injury was likely to occur when demands were made of the child and unlikely to occur when the child was told amusing stories. It appeared that the self-injury represented an escape response to an aversive demand situation. They decided to introduce amusing stories into the demand situation to reduce the aversiveness of that situation. This manipulation of antecedent stimuli produced a dramatic decline in the frequency of self-injury. In their subject, it appeared to be possible to control self-injury by carefully examining the stimuli that preceded the occurrence or nonoccurrence of the behavior, and altering these antecedents.

Other treatment procedures concentrate on strengthening response alternatives that compete with and eventually replace the deviant behavior. The use of *differential social reinforcement* is one such procedure. This technique is based on the assumption that when social reinforcement is provided only for appropriate behaviors and not provided for self-injurious behavior, the latter should become considerably less frequent. This outcome has been demonstrated (52).

A second method for strengthening response alternatives is referred to as *differential reinforcement of other behaviors (DRO)*. In the DRO procedure, the child receives social reinforcement contingent on the *absence* of self-injury for a period of time. Any behavior, other than self-injury, which occurs at the end of the time period is reinforced. This technique has proven effective in reducing self-injury in a number of cases (28, 57, 63). In an interesting extension of the DRO procedure, Favell, McGimsey, and Jones (23) used physical restraint as the reinforcer. It has been observed that many children with self-injurious behaviors will attempt to restrain their own limbs with clothes, ropes, or anything else that they can find in the environment (29, 53). Usually, when these children have their restraints removed, they become upset and try to restrain themselves again. Favell et al. demonstrated that physical restraint could be used as a reinforcer to reduce the frequency of self-injury. In their experiment, children were released from restraints and permitted to get back into them contingent upon periods of no self-injury (DRO). They enhanced the effectiveness of this procedure by introducing toys and other pleasurable activities during the periods of non-restraint.

These studies suggest that controlling self-injury by strengthening alternative responses is an ethical, effective treatment approach (13). Russo, Cataldo, and Cushing (71) applied these principles to compliance training for the simultaneous reduction of multiple deviant behaviors including self-injury. In this study, alternative response and response-response relationship (59, 83) procedures were integrated to produce multiple changes in nontargeted deviant behaviors. Three retarded children who exhibited self-injury, aggression, and crying were treated. The children were primarily reinforced for complying with adult demands. As compliance was strengthened over time, the rate of deviant behaviors, including self-injury, decreased to low levels. In this study, deviant behaviors appeared to function as a response class inversely covarying with compliance. The strategy outlined by Russo et al. is of potential clinical significance since the procedure allows the development of a specific beneficial response, such as compliance, which may be *functionally* incompatible with deviant behaviors; the efficient reduction of deviant responses through indirect means; and the modification of deviant behavior in an ethically acceptable manner.

SOME ADDITIONAL CONSIDERATIONS

The procedures reviewed in this chapter have been empirically validated in a variety of clinical settings and have proved effective. With these disorders, many issues other than treatment effectiveness must be considered; for example, *early* treatment of self-injury is desirable for medical and educational reasons. It is necessary to make a differential assessment of motivation for self-injurious behaviors so an appropriate treatment program can be prescribed. Carr (10) outlines a simple screening procedure to facilitate the medical and behavioral analysis of self-injurious behavior.

Table 1. A Screening Sequence to Determine the Motivation of Self-Injurious Behavior*

Step 1

Screen for genetic abnormalities (e.g., Lesch-Nyhan and de Lange syndromes), particularly if lip, finger, or tongue biting is present.
Screen for nongenetic abnormalities (e.g., otitis media), particularly if head banging is present.
If screening is positive, motivation may be organic.
If Step 1 is negative, proceed to Step 2.

Step 2

Does self-injurious behavior increase under one or more of the following circumstances:
(a) When the behavior is attended to?
(b) When reinforcers are withdrawn for behaviors other than self-injurious behavior?
(c) When the child is in the company of adults (rather than alone)?
If Yes, motivation may be positive reinforcement.
Does self-injurious behavior occur primarily when demands or other aversive stimuli are presented?
If Step 2 is negative, proceed to Step 3.

Step 3

Does self-injurious behavior occur primarily when there are no activities available and/or the environment is barren?
If yes, motivation may be self-stimulation.

*© Copyright 1977 by the American Psychological Association. Reprinted with permission.

Taken in conjunction with other factors, such as the ethics of the suggested treatment, the empirical documentation of treatment effectiveness, and the continued joint review of the program by both behavioral and medical specialists, this outline helps direct an inquiry into the causes and treatments of self-injury in any specific case.

Concluding Comment

In this chapter, we have reviewed theories of etiology, motivation, and treatment of self-injurious behaviors. Treatment of these disorders requires a joint effort by behavioral clinicians and medical practitioners. Research on both the physiological and the behavioral aspects of this problem has produced a sophisticated understanding of this clinically significant deviant behavior. Continued collaborative effort will undoubtedly lead to even more effective treatment programs for children with these disorders.

ACKNOWLEDGMENTS

Manuscript preparation support by Project #917, Maternal and Child Health Service, U.S. Department of Health, Education and Welfare and Grant No. MH 11440 from the National Institute of Mental Health.

REFERENCES

1. Anderson, L.T., and Hermann, L. Lesch-Nyhan disease: A specific learning disability. Paper presented at the meeting of the Association for Advancement of Behavioral Therapy, San Francisco, December 1975.
2. Azrin, N.H., and Foxx, R.M. A rapid method of toilet training the institutionalized retarded. *J. Appl. Behav. Anal.* 4:89-99, 1971.
3. Azrin, N.H., Gottlieb, L., Hughart, L., Wesolowski, M.D., and Rahn, T. Eliminating self injurious behavior by educative procedures. *Behav. Res. and Ther.* 13:101-111, 1975.
4. Bachman, J.A. Self-injurious behavior: A behavioral analysis. *J. Abnorm, Psychol.* 80:211-244, 1972.
5. Baumeister, A.A., and Forehand, R. Stereotyped acts, in N.R. Ellis (ed.), *International Review of Research in Mental Retardation,* vol. 6. New York: Academic Press, 1973.
6. Berkson, G., and Mason, W.A. Stereotyped movements of mental defectives: IV. The effects of toys and the character of the acts. *Am. J. Ment. Defic.* 68:511-524, 1964.
7. Boe, R.B. Economical procedures for the reduction of aggression in a residential setting. *Ment. Retard.* 15:25-28, 1977.
8. Bryson, V., Sakati, N., Nyhan, W.L., and Fish, C.H. Self-mutilative behavior in the Cornelia de Lange syndrome. *Am. J. Ment. Defic.* 76:319-324, 1971.
9. Bucher, B., and Lovaas, O.I. Use of aversive stimulation in behavior modification, in M. Jones (ed.), *Miami Symposium on the Prediction of Behavior, 1967: Aversive Stimulation.* Coral Gables, Fla.: University of Miami Press, 1968.
10. Carr, E.G. The motivation of self-injurious behavior: A review of some hypotheses. *Psychol. Bull.* 84:800-816, 1977.
11. Carr, E.G., and McDowell, J.J. Unpublished data, 1978.
12. Carr, E.G., Newsom, C.D., and Binkoff, J.A. Stimulus control of self-destructive behavior in a psychotic child. *J. Abnorm. Child Psychol.* 4:139-153, 1976.
13. Cataldo, M.F., and Russo, D.C. Developmentally disabled in the community: Behav-

ioral/medical considerations, in L.A. Hamerlynck (ed.), *Behavioral Systems for the Developmentally Disabled: II. Institutional, Clinic, and Community Environments.* New York: Brunner/Mazel, in press.

14. Corte, H.E., Wolf, M.M., and Locke, B.J. A comparison of procedures for eliminating self-injurious behavior of retarded adolescents. *J. Appl. Behav. Anal.* 4:201-213, 1971.

15. Davenport, R.K., and Berkson, G. Stereotyped movement of mental defectives: II. Effects of novel objects. *Am. J. Ment. Defic.* 67:879-882, 1963.

16. de Lange, C. Sur un type nouveau de degeneration (Typus Anstelodamensis). *Archives Medicin des Enfants* 36:713, 1933.

17. de Lissovoy, V. Head banging in early childhood: A suggested cause. *J. Genet. Psychol.* 102:109-114, 1963.

18. Dizmang, L.H., and Cheatham, C.F. The Lesch-Nyhan syndrome. *Am. J. Psychiatry* 127:671-677, 1970.

19. Duker, P. Behavioral control of self-biting in a Lesch-Nyhan patient. *J. Ment. Defic. Res.* 19:11-19, 1975.

20. Epstein, L.H., Doke, L.A., Sajwaj, T.E., Sorrell, S., and Rimmer, B. Generality and side effects of overcorrection. *J. Appl. Behav. Anal.* 4:201-213, 1974.

21. Fabish, W., and Darbyshire, R. Report on an unusual case of self-induced epilepsy with comments on some psychological and therapeutic aspects. *Epilepsia* 6:335-340, 1965.

22. Favell, J.E., and McGimsey, J.F. The control of self-injury by a combination of positive procedures. Paper presented at meeting of the American Psychological Association, Washington, D.C., 1976.

23. Favell, J.E., McGimsey, J.F., and Jones, M.L. The use of physical restraint in the treatment of self-injury and as positive reinforcement. *J. Appl. Behav. Anal.,* in press.

24. Ferster, C.B. Positive reinforcement and behavioral deficits of autistic children. *Child Dev.* 32:437-456, 1961.

25. Fordyce, W.E. *Behavioral Methods for Chronic Pain and Illness.* St. Louis: C.V. Mosby, 1976.

26. Foxx, R.M., and Azrin, N.H. Resitition: A method of eliminating aggressive-disruptive behavior of retarded and brain damaged patients. *Behav. Res. and Ther.* 10:15-27, 1972.

27. Foxx, R.M., and Azrin, N.H. The elimination of autistic self-stimulatory behavior by overcorrection. *J. Appl. Behav. Anal.* 6:1-14, 1973.

28. Frankel, F., Moss, D., Schofield, S., and Simmons, J.Q. Case Study: Use of differential reinforcement to suppress self-injurious and aggressive behavior. *Psychol. Rep.* 39:843-849, 1976.

29. Frankel, F., and Simmons, J.Q. Self-injurious behavior in schizophrenic and retarded children. *Am. J. Ment. Defic.* 80:512-522, 1976.

30. Galbraith, D.A., Byrick, R.J., and Rutledge, J.T. An aversive conditioning approach to the inhibition of chronic vomiting. *Can. Psychiatr. Assoc. J.* 15:311-313, 1970.

31. Gardner, W.I. Use of punishment procedures with the severely retarded: A review. *Am. J. Ment. Defic.* 74:86-103, 1969.

32. Goldfarb, W. Pain reactions in a group of institutionalized schizophrenic children. *Am. J. Orthopsychiatry* 28:777-785, 1958.

33. Green, A.H. Self destructive behavior in physically abused schizophrenic children. *Arch. Gen. Psychiatry* 19:171-179, 1968.

34. Hamilton, J., Stephens, L., and Allen, P. Controlling aggressive and destructive behavior in severely retarded institutionalized residents. *Am. J. Ment. Defic.* 71:852-856, 1967.

35. Harkness, J.E., and Wagner, J.E. Self-mutilation in mice associated with otitis media. *Lab. Anim. Sci.* 25:315-318, 1975.

36. Harlow, H.F., and Griffin, G. Induced mental and social deficits in rhesus monkeys, in

S.F. Osler and R.E. Cooke (eds.), *The Biosocial Basis of Mental Retardation*. Baltimore: Johns Hopkins Press, 1965.

37. Harlow, H.F., and Harlow, M.K. Psychopathology in monkeys, in H.D. Kimmel (ed.), *Experimental Psychopathology*. New York: Academic Press, 1971.

38. Harris, S.L., and Romanczyk, R.G. A brief report on treating self-injurious behavior with overcorrection. *Behav. Ther.* 7:237, 1976.

39. Hoefnagel, D. The syndrome of athetoid cerebral palsy, mental deficiency, self-mutilation, and hyperuricemia. *J. Ment. Defic. Res.* 9:69-74, 1965.

40. Hoefnagel, D., Andrew, E.D., Mireault, N.G., and Berndt, W.O. Hereditary choreo-athetosis, self-mutilation, and hyperurecemia in young males. *New England J. Med.* 273:130-135, 1965.

41. Holz, W.C., and Azrin, N.H. Discriminative properties of punishment. *J. Exper. Anal. Behav.* 4:225-232, 1961.

42. Ilg, F.L., and Ames, L.B. *Child Behavior*. New York: Harper, 1955.

43. Jervis, G.A., and Stimson, C.W. De Lange syndrome. *J. Pediatrics* 63:634-645, 1963.

44. Jones, F.H., Simmons, J.Q., and Frankel, F. An extinction procedure for eliminating self-destructive behavior in a 9-year-old autistic girl. *J. Autism Child Schizo.* 4:241-250, 1974.

45. Kanner, L. *Child Psychiatry*, 3rd ed. Springfield, Ill.: C.C. Thomas, 1957.

46. Landwirth, J. Sensory radicular neuropathy and retinitis pigmentosa. *Pediatrics* 34:519, 1964.

47. Lesch, M., and Nyhan, W.L. A familial disorder of uric acid metabolism and central nervous system function. *Am. J. Med.* 36:561-570, 1964.

48. Lichstein, K.L., and Schreibman, L. Employing electric shock with autistic children. *J. Autism Child Schizo.* 6:163-174, 1976.

49. Linscheid, T.R. Disturbances of eating and feeding, in P.R. Magrab (ed.), *Psychological Management of Pediatric Problems (Vol. 1): Early Life Conditions and Chronic Diseases*. Baltimore: University Park Press, 1978.

50. Lovaas, O.I., Freitag, G., Gold, V.J., and Kassorla, I.C. Experimental studies in childhood schizophrenia. I. Analysis of self-destructive behavior. *J. Exper. Child Psychol.* 2:67-84, 1965.

51. Lovaas, O.I., and Newsom, C.D. Behavior modification with psychotic children, in H. Leitenberg (ed.), *Handbook of Behavior Modification and Behavior Therapy*. New York: Appleton-Century-Crofts, 1976.

52. Lovaas, O.I., Schaeffer, B., and Simmons, J.Q. Experimental studies in childhood schizophrenia: Building social behavior by use of electric shock. *J. Exper. Studies in Personality* 1:99-109, 1965.

53. Lovaas, O.I., and Simmons, J.Q. Manipulation of self-destruction in three retarded children. *J. Appl. Behav. Anal.* 2:143-157, 1969.

54. Marks, J.F., Baum, J., Keele, D.K., Kay, J.L., and MacFarlen, A. Lesch-Nyhan syndrome treated from the early neonatal period. *Pediatrics* 42: 357-359, 1968.

55. Measel, C.J., and Alfieri, P.A. Treatment of self-injurious behavior by a combination of reinforcement for incompatible behavior and overcorrection. *Am. J. Ment. Defic.* 81:147-153, 1976.

56. Mizuno, T., and Yugari, Y. Prophylactic effect of 5-hydroxytryptophan on self-mutilation in the Lesch-Nyhan syndrome. *Neuropaediatrie* 6:13-23, 1975.

57. Myers, D. Extinction, DRO, and response cost procedures for eliminating self-injurious behavior: A case study. *Behav. Res. and Ther.* 13:190, 1975.

58. Myerson, L., Kerr, N., and Michael, J.L. Behavior modification in rehabilitation, in S.W. Bijou and D.M. Baer (eds.), *Child Development: Reading in Experimental Analysis*. New York: Appleton-Century-Crofts, 1967.

59. Nordquist, V.M. The modification of a child's enuresis: Some response-response relationships. *J. Appl. Behav. Anal.* 4:241-247, 1971.
60. Nyhan, W.L. Lesch-Nyhan syndrome: Summary of clinical features. *Fed. Proc.* 27:1034-1041, 1968.
61. Nyhan, W.L. Behavior in the Lesch-Nyhan syndrome. *J. Autism Child Schizo.* 6:235-252, 1976.
62. Nyhan, W.L., Pesek, J., Sweetman, L., Carpenter, D.G., and Carter, C.H. Genetics of an X-linked disorder of uric acid metabolism and cerebral function. *Pediatr. Res.* 1:5-13, 1967.
63. Peterson, R.F., and Peterson, L.R. The use of positive reinforcement in the control of self-destructive behavior in a retarded boy. *J. Exper. Child Psychol.* 6:351-360, 1968.
64. Phillips, R.H., and Alkan, M. Some aspects of self-mutilation in the general population of a large psychiatric hospital. *Psychiatric Q.* 35:421-423, 1961.
65. Rincover, A., and Koegel, R.L. Research on the education of autistic children: Recent advances and future directions, in B.B. Lahey and A.E. Kazdin (eds.), *Advances in Clinical Child Psychology,* vol. 1. New York: Plenum Press, 1977.
66. Risley, T.R. The effects and side effects of punishing the autistic behaviors of a deviant child. *J. Appl. Behav. Anal.* 1:21-34, 1968.
67. Risley, T.R. Certify procedures not people, in W.S. Wood (ed.), *Issues in Evaluating Behavior Modification.* Champaign, Ill.: Research Press, 1975.
68. Romanczyk, R.G. Punishment of self-injurious behavior: Guarded optimism. Paper presented at meeting of Association for Advancement of Behavior Therapy, San Francisco, December 1976.
69. Romanczyk, R.G. Personal communication, 1978.
70. Romanczyk, R.G., and Goren, E.R. Severe self-injurious behavior: The problem of clinical control. *J. Consult. Clin. Psychol.* 43:730-739, 1975.
71. Russo, D.C., Cataldo, M.F., and Cushing, P.C. Compliance training and response-response relationships in the treatment of multiple behavior problems. Unpublished manuscript.
72. Schaeffer, H.H. Self-injurious behavior: Shaping head-banging in monkeys. *J. Appl. Behav. Anal.* 3:111-116, 1970.
73. Seegmiller, J.E. Diseases of purine and pyrimidine metabolism, in P.K. Bondy (ed.), *Duncan's Diseases of Metabolism,* 6th Ed. Philadelphia: Saunders, 1969.
74. Seegmiller, J.E. Lesch-Nyhan syndrome and the X-linked uric acidurias. *Hospital Practice* 7:79-90, 1972.
75. Seegmiller, J.E., Rosenbloom, F.M., and Kelley, W.N. Enzyme defect associated with a sex-linked human neurological disorder and excessive purine synthesis. *Science* 155:1682-1684, 1967.
76. Shear, C.S., Nyhan, W.L., Kirman, B.H., and Stern, J. Self-mutilative behavior as a feature of the de Lange syndrome. *J. Pediatrics* 78:506-509, 1971.
77. Shintoub, S.A., and Soulairac, A. L'enfant automutilateur. *Psychiatrie de l'Enfant* 3:111-145, 1961.
78. Simmons, J.Q., and Lovaas, O.I. The use of pain and punishment as treatment techniques with childhood schizophrenics. *Am. J. Psychotherapy* 23:23-26, 1969.
79. Smolev, S.R. Use of operant techniques for the modification of self-injurious behavior. *Am. J. Ment. Defic.* 76:295-305, 1971.
80. Solnick, J.V., Rincover, A., and Peterson, C.R. Some determinants of the reinforcing and punishing effects of timeout. *J. Appl. Behav. Anal.* 10:415-424, 1977.
81. Stokes, T.F., and Baer, D.M. An implicit technology of generalization. *J. Appl. Behav. Anal.* 10:349-367, 1977.

82. Tate, B.G., and Baroff, G.S. Aversive control of self-injurious behavior in a psychotic boy. *Behav. Res. and Ther.* 4:281-287, 1966.
83. Wahler, R.G. Some structural aspects of deviant child behavior. *J. Appl. Behav. Anal.* 8:27-42, 1975.
84. Weisberg, P. Operant procedures with the retardate: An overview of laboratory research, in N.R. Ellis (ed.), *International Review of Research in Mental Retardation,* vol. 5. New York: Academic Press, 1971.
85. White, J.C., and Taylor, D.J. Noxious conditioning as a treatment for rumination. *Ment. Retard.* 5:30-33, 1967.
86. Wolf, M.M., Risley, T., Johnston, M., Harris, F., and Allen, E. Application of operant conditioning procedures to the behavior problems of an autistic child: A follow-up and extension. *Behav. Res. and Ther.* 5:103-111, 1967.
87. Wolf, M.M., Risley, T., and Mees, H. Application of operant conditioning procedures to the behavior problems of an autistic child. *Behav. Res. and Ther.* 1:305-312, 1964.
88. Wright, L. Aversive conditioning of self-induced seizures. *Behav. Ther.* 4:712-713, 1973.
89. Yeakel, J.A., Salisbury, L.L., Greer, S.L., and Marcus, L.F. An appliance for autoinduced aversive control of self-injurious behavior. *J. Exper. Child Psychol.* 10:159-169, 1970.

Introduction to
Geriatric Disorders

Behavioral approaches to geriatric problems have focused on the treatment of diseases occurring in this population (see Chapter 3) or on the management of nursing homes in which progressively larger numbers of geriatric patients are forced to live. As Edwards notes, "nursing homes, developed as cheap alternatives to hospitals, have become poor alternatives to living." The situation is particularly pathetic for geriatric psychiatric patients, who often have been discharged from state mental hospitals after a lengthy stay to return to their community. Instead they are placed in a downtrodden, poorly maintained environment, they are overmedicated, understimulated, and largely neglected. Todd Risley's Living Environments in Kansas should be credited with undertaking a number of studies to help develop better treatment programs for patients in nursing homes. In his chapter, Edwards presents some findings from this group relevant to nursing homes and more generally relevant to treating senility.

The treatment of senile patients must begin with appropriate medical diagnosis and treatment. Despite the apparent obsession of many physicians with medicating older patients, the limits of these medications and the limitations of their use in this population are well known. Operant techniques have been shown to be useful in promoting self-control and social behavior in senile patients. Simple environmental manipulation like providing roommates, cueing, activity programs, and consistently orienting patients to reality often markedly alleviates symptoms of senility without medication.

Most "senile" patients are cared for in nursing homes, and the problem of patient management often lies more with the treatment setting than with the patient's symptoms. Appropriately treating patients may require restructuring existing nursing homes; for example, staff must be taught to reinforce appropriate behaviors and not attend to inappropriate behaviors, to not reinforce sitting in a corner, and to reward active interaction between patients. Many studies have shown that under such contingencies patients can be toilet trained, can engage in self-care, and can interact with appropriate social behaviors.

Although there is little outcome data in the area of rehabilitation of this population, it is of extreme importance for society. The percentage of our population falling into this diagnostic category is increasing as the average age of our population increases. In this population, outcome cannot be assessed in terms of cure, but in terms of life quality. The return to sociability after seclusion because of sloppy eating habits, or lack of toilet training, can be considered a major therapeutic achievement in most nursing-home situations.

Other chapters contain material relevant to the geriatric population. Rosenzweig and Bennett (Chapter 9, Volume 1) describe possible neuroanatomical explanations for positive changes seen in some senile patients, who have been placed in stimulating environments, and offer an anatomical basis for hope that some retraining and recovery of intellectual function is possible in this population. Poon's chapter on memory dysfunction provides useful information for dealing with memory disturbance, common in this population. Since most nursing-home patients suffer from chronic diseases, the chapters on chronic pain disorders are especially relevant. For general medical problems that are common in this population, the chapters on cardiovascular problems and treatment of fecal incontinence are especially relevant.

CHAPTER 3

Restoring Functional Behavior of "Senile" Elderly

K. Anthony Edwards

In all nursing homes there is a group of residents labeled "senile" or "confused" (30). Typically, they are nonambulatory, incontinent, incapable of interacting socially, and require assistance with self-help behaviors. Their condition is termed *senile dementia,* a behavioral disorder caused by brain damage or loss of functional brain capacity. They usually demonstrate the following symptoms: 1) alterations in personality, 2) dysmesia, or memory disturbance, 3) disorientation, 4) impairment of judgment, and 5) deterioration of other intellectual functioning (77). In some nursing homes, patients of this type spend most of the time in their own rooms with few visitors and fewer changes in daily routine.

In 1963, about half of the five hundred thousand residents in nursing homes were diagnosed as mentally disordered or senile (47). Nearly all were 65 years of age or older. Almost twice this number of beds were filled in 1973 (62); and presumably about half of these—one-half million residents—were also diagnosed as mentally disordered or senile. A recent study of skilled-care nursing facilities found that 78% of this population was over 64 years old, 33% were considered to have chronic brain disease, 10% neurological disease, and 10% neuroses or psychoses (81). Estimates of the incidence of senility in this population range from 10% to 60% (50). Chronic brain disease is the second most common primary diagnosis, and second most diagnosed condition of any type for patients over 64 years old at the time of admission (81).

In recent years the number of elderly persons in the general population has increased more rapidly than the number in other age groups (33, 34, 47). This increase has been brought about in part by an increase in longevity. Unfortunately, with an increase in life span there is also an increase in the number of elderly people with infirmities (34), including the chronic brain syndromes and senility. Methods for minimizing patients' disabilities and maximizing their functioning must be developed. Of the methods available, behavioral management is particularly promising. Research in this area has been limited, perhaps because of the unduly pessimistic belief that restoration of functional capacity is impossible with this population of elderly individuals (19).

In this chapter we will present behavioral and environmental strategies for restoring functional behaviors in elderly nursing-home residents who at one time in their lives were fully capable of successfully interacting with their environment. First, we will describe some of the problems of treating the elderly in nursing homes. Next, we will describe the theory behind behavioral caregiving routines in nursing homes and review the data from several studies which explored an environmental-change (eco-behavioral) approach for preventing senilelike behaviors. Finally, we will discuss the implications of our work in nursing homes and speculate on future applications.

A STATEMENT OF THE PROBLEM

Treating the Elderly in Nursing Homes

The medical profession has provided the overall guidelines for treating the elderly. It is usually recommended that these patients be placed in "homes" because they are "sick" and need "nursing" care. Often this assignment is made out of frustration. Although often no specific disease process can be diagnosed, the patients often have many somatic complaints, and "nursing" care will at least get them out of the doctor's office and their family's home. Nursing homes are a logical extension of the national medical care system, and a response to rising costs of hospitalization. However, although medically they are both logical and necessary, their organization and care from a behavioral perspective are often disastrous. They are usually organized on an acute treatment model where experts periodically treat the patients and send them home to rest and recover. Although this is appropriate for acute illness, only a few patients in nursing homes fit this model. Most "patients" are long-term residents where the emphasis should be shifted from "nursing" to "home" and where "cure" can only be achieved by activity, not by inactivity.

Nursing homes as they are presently organized and managed are not satisfactory places for the elderly. Medical schools have failed to produce enough physicians interested in treating this population and taking responsibility for designing better treatment strategies. This burden has fallen to nursing professionals who lack the training, skills, and authority for implementing the necessary environmental changes. Their responsibilities are clearly defined as medical, and they rarely have the necessary supervisory training to direct the staff who directly interact with patients. In addition, nursing-home administrators usually lack the skills required to manage people-oriented long-term care systems.

A good deal of support for a social-environmental model of nursing home geriatric patient care has developed (1, 15, 21, 24, 25, 44, 45, 46, 48, 50, 51). Kramer and Kramer (44, 45, 46) recently concentrated their efforts on developing a management program for therapeutic care at a "total" facility. Ample evidence shows that even the most demented elderly can benefit from well-managed environmental change (60). Miller (60) outlined two basic approaches to the treatment of dementia. One is an attempt to alter the individual to help him cope with the environment more effectively; the other is modification of the environment to meet the individual's needs. The latter, a prosthetic environmental approach, was first proposed by Lindsley (49). Evidence that environmentally based motivational change programs are effective for the elderly nursing-home population is provided in the behavioral literature below.

To summarize, the organization and staff management of nursing homes often accentuates any preexisting "senile" problems in the elderly. It is often a foregone conclusion that a patient with, or often without, signs of senility will rapidly become institutionalized and deteriorate in a nursing home (cf. 13, 31, 64). Ironically, the best protection against the system is the patient's own refusal—or the refusal of a relative—of placement in a "home."

Defining and Treating Senility

"Senile" is a label often given to a group of patients with a wide variety of problems of various etiologies (74). Organic brain syndrome associated with senile brain disease is usually accompanied by intellectual impairment, disorientation, disorganization of thought processes, loss of ability to perform basic self-care and social functions, social withdrawal, and disturbed nocturnal behavior (15, 80). These behavioral symptoms can also result from nonsenile conditions such as dehydration, starvation, viral infection, and medication; all of these symptoms can be markedly exacerbated by depression, a common condition in the nursing-home environment.

Chronic brain disorders leading to senility have received pathological definition and some medical attention, although it has not yet become clear whether they are diseases caused by aging or diseases that accompany aging (75). Despite any neuropathological substrate, there is ample evidence that psychosocial deterioration results from inactivity (40), which is the hallmark of most institutional settings for the elderly. Patients learn to withdraw from their environment and activity, become passive and dependent (23, 36), exhibit few motor behaviors and few social interactions, and stop participating in activities (42, 55, 66). This social withdrawal and nonparticipation is accompanied by a wide range of physiological and behavioral changes. For example, the circulatory, respiratory, and digestive systems function less effectively and muscles atrophy (12), and their metabolism is slowed (76). Impairment of cognitive functions is generally correlated with lowered oxygen concentration which accompanies the reduced blood flow in patients with cerebral arteriosclerosis and other chronic brain syndromes (40). These patients behave more slowly, engage in fewer behaviors, and show a decreased variety of behaviors (18).

Butler and Lewis (15) describe two groups of older patients in mental hospitals or nursing-home facilities. One includes people who were admitted to mental hospitals early in life and aged there; the other consists of those who developed socially unacceptable behavior after becoming old. Reversible brain disorders were found in 13% of the patients in a large municipal hospital, and 33% were found to have mixed reversible and chronic disorders. Diagnostic failure often results in recoverable people being sent to long-term care facilities when home care would have been more beneficial to them.

Diagnostic mislabeling is recognized as a major problem with the elderly (14, 15, 16, 21, 50, 78, 82). Tomlinson (82) argues convincingly that the term "senile" is misleading since physiological evidence shows that the changes commonly described as senile are present in middle-aged as well as old people. Carp (16) describes a study that failed to show differences between the elderly and college students on a commonly used measure of senility. MacDonald (50) lists three nonneurological causes for senilelike behaviors which often lead to a diagnostic label of senility: 1) the general social expectancy for senility to accompany old age, 2) an infirmity or a group of preventable and reversible infirmities that occur with accompanying confusion, and 3) the senilelike confusion resulting from environmental change, deprivation, or input.

"Senility" as a result of institutional care is not unknown (50). Social learning theory suggests that improperly given assistance may produce these behaviors and further deterioration in self-help behavior with a result that the recipient of the "care" becomes increasingly passive and more dependent on caregivers. For example, a nursing-home resident who can feed himself, but whose table manners have deteriorated, is often served meals in his own room because the caregiver wants to maintain a more pleasant dining condition for other residents. The isolated individual then deteriorates, losing his ability to feed himself; social attention is restored in the form of a nurses aide feeding him. This attention reinforces the failure to feed himself, and the patient becomes progressively more helpless. These patients' days are characterized by little stimulation. Activities and programs are usually nonexistent in the "homes" for them since it is generally assumed that those patients are incapable of participating. Since there are no opportunities to participate, they are not likely to exhibit any signs showing an ability to participate, and the assumption is perpetuated. If activity is offered, and the patients refuse to participate or if the offer is ignored, the assumption that they won't participate is strengthened. This cycle continues until there is a complete breakdown of social and motor skills resulting in irreversible physical and neurological functioning (57).

Diagnostic instruments are often used to differentiate acute (reversible) and chronic (irreversible) brain syndromes. Unfortunately, they are designed to define the "disease process," but usually ignore the person's behaviors, or specify behaviors that need to be—or could be (15). The medical diagnostic system often leads to a therapeutic nihilism (65). For example, if a patient is determined to have a chronic brain disorder, his condition is often considered irreversible and thus untreatable. His behaviors continue to demonstrate incompetence, he is segregated from society into a nursing home, and further decline is witnessed. It is clear that some old people behave quite capably despite brain damage (15, 35) and that inactivity produces a wide variety of degenerative disorders (12, 20). Brain damage does not necessarily "cause" behavioral disorders, despite often coexisting with them. In practice, irreversibility and reversibility can be best determined by treatment; if the treatment is successful, the patient's syndrome is reversible. If it is not successful, the disease may be irreversible or the treatment may be inadequate or inappropriate. Different treatments should be considered before writing off the patient. Ecological assessment techniques, which assess the interactions of the patient with his environment, may be helpful in planning relevant treatment strategies that consider the patient's skill levels and rehabilitation potential (11).

Few medications are useful in treating the "confusion" of the elderly patient. In most cases medications exacerbate or cause confusion (14, 25, 80). Elderly patients are most sensitive to most drug effects and especially to their side effects, a problem that is compounded by medication compliance "errors" such as taking too much medication or medications at the wrong time of day, and medication prescription "errors" such as prescribing cardiac drugs known to cause depression (alpha methyldopa and reserpine) for a cardiac condition, and other medications to correct the behavioral change caused by the cardiac drugs. Although acute organic brain syndromes can usually be treated after appropriate diagnosis—for example, apathetic hyperthyroidism or pernicious anemia with dementia—no definitive treatment exists for dementias caused by a variety of cerebral atrophies, cerebral arteriosclerosis, or other organic degenerative disorders (15, 83). However, social prosthetics and social-environmental strategies are successful techniques for reducing the behavioral problems occurring from these conditions and markedly improving the quality of life of these patients once they are institutionalized (1, 15, 35, 83).

From a behavioral viewpoint, the nursing-home resident's confusion is caused by many factors, including a lack of environmental feedback and/or pain avoidance. Incontinence can result from avoidance of painful movement or simply "miscueing." Dehydration may result from avoiding painful movement or a lack of thirst cues. A resident may be inactive because it is painful to move or simply because there is nothing to do within reach. Residents may be nonambulatory because it is painful to move or simply because there is nowhere interesting to go. The attitude that commonly develops is, "Why bother doing anything when there always is someone who eventually will do it for me?" The simplest way to prevent symptoms of senility is to maintain self-help and self-care skills.

To the staff who deals directly with nursing-home patients every day, it is irrelevant which patients have medically defined disorders and which have psychologically defined disorders. The staff need to know the best available technology for treating these problems effectively, efficiently, and humanely regardless of cause. It is important that they are aware when debilitation is related to environmental variables that can be identified and manipulated rather than, or in addition to, intrinsic neurological processes so an appropriate environmental milieu for each patient can be designed (43).

Several studies have shown that intervention programs that reinforce high activity levels can delay the physical and behavioral deterioration associated with aging and can help to maintain patients' social and motor skills (32, 41, 52, 54, 66, 71). The question has been raised whether or not a physical environment can be created which maximizes both the happiness of the geriatric patient and his longevity and what kinds of prosthetics and reinforcements can be used in this type of program (19). We would like to suggest that such a program can be created and point out some physical changes and the types of interactions of the individuals with his physical and behavioral environment which aid in the formation of this type of program.

BEHAVIORAL CAREGIVING ROUTINES IN NURSING HOMES

What to Change

When one considers possible areas of environmental manipulation for these living groups, the list of important factors includes the physical properties of the setting, staff characteristics, equipment and materials, staff-resident relationships, measures of resident participation and staff performance, training and supervision of paraprofessional staff, and program packaging and dissemination (cf. 22). Often, before any change in patient treatment priorities can be made, a nearly complete restructuring of the environment is necessary. Although the residents' behaviors are constrained and prompted by the evironmental structure, so are those of the staff. The care provided by the staff—including nursing, dietary, housekeeping, activities, physical therapy, and recreation—depends on available equipment, usable space, and staff assignments. For example, hand-carrying large amounts of equipment long distances may be exhausting and hinder the staff's capacity for caregiving. Many of the elements necessary for a high quality of life, such as a friendly social interaction with residents, may be dropped in a hectic, trying schedule, and it may become more important to the nursing-home geriatric aide to suppress spontaneous resident activity than to generate it. Staff respond to criticism for overemphasis on systematic routines by pointing out that these are assigned tasks and, unlike their interactions with residents, are regularly monitored for completion. Staff turnover in nursing homes is generally high, over 80% nationally (61), requiring expensive training of replacements. This "training" often consists of only two or three days on the job with little supervision before the aides are permitted to "care" for residents on their own without supervision.

In considering the total environment of nursing-home residents, it is first necessary to look at the activities of the staff to determine exactly what they do in an average day. The next step is to restructure staff activities so minimal time and energy are lost in nonessential activities and maximum time and energy are spent in assisting residents in self-help and self-care and improving the quality of their lives. The nursing home is ideally a place for the elderly person to live a full social and active life in the years during which expected infirmities no longer allow the independence that was once available. We have developed a good environmental technology for preschool children in day-care centers; a nearly identical technology can provide a good environment for the elderly in the nursing home.

Activities of aides and residents can be assigned to employee-patient units of three aides for 20 to 30 residents requiring skilled and intermediate care. One aide can be made responsible for assisting residents with routines including fluid intake, bowel-and-bladder care, and recreational equipment (70). This system can include assisting patients who are bedridden to turn over, taking routine tests for diabetes and dehydration, taking care of catheter bags, and performing other tasks that can be accomplished at the same time. The two additional aides can assist residents in other behaviors that are routine but not as easily performed within the context of the resident's room, such as assistance with showers or help in eating, which require more time for each visit. The latter "ancillary" or "personal care" self-help assistance routines, and the former system, can be conducted using carts loaded with all equipment necessary for each care cycle, thus reducing unnecessary movement.

Systematic behavioral interventions often reduce the incidence of symptoms usually attributed to "senility." For example, incontinence may be eliminated by assisting patients to the bathroom on a regular schedule; inactivity can be eliminated by offering recreational equipment and prompting its use, which enables "senile" patients to engage and interact with their environment; and dehydration, another consequence of senility, can be counteracted by periodically offering and assisting with fluid intake. Additional examples can be found in the dining room where residents tend to be "withdrawn" and "nonsocial." Prompts for engaging other patients in social activities often eliminates this "withdrawal" and "nonsocial" behavior. Concern for the residents should begin at the time of referral; evidence has indicated that even moving from one room to another in the same nursing home can be traumatic enough to increase mortality (64).

Historical Antecedents

Although behavioral management techniques seem to offer great promise in helping the elderly, their use is only recent (7). Berger and Rose (10) found only three reports describing the application of the social learning model to the elderly prior to 1968, and 18 reports betwen 1968 and 1977, Wisocki and Mosher (85) listed 31 published articles describing the application of behavior modification strategies with the elderly. Cautela and Mansfield (19) also noted the paucity of behavioral work in geriatric populations in their review. Since Lindsley's (49) report suggesting prosthetic additions to behavioral strategies with geriatric patients, interest in applied behavior analysis with these patients has dramatically increased. An answer to the question whether a physical environment that provides happiness can be established, and which kinds of prosthetics and consequences can be utilized to this end, may be in sight.

Classical conditioning procedures to help geriatric patient care were proposed as early as 1966 (17). Since then, important demonstrations of operant learning strategies with the elderly have taken place. For example, Baltes and Zerbe (9) retrained a 67-year-old nursing-home resident to feed herself using a variety of foods as reinforcers. The training was begun in the patient's room and, when stabilized, was continued in the dining room. An ABA experimental design demonstrated operant control of her self-feeding behaviors. Baltes and Lascomb (8) also used an ABA experimental design with social and tangible reinforcers (tokens) to reduce the frequency of screaming in an 80-year-old geriatric patient. They noted that it is important for nurses to recognize their inherent social reinforcing value for patients and to use it wisely.

MacDonald (51), using behavior modification strategies, dramatically increased the mean rate of verbalization for three socially isolated geriatric patients with environmental engineering techniques. Using an ABAB design, the experimenter either prompted and socially reinforced verbalization (B) or ignored patients and read to them from a book (A). She concluded that prompts generated verbalizations, and social reinforcement maintained higher levels of verbalization than passive activity like listening to readings. With increased verbal behavior there is less incidence of senile symptoms.

Environmental change can even affect sleeping and waking time and letter writing in this population. Will and Cone (84), for example, reported a case study in which they reduced daytime sleeping in a resident whose baseline was zero time awake during daylight hours. Providing a roommate increased his waking time to about 25% of the day. When reinforcements, orange quarters, and experimenter attention were systematically provided to the patient, waking time increased to 37%, which was comparable to the median waking time of the other residents during baseline (36%). Compared with the group median (29%) during the reward condition, reinforcement did little to affect waking time. The authors concluded that reinforcement had virtually no influence, but environmental change provided by a roommate, and perhaps the relocation of the bed nearer the door, had a powerful effect. The patient exhibited less "withdrawal" and had more interaction with his enviromment. In another example, an interesting display of increasing behavior through prompts to facilitate naturally occurring reinforcers, Goldstein and Baer (28) trained and prompted letter writing in three nursing-home residents. With the increased letter writing, more letters were received in turn by the residents. They concluded that this was a relatively inexpensive way to maintain resident's contact with their social environment.

McClannahan and Risley (58) interrupted the "vicious degenerative cycle" by placing recreational equipment on the geriatric table and comparing levels of engagement with and without the materials. Interaction of the resident with the environment was consistently higher when equipment was available than when it was not. It was concluded that "patients' levels of participation with their environment can be greatly increased by providing recreation materials,...some types of recreation equipment are used significantly more than others,...[and that] individual patients differ markedly in their usage of recreation materials." Recreation is not the only way to generate involvement with the environment for nursing–home residents. McClannahan and Risley (55) examined the shopping behavior of nursing–home elderly by setting up a store in the nursing home. During a one-hour shopping time one day each week, observers recorded residents in the area, residents participating, quantity purchased, item description, item cost, and purchaser's name. Data from the store-open hour were compared with another day at the same time when the store was closed. Substantial increases in participation and attendance in the store area were noted during the open hour compared with the store-closed hour. They concluded that with the store available, residents were encouraged to leave their own rooms and go into the public areas of the home where they were more likely to engage in activities in the environment. The store contributed to maintenance of patients' self-care skills and set the occasion for social and recreational engagement during the week. In a similar program, one resident has taken responsibility for operating a store in another nursing home. Dealing with small change, opening and closing the store, and obtaining small items for buyers permits him to engage in fine-motor skills. Previously a physical therapist was unable to interest him in exercises.

In one of our recent studies (69), we selected 16 alert residents to participate in two experiments, eight residents in each. In each experiment, four residents at one table were served family-style meals. Independent observers counted social interactions at intervals using a time-sampling technique. Counterbalancing the experiment, we first served one table family style, then at the next meal the same table was served institutional style. Interpersonal interactions while served family style more than doubled for 9 of 16 residents, and social interactions increased for nearly all residents. The simple intervention of serving a meal that required residents to pass food to one another markedly increased levels of social interaction. Additionally, residents reported that they enjoyed the meal more, and they seemed to recall it better when served family style than when served in an institutional style. This improvement in ability to recall meals is contradictory to reports of senile behaviors in elderly nursing-home residents.

Once the quality of care—assistance in maintaining or restoring self-help—is ensured, the resident's quality of life needs to be considered. Elderly persons tend to require prompting before they will attend activities (2), and reinforcement seems necessary for maintaining attendance (29). McClannahan and Risley (56) found that announcement of activities was needed to recruit attendance at activities; announcing activities increased attendance levels to more than twice that of unannounced activites. Although three different types of announcements, public address, signs, and dinner table, were not different in effectiveness, a slightly larger number of residents were recruited when all three types of announcements were made for an activity. Patients in nursing homes need meaningful activities to fill their time. McClannahan found that more residents attended group activities with prompting and reinforcement and that participation was closely related to attendance; i.e., the greater the attendance, the greater the participation (54). A higher percentage of attending residents participated in dance than in other exercises during the exercise activity, and a higher percentage of attending residents participated in the use of rhythm instruments than with singing or kazoos during music activities.

Salter and Salter (72), in an elaborate reality-orientation and daily-living-activities strategy, trained staff over a two-month interval. Male patients in the study (N = 45) ranged in age from 60 to 86 ($\bar{x}$ = 68). All were diagnosed as having an organic brain syndrome in addition to other disorders. At the start of the study, 86% were disoriented, confused, and lacking in motivation. The remainder would participate in some activities. Following evaluation of each resident's capabilities, a staff member was assigned to carry out a certain number of activities with a small group of patients. Checklists were filled out daily to evaluate the patients' behaviors. These behaviors were shaped to increase participation in reality orientation, activities of daily living, and recreational activities, using as reinforcers social approval, candy, and cigarettes. After four months, the number of patients considered motivated rose to 76%. Marked improvements in physical condition were also noted. The most useful educational tool, they found, was several posters placed in a large number of places on the ward which prompted aides to attend to the reality-orientation task.

Hoyer et al. (38) used exchangeable tokens, candy, or cigarettes as reinforcers to increase verbal responses to questions. In two experiments using an ABAB design, their elderly mental patients showed increased frequencies of verbal response under reinforcement conditions. Geiger and Johnson (26) demonstrated that some elderly patients are subject to reinforced food-eating behavior through the administration of readily available events and objects of their own choosing. We recently examined procedures designed to train geriatric aides to assist residents in regaining self-feeding skills. Observers watched each feeding event, e.g., bites of food or sips of a beverage, and recorded the eating behavior, e.g., scooping, cutting, and drinking, and level of independence, e.g., amount of instruction provided by the aide, independent food choice, who paces the action, and any "errors," e.g., spills, use of hands for utensil items. After a meal, the number of feeding events is divided into the number scored under each category to give an indication of the patient's participation and independence. All three patients trained with this procedure were previously spoonfed by aides; after proper aide training, there were dramatic increases in the patients' participation in their own feeding.

Baltes and Baltes (5, 6) have proposed joining behavioral-ecological approaches to life-span developmental approaches. While behavioral management should continue to expand response repertoires, behavioral research with the elderly should focus increased attention on maintaining and generalizing competencies and stabilizing these competencies at community and individual levels (63).

Practice*

Recently our group structured the environment of a Tennessee nursing home as construction was being completed and staff hired. Using a set of procedures similar to those developed by Risley and Favell for working with profoundly

---

*The information provided here has been summarized in greater detail in Risley, T.R., and Edwards, K.A. *Behavioral technology for nursing home care: Toward a system of nursing home organization and management.* Paper presented at the Nova Behavioral Conference on Aging, Port St. Lucie, Florida, May 1978.

retarded children (68), we armed ourselves with a set of materials based on several years' work at the University of Kansas by many students and researchers working in the Living Environments Group under the supervision of Todd R. Risley. All data are not yet in, but in this section we will describe the work leading to the Tennessee trip.

Research at LEG is directed toward developing complete environments which serve to continuously maintain behaviors appropriate to the setting, and is concerned with the description, selection, and organization of facilities, equipment, materials, and personnel. Additionally, the group attends to the usual behavior intervention variables of applied psychology. This research has been conducted in a wide variety of settings including infant and toddler day care centers. One notable finding has been the amazing amount of resemblance among settings and their effects on behavior. Our goal, then, has been to provide a complete nursing home environment that would restore and maintain functional behaviors with nursing home elderly including the so-called "senile."

In our previous work, we have observed staff in nursing homes perform their normal functions throughout the day. Program activities, storage, traffic, and equipment used were also evaluated. We prepared introductions to therapeutic routines for the staff which described the rationale. In restructuring the environment our priority was patient *care,* or more specifically, assistance in regaining self-help skills. Therefore, we attempted to remove time-wasting activities that focused on anything other than this.

After the necessary information about the environment and patient and staff activity was obtained, the sequence of resident activities was restructured. Since most of the day in a skilled-nursing facility is spent in physical-care activities such as bathing, feeding, or waking and dressing, much of the time aides spend with residents is basically custodial care. In an effort to decrease the emphasis on custodial care and introduce some additions to the resident's quality of life, we previously (70) developed a simple nursing-home treatment routine. To reduce dehydration and incontinence and to increase activity levels, a "health-care technician" circulated through nonambulatory patients' rooms every hour with a cart equipped with liquids, diapers, linens, and recreational materials. During each visit, he offered bathroom assistance, helped the patient clean himself if soiled, prompted the consumption of liquids, and gave the patient his choice of recreational equipment. Prior to introducing the care routines, 25% of patients were considered dehydrated. Subsequent to its use, none were found to be dehydrated. Soiling was reduced 50%, and engagement with the environment was increased for nearly all residents. This type of well-structured "custodial" care has social-care components that generate a side effect of improved physical condition.

Training aides in these tasks was accomplished by preparing checklists for routines and subroutines including instructions stating the necessary and sufficient steps for completing each routine and maximizing social contact and quality of care. Training aides can be accomplished in three steps: 1) the trainee reads the checklist and practices the suggested steps, 2) another aide checks the first aide, and 3) the trainee informs the supervisor when he is ready for a "mastery" test. For each activity it may be necessary to conduct an informal time-and-motion study to determine which efforts are minimal and at the same time bring about the greatest amount possible of contact with residents. A great deal of institutional reorganization may be necessary, since staff may resist or have difficulty adjusting to instructions that require longer meal times or less time to be spent making beds.

Monitoring and maintaining performance can be done by nursing staff using checklists to periodically examine either the process or products of an aide's performance. The supervisor then can give feedback to the staff member to help correct performances and/or reward good performances. Further quality control can be provided by an external monitor who can provide feedback to aides as well as to their supervisor for work well or poorly done.

Our initial work with elderly nursing-home residents has produced some restoration of functional behavior in senile and senilelike patients (55, 56, 57, 69, 70). Strategies for staff training in skills promoting self-help appear to be more successful than those focusing directly on patient care (30). Most important, once the training has been completed, its maintenance through supervision is imperative. An external monitoring system guarantees that supervision is maintained at a high level. Tying this together with a quality assurance measure of patient care and an assessment of patient self-help skills completes the total environmental package for a nursing home.

IMPLICATIONS AND SPECULATIONS FOR FUTURE APPLICATIONS

The physical environment of the elderly nursing-home resident is often neglected despite the evidence presented by Sommer (79) and others (59, 67, 86) that the quality of the space surrounding us has more effect on behavior than the way people behave toward one another. Ideally, a nursing home would provide an environment specifically suited for elderly men and women. Its residents are equal-aged peers with similar interests and interesting experiences that could be shared. It could have a large store of materials and equipment to be used for recreation. There can be interested and devoted nurses and nursing aides, cooks and cook's assistants, housekeepers and housekeeping assistants, and skilled activity directors, physical therapists, and recreational programmers. Many nursing-home personnel are warm, loving, and responsive to the patient's needs. There are some who are skilled at arranging activities that engage patients' interest, answering questions when needed, comforting when physically or emotionally hurt, and encouraging alternative ways of dealing with conflicts. Residents in some facilities participate in conducting their own government, and their demands are met by a responsive administration which is sensitive to the residents' needs. Some nurses and aides are perceptive, quick to pick out a resident who needs special help with some portion of his daily living, and ready to accept every resident for the things that make him lovable, while trying to change those things that are causing discomfort and hampering his quality of life (3).

Nursing homes often contain a wide variety of equipment and rehabilitation materials that few individuals could afford. When properly motivated, residents can regain their large muscle skills, walk in hallways or in neighborhoods, play games designed for their skill levels, and even dance; and they can redevelop fine motor skills and manual dexterity. They can live socially with their peers in rewarding ways (37) and take responsibility for sharing their experiences with others. The presence of many residents engaging in a wide range of activities and pursuing a variety of special interests allows them to remain a member of an active community and to enjoy many of their remaining years without being alone.

It is hard to imagine an environment more suited to aiding both normal and abnormal elderly in training and retraining than the nursing home. The home described above, however, is an ideal setting in which the elderly receive concerned and skilled behavioral care. All nursing homes undoubtedly have one or more of the components necessary for conducting or maintaining an ideal setting. It is these components that keep nursing homes running and nursing-home administrators from being tarred and feathered. Ideally, what we are working for is an increase in the number of these components in each nursing home. We have not yet seen the ideal nursing home, but attention has been focused in that direction. A description of the development of an ideal setting leading to the restoration of functional behavior in geriatric, "senile" patients has begun.

CONCLUSIONS

Medical treatments for the various disorders commonly collected under the heading "senility" are generally unsatisfactory. The nursing homes, originally developed as cheap alternatives to hospitals, have become poor alternatives to living. Behavioral treatments do not "cure" brain damage or restore the neural functioning of the elderly, but they can restore behavioral functioning and remove many of the symptoms that cause the elderly to be labeled "senile." By concentrating on appropriate models, we may be far more successful in treatment of the elderly, and these successes would make the elderly a far more pleasurable population to work with. Behavioral techniques may be especially useful for making nursing homes into *homes* rather than repositories for the sick and aged.

ACKNOWLEDGMENTS

This report is one in a series of studies by the Living Environments Group at the University of Kansas, supported in part by a grant from the Department of Health, Education and Welfare, National Institutes of Health #R01 HS 02510, Todd R. Risley, principal investigator. Requests for reprints should be sent to the author at the Human Services Program, Department of Allied Health and Nursing, Northern Kentucky University, Highland Heights, Ky. 41076.

REFERENCES

1. Albrecht, R. Social roles in the prevention of senility. *J. Gerontology* 6:380-386, 1951.
2. Anderson, J.E. Environment and meaningful activity, in F.G. Scott and R.M. Brewer (eds.), *Perspectives in Aging. I: Research Focus.* Corvallis, Or.: Oregon Center for Gerontology, 1971, pp. 178-190.
3. Armstrong, P.W. More thoughts on senility. *Gerontologist* 18:315-316, 1978.
4. Azrin, N.H. A strategy for applied research: Learning based but outcome oriented. *Am. Psychol.* 32:140-149, 1977.
5. Baltes, M.M. Health care from a behavioral-ecological viewpoint, in M. Keininger (ed.), *Transcultural Health Care Issues and Condition.* Philadelphia: David Company, 1976.
6. Baltes, M.M., and Baltes, P.B. The ecopsychological relativity and plasticity of psychological aging: Convergent perspectives of cohort effects and operant psychology. *Zeitschrift fur Experimentelle und Angewandte Psychologie* 24:179-197, 1977.
7. Baltes, M., and Barton, E.M. New approaches toward aging: A case for the operant model. *Educational Gerontology* 2:383-405, 1977.
8. Baltes, M.M., and Lascomb, S.L. Creating a healthy institutional environment for the elderly via behavior management: The nurse as a change agent. *Internat. J. Nursing Studies* 12:5-12, 1975.
9. Baltes, M.M., and Zerbe, M. Behavior management and self maintenance in nursing homes. *Nursing Research* 25:24-26, 1976.
10. Berger, R.M., and Rose, S.D. Interpersonal skill training with institutionalized elderly patients. *J. Gerontology* 32:345-353, 1977.
11. Bernal, G.A.A., Brannon, L.J., Belar, C., Lavigne, J., and Cameron, R. Psychodiagnostics of the elderly, in W.D. Gentry (ed.), *Geropsychology: A Model of Training and Clinical Service.* Cambridge, Mass.: Ballinger, 1977, pp. 43-77.
12. Bonner, O.D. Rehabilitation instead of bed rest? *Geriatrics* 24:109-118, 1969.
13. Bush, S. A change of scene can be fatal. *Psychol. Today* 10 (9):32, 1977 (Summary).
14. Butler, R.N. *Why Survive? Being Old in America.* New York: Harper & Row, 1975.
15. Butler, R.N., and Lewis, M.I. *Aging and Mental Health: Positive Psychosocial Approaches.* Sant Louis: C.V. Mosby, 1973.
16. Carp, R.M. Senility or garden-variety maladjustment?, in F.G. Scott and R.M. Brewer (eds.), *Perspectives in Aging. I: Research Focus.* Corvallis, Or.: Oregon Center for

Gerontology, 1971, pp. 78-84.

17. Cautela, J.R. Behavior therapy and geriatrics. *J. Genetic Psychol.* 108:9-17, 1966.

18. Cautela, J.R. A classical conditioning approach to the development and modification of behavior in the aged. *Gerontologist* 9:109-113, 1969.

19. Cautela, J.R., and Mansfield, L. A behavioral approach to geriatrics, in W.D. Gentry (ed.), *Geropsychology: A Model of Training and Clinical Service.* Cambridge, Mass.: Ballinger, 1977.

20. Comstock, R.L., Mayers, R.L., and Folsom, J.C. Simple physical activities for the elderly. *Hospital and Community Psychiatry* 20:377-380, 1969.

21. Cosin, L.Z., Mort, M., Post, F., Westropp, C., and Williams, M. Experimental treatment of persistent senile confusion. *Internat. J. Soc. Psychiat.* 4:24-42, 1958.

22. Davis, S., and Cayan, P. Personnel selection and training, in S.M. Schneeweiss and S.W. Davis (eds.), *Nursing Home Administration.* Baltimore: University Park Press, 1974, pp. 19-43.

23. Donahue, W. Rehabilitation of long-term aged patients, in R.H. Williams (ed.), *Processes of Aging.* New York: Atherton, 1963.

24. Eisdorfer, C. The implications of research for medical practice, in F.G. Scott and R.M. Brewer (eds.) *Perspectives in Aging, I: Research Focus.* Corvallis, Or.: Oregon Center for Gerontology, 1971, pp. 48-53.

25. Ford, C.S. Confused and disoriented elderly, in Health Resources Administration (eds.), *Working with Older People: A Guide to Practice. Volume III: The Aging Person: Needs and Services.* (DHEW Publication No. [HRA] 74-3118). Rockville, Md.: U.S. Dept. of Health, Education and Welfare, 1974, pp. 50-51.

26. Geiger, O.G., and Johnson, L.A. Positive education for elderly persons: Correct eating through reinforcement. *Gerontologist* 14:432-436, 1974.

27. Goldfarb, A.I., Hochstadt, N.J., Jacobson, J.H., and Weinstein, E.A. Hyperbaric oxygen treatment of organic mental syndrome in aged persons. *J. Gerontology* 27:212-217, 1972.

28. Goldstein, R.S., and Baer, D.M. R.S.V.P.: A procedure to increase the personal mail and number of correspondents for nursing home residents. *Behav. Ther.* 7:348-354, 1976.

29. Gottesman, L.E. Behavior change and therapy for geriatric mental patients, in D.K. Heyman (ed.), *Duke University Council on Aging and Human Development: Proceedings of Seminars, 1970-1976.* Durham, N.C.: Center for the Study of Aging and Human Development, Duke University, 1976, pp. 155-171.

30. Gottesman, L.E., and Hutchinson, E. Characteristics of institutionalized elderly, in E.M. Brody (ed.), *A Social Work Guide for Long-Term Care Facilities.* (DHEW Publication No. [ADM] 75-177). Rockville, Md.: National Institute of Mental Health, 1974, pp. 27-45.

31. Haberkorn, S.B., Davis, L.J., and Pastalan, L.A. The Pennsylvania nursing home relocation program: Process and impact. *Gerontologist* 17:70, 1977. (Abstract)

32. Havighurst, R.J. Successful aging, in R.H. Williams (ed.), *Processes of Aging.* New York: Atherton, 1963.

33. Health Resources Administration. *Working with Older People: A Guide to Practice. Volume II: Biological, Psychological, and Sociological Aspects of Aging.* (DHEW Publication No. [HRA] 74-3117). Rockville, Md.: Department of Health, Education and Welfare, 1974.

34. Health Resources Administration. *Health: United States, 1975.* (DHEW Publication No. [HRA] 76-1232). Rockville, Md.: U.S. Department of Health, Education and Welfare, 1976.

35. Hellebrandt, F.A. The senile dement in our midst: A look at the other side of the coin. *Gerontologist* 18:67-70, 1978.

36. Henry, J. Personality and aging—with special reference to hospitals for the aging poor, in J.C. McKinney and F.T. deVyver (eds.), *Aging and Social Policy*. New York: Appleton-Century-Crofts, 1966.
37. Hirsch, K., and Linn, M.W. How being helpful helps the elderly helper. *Gerontologist* 17:75, 1977. (Abstract)
38. Hoyer, W.J., Kafer, R.A., Simpson, S.C., and Hoyer, F.W. Reinstatement of verbal behavior in elderly mental patients using operant procedures. *Gerontologist* 14:149-152, 1974.
39. Jarvik, L.F. Thoughts on the psychobiology of aging. *Am. Psychol.* 30:576-583, 1975.
40. Jarvik, L.F., and Cohen, D. A biochemical approach to intellectual changes with aging, in C. Eisdorfer and M.P. Lawton (eds.), *The Psychology of Adult Development and Aging*. Washington, D.C.: American Psychological Association, 1973, pp. 220-280.
41. Jeffers, F., and Nichols, C.R. The relationship of activities and attitudes to physical well-being in older people. *J. Gerontology* 16:67-70, 1969.
42. Kart, C.S., and Manard, B.B. Quality of care in old-age institutions. *Gerontologist* 16:250-256, 1976.
43. Kastenbaum, R. Perspectives on the development and modification of behavior in the aged: A developmental-field perspective. *Gerontologist* 8:280-283, 1968.
44. Kramer, C.H., and Kramer, J.R. The nursing home as a total therapeutic situation: Some basic assumptions. *J. Geriatric psychiatry* 1:179-220, 1968.
45. Kramer, C.H., and Kramer, J.R. Basic Principles of Long-Term Patient Care: Developing a Therapeutic Community. Springfield, Ill.: Charles C. Thomas, 1976.
46. Kramer, J.R. Organizing a therapeutic milieu for long term care, in D.K. Heyman (ed.), *Duke University Council on Aging and Human Development: Proceedings of Seminars, 1970-1976*. Durham, N.C.: Center for the Study of Aging and Human Development, Duke University, 1976, pp. 129-141.
47. Kramer, M., Taube, C.A., and Redick, R.W. Patterns of use of psychiatric facilities by the aged: Past, present, and future, in C. Eisdorfer and M.P. Lawton (eds.), *The Psychology of Adult Development and Aging*. Washington, D.C.: American Psychological Association, 1973, pp. 428-528.
48. Lawton, M.P. Some beginnings of an ecological psychology of old age, in D.K. Heyman (ed.), *Duke University Council on Aging and Human Development: Proceedings of Seminars, 1970-1976*. Durham, N.C.: Center for the Study of Aging and Human Development, Duke University, 1976, pp. 183-192.
49. Lindsley, O.R. Geriatric behavioral prosthetics, in R. Kastenbaum (ed.), *New Thoughts on Old Age*. New York: Springer, 1964, pp. 41-60.
50. MacDonald, M.L. The forgotten Americans: A sociopsychological analysis of aging and nursing homes. *Am. J. Community Psychology* 1:272-294, 1973.
51. MacDonald, M.L. Environmental programming for the socially isolated aging. *Gerontologist* 18:350-354, 1978.
52. McClannahan, L.E. Recreation programs for nursing home residents: The importance of patient characteristics and environmental arrangements. *Therapeutic Recreation J.* 7:26-31, 1973.
53. McClannahan, L.E. Therapeutic and prosthetic living environments for nursing home residents. *Gerontologist* 13:424-429, 1973.
54. McClannahan, L.E. Design of living environments for nursing home residents. Unpublished doctoral dissertation, University of Kansas, 1973.
55. McClannahan, L.E., and Risley, T.R. A store for nursing home residents. *Nursing Homes* 22:10-11, 29, 1973.
56. McClannahan, L.E., and Risley, T.R. Design of living environments for nursing home

residents: Recruiting attendance at activities. *Gerontologist* 14:236-240, 1974.

57. McClannahan, L.E., and Risley, T.R. Design of living environments for nursing home residents: Increasing participation in recreation activities. *J. Appl. Behav. Anal.* 8:261-268, 1975.

58. McClannahan, L.E., and Risley, T.R. Activities and materials for severely disabled geriatric patients. *Nursing Homes* 24:10-13, 1975.

59. McCue, G.M., and Ewald, W.R. *Creating the Human Environment.* Urbana: University of Illinois Press, 1970.

60. Miller, E. The management of dementia: A review of some possibilities. *Br. J. Soc. Clin. Psychol.* 16:77-83, 1977.

61. Molberg, E., and Brothen, T. Factors affecting nursing home assistants' intentions to seek new employment. *J. Gerontology,* submitted.

62. National Center for Health Statistics. *Selected Operating and Financial Characteristics of Nursing Homes.* (DHEW Publication No. [HRA] 76-1773). Rockville, Md.: Health Resources Administration, 1975.

63. Nietzel, M.T., Winett, R.A., MacDonald, M.L., and Davidson, W.S. *Behavioral Approaches to Community Psychology.* New York: Pergamon Press, 1977.

64. Pablo, R.Y. Intra-institutional relocation: Its impact on long-term care patients. *Gerontologist* 17:426-435, 1977.

65. Pfeiffer, E. Psychopathology and social pathology, in J.E. Birren and K.W. Schaie (eds.), *Handbook of the Psychology of Aging.* New York: Van Nostrand, 1977, pp. 650-671.

66. Quilitch, H.R. Purposeful activity increased on a geriatric ward through programmed recreation. *J. Am. Geriatrics Society* 22:226-229, 1974.

67. Risley, T.R. The ecology of applied behavior analysis, in A. Rogers-Warren and S. Warren (eds.), *Ecological Perspectives in Behavior Analysis.* Baltimore, Md.: University Park Press, 1977, pp. 149-163.

68. Risley, T.R., and Favell, J. Constructing a living environment in an institution, in L. Hamerlynck (ed.), *History and Future of Behavior Modification for the Developmentally Disabled.* New York: Brunner/Mazel, in press.

69. Risley, T.R., Gottula, P., and Edwards, K.A. Family- and institutional-style meal service in a nursing home dining room. Paper presented at the Nova Behavioral Conference, Port St. Lucie, Florida, May 1978.

70. Risley, T.R., Spangler, P., and Edwards, K.A. Care of non-ambulatory geriatric patients: A routine to reduce incontinence, dehydration, and inactivity. Paper presented at the Nova Behavioral Conference, Port St. Lucie, Florida, May 1978.

71. Roth, M. Chairman's closing remarks, in G.E.W. Wolstenholme and M. O'Connor (eds.), *Alzheimer's Disease and Related Conditions.* London: J.&A. Churchill, 1970, pp. 301-305.

72. Salter, C. de l., and Salter, C.A. Effects of an individualized activity program on elderly patients. *Gerontologist* 15:404-406, 1975.

73. Schwab, M. Issues in long-term care and implications for the nursing profession, in U.S. Department of Health, Education and Welfare, *Assessing Health Care Needs in Skilled Nursing Facilities: Health Professional Perspectives.* (DHEW Publication No. [OS] 77-50049). 1977, pp. 1-3.

74. Settin, J.M. Some thoughts about diseases presenting as senility. *Gerontologist* 18:71-72, 1978.

75. Shelanski, M.L. The aging brain: Alzheimer's disease and senile dementia, in A.M. Ostfeld, D.D. Gibson, and C.P. Donnelly (eds.), *Epidemiology of Aging.* Bethesda, Md.: National Institute of Child Health and Human Development, 1972, pp. 113-127.

76. Shock, N.W. Energy metabolism, calorie intake and physical activity of the aging, in L.A.

Carlson (ed.), *Nutrition in Old Age*. Uppsala, Sweden: Almquist & Wiksell, 1972.

77. Slaby, A.E., and Wyatt, R.J. *Dementia in the Presenium*. Springfield, Ill.: Charles C. Thomas, 1974.

78. Slater, R., and Lipman, A. Staff assessments of confusion and the situation of confused residents in homes for old people. *Gerontologist* 17:523-530, 1977.

79. Sommer, R. Looking back at personal space, in J. Lang, C. Burnette, W. Moleski, and D. Vachon (eds.), *Designing for Human Behavior: Architecture and the Behavioral Sciences*. Stroudsburg, Pa.: Dowden, Hutchinson, & Ross, 1974, pp. 202-209.

80. Stotsky, B.A. *The Nursing Home and the Aged Psychiatric Patient*. New York: Appleton-Century-Crofts, 1970.

81. Subcommittee on Health of the Committee on Ways and Means. *National Health Insurance Resource Book*. Washington, D.C.: U.S. Government Printing Office, 1976.

82. Tomlinson, B.E. Senile brain changes in middle and late life, in D.K. Heyman (ed.), *Duke University Council on Aging and Human Development: Proceedings of Seminars, 1970-1976*. Durham, N.C.: Center for the Study of Aging and Human Development, Duke University, 1976, pp. 97-113.

83. Wershow, H.J. Reality orientation for gerontologists: Some thoughts about senility. *Gerontologist* 17:297-302, 1977.

84. Will, J.A., and Cone, J.D. Reducing daylight sleeping in an elderly man. Paper presented at the meeting of the Midwestern Association of Behavior Analysis, Chicago, May 1976.

85. Wisocki, P.A., and Mosher, P.M. Behavior modification with the elderly. Workshop presented at the Annual Meeting of the Association for Advancement of Behavior Therapy, Atlanta, Georgia, December 1977.

86. Zeisel, J. Fundamental values in planning with the nonpaying client, in J. Lang, C. Burnette, W. Moleski, and D. Vachon (eds.), *Designing for Human Behavior: Architecture and the Behavioral Sciences*. Stroudsburg, Pa.: Dowden, Hutchinson, & Ross, 1974, pp. 293-301.

Treatment of
Chronic Disorders

Chronic medical disorders are common and will become increasingly so as the average age of our population rises and death from the complications of chronic disease declines. For example, mortality from myocardial infarction has declined significantly, partly because of advances in coronary care and partly because of the wide dissemination of information about cardiac resuscitation.

The cost of providing care for chronic disorders is very large at present, both for individuals and for society. Unfortunately, this cost is escalating at an alarming rate. Treatment strategies for the prevention and remediation of these conditions are urgently needed. The authors present three chronic disorders: seizures, movement disorders, and pain in children. These examples are explored in detail to illustrate the application of behavioral technology to chronic medical disorders in general. The authors' behavioral approach is in many ways similar to the medical approach: a detailed history is obtained with specific reference to exacerbation, remissions, antecedent events, and apparent reinforcing environmental events. The behavioral analysis and treatment program can often lessen the symptoms of these diseases when properly implemented, and appears to be a very cost-effective way of dealing with chronic disorders.

CHAPTER 4

Assessment and Management of Chronic Disorders

Michael F. Cataldo
Dennis C. Russo
Bruce L. Bird
James W. Varni

The advances in biomedical science applied to medical care in this country are unequalled in recorded history. In a recent speech to the American College of Surgeons, Dr. George R. Dunlop (University of Massachusetts Medical School) said: "Today, medicine stands at the highest peak of its achievements. Infant mortality has declined 12.7 percent since 1950. The death rate from heart disease has declined 15 percent in the last six years." In part because of the successes in solving problems of acute care, infectious diseases, and threats to public health through improvements in sanitation, food processing, etc., increasing emphasis is being placed on the problems of chronic disorders.

This chapter will: 1) briefly explore the demography of chronic disorders, their extent, age factors, etc.; 2) identify cost factors that portend changes in our health-care system; 3) discuss the approach of behavioral medicine to chronic disorders, with examples of application to specific diseases; and 4) identify some unique areas in which behavioral approaches can aid with the problem of chronicity, independent of the particular disorder.

DEMOGRAPHICS OF CHRONIC DISORDERS

Approximately one out of every ten persons in the United States suffers from a chronic disorder or disability severe enough to limit activity. Comprehensive statistics available for 1972 (46) and 1974 (98) indicate an increase of 13% in chronic disorders and disabilities in that two-year period, from 25.8 to 29.2

million Americans. This percentage increase is above the population growth rate for the same two-year period. Although the exact degree of increase may be affected by different reporting and sampling techniques, the assumption is that the number of persons with chronic activity-limiting conditions is increasing, and at a rate greater than that accounted for by general population increases.

Analysis by age indicates, as would be expected, that limitations in daily living affect a greater percentage of individuals 65 years of age and over. However, as shown in Figure 1, the number of individuals in the 44–65-year age group is closely comparable to the 65-and-over group.

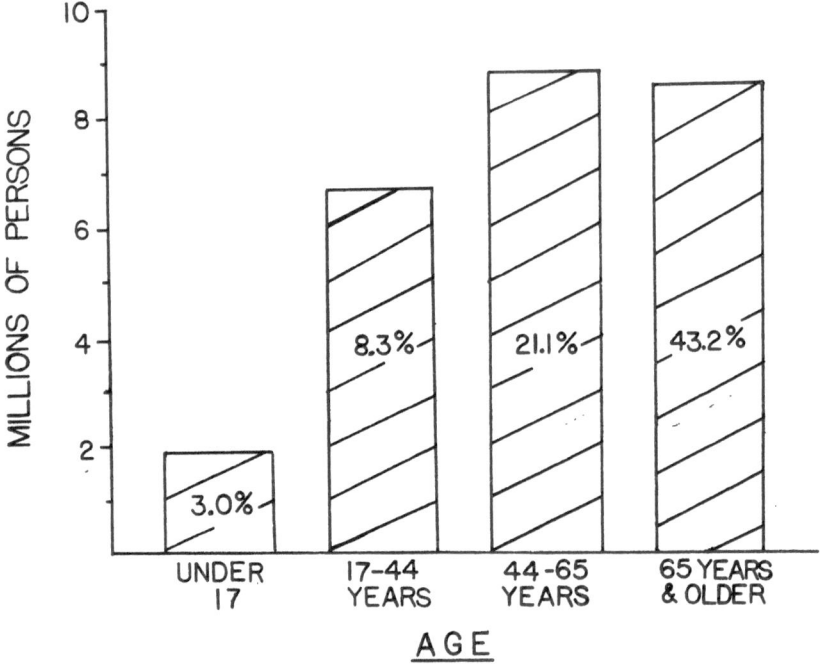

Fig. 1. Number of persons with activity limitations of all degrees, by age group. Within each bar is the percentage of persons in that group with activity limitation.
Source: "Limitation of Activity and Mobility Due to Chronic Conditions: United States, 1972." Health Resources Administration. DHEW Publication No. (HRA) 75-1523.

In all, approximately 68% of noninstitutionalized individuals with activity limitations due to chronic conditions are over 45 years of age (46). Comparison data by race and financial status using age-adjusted statistics for activity limitations are presented in Table 1. For all age categories, there is a race difference, with whites tending toward lower rates of chronic disorders than other races. Income is also a factor, irrespective of race, with activity limitations

Table 1. Age-Adjusted Percents of Population with Activity Limitation by Race, Family Income, and Age

Characteristic	All Ages	Under 17 years	17-44 years	45-64 years	65 years and older
Total White	12.4	3.0	8.0	20.6	42.4
Income less than $5000	19.5	4.0	13.2	41.4	48.2
Income greater than $5000	10.8	2.9	7.3	17.1	36.7
Total Other Races	15.2	2.8	10.2	26.1	51.8
Income less than $5000	21.0	3.2	15.0	42.6	55.9
Income greater than $5000	10.9	2.7	7.7	15.7	39.3

Source: Abstracted from "Limitation of Activity and Mobility Due to Chronic Conditions: United States, 1972." Health Resources Administration, National Center for Health Statistics, U.S. Department of Health, Education and Welfare, U.S. Gov't. Printing Office, 1974. (DHEW Publication No. [HRA] 75-1523).

,ccurring in far greater numbers for persons with family incomes under $5000.

Categorization of chronic disorders depends a great deal on the choice of classification system. For example, according to the categorization presented in Table 2 from an analysis published by the Department of Commerce (98), heart conditions and arthritis and rheumatism account for the highest percentage of chronic conditions resulting in activity limitation. The table also indicates that while the overall prevalence of chronic conditions is similar for both sexes, specific disabilities occur with greater frequency in one sex or the other; e.g., males are more often affected by heart conditions than females, while females are proportionately more limited by arthritis and rheumatism.

On the other hand, an analysis by the Health Resources Administration (46) indicates that while heart disease, arthritis, and hypertension are the major diseases causing chronic disorders, evaluation by the area of the body afflicted indicates that musculoskeletal disorders represent a significant proportion of chronic disabilities, particularly those of the lower extremities, back, and spine.

Costs Related to Chronic Disorders

Chronic conditions, particularly those resulting in disabilities, cause an inestimable amount of suffering and emotional cost. Such conditions also directly impact family, corporate, and national income. In 1975, working Americans suffering from all disorders spent 3.7 billion days in restricted activity, 1.37 billion of which were days restricted to bed, *and* an estimated 433 million work days were lost because of disability (98). Arthritis and rheumatism alone account for 238 million days of restricted activity each year and 14.2 million days

Table 2. Total Number and Percentages of Individuals in the U.S. with Selected Chronic Conditions, by Sex

Disorder	BOTH SEXES All Ages	Over 65	MALE All Ages	Over 65	FEMALE All Ages	Over 65
Total persons with limitation	29,292,000	9,511,000	14,275,000	4,263,000	15,017,000	5,247,000
Percent with:						
Heart conditions	16.2	23.5	18.0	25.2	14.5	22.2
Arthritis & rheumatism	15.0	23.2	10.1	15.6	19.6	29.4
Visual impairments	5.9	9.8	5.9	8.6	5.9	10.7
Hypertension without heart involvement	6.7	8.7	4.5	6.0	8.9	10.9
Mental & nervous conditions	5.1	3.4	4.8	3.0	5.5	3.8

Source: Adapted from "Statistical Abstract of the United States—1977." U.S. Department of Commerce, U.S. Bureau of the Census. U.S. Government Printing Office, 1977.

lost from work. This costs the nation $9.2 billion dollars annually; included in this figure are $3.5 billion in wages and salaries lost by persons unable to work, $3.8 billion in annual medical costs, and $773 million lost from income and excise taxes on wages and salaries (71).

During 1975, of the $17.4 billion spent on federally funded health and medical programs, $4.2 billion went for direct hospital and medical care (98), $972 million in Medicare money for treatment of disabled individuals, and over $1 billion in Medicaid payments.

In addition, 1.9 million individuals judged permanently disabled each received an average of $141 in monthly cash payments, and $3.76 billion was paid as workmen's compensation from private carriers, state funds, and self-insurance (98). Clearly, programs to reduce chronic conditions or remediate their disabling effects could provide potential savings in personal and public costs. However, methods for direct treatment or research to develop new treatments must be considered in the perspective of the current health-care costs.

Health-Care Costs and the Need for Alternative Health-Care Strategies

Health-care costs are increasing rapidly, and much of this increase represents treatment of chronic disorders. From 1976 to 1977 alone, hospital charges have increased 11.8% and physician costs 10.7%, while the cost of living has risen only 4.5%. Today, hospital costs are $154–$175 per day, as opposed to $48 per day in

1966 and $16 per day in 1950. This increase of 1000% in one generation is seven times greater than the rate of inflation for the rest of the economy over the same period (62).

According to these figures, approximately $1 out of every $9 earned is spent on health care. This means that on the average, health care is costing every American, regardless of age, approximately $650 per year. Most of this cost is hidden. Three-quarters is accounted for through taxes, insurance premiums, and overall wage inflation. The cost to the federal government (the repository of our tax dollars) is equally disturbing. In the past four years, outlays for health care have more than doubled to $39.5 billion—almost 1/10 of the federal budget (46).

The 1977 estimate for total private and public outlays for health care and services exceeds $155 billion. This amount represents 8.6% of the nation's total output of goods and services (as compared to 5.9% in 1966 and 4.5% in 1950), and is expected to double within six years.

Providing such high-cost medical care increasingly becomes financially impractical. While there are many causes for this high cost, one solution is to look to the behavioral sciences for new treatment approaches for chronic medical problems. The potential contributions of behavioral science are many (65, 83). Goldiamond (42) has described the behavioral excursion into health care as tripartite: 1) individual health problems affected by societal contingencies (e.g., Medicaid and health benefits) for which the most appropriate solution is a change at the societal level; 2) individual health problems based on societal variables that can be addressed by direct contingency management at the level of the individual, e.g., smoking; and 3) individual health problems that are traceable to the idiosyncratic contingency histories of the individual, e.g. environmentally exacerbated asthma.

This volume provides examples of behavioral approaches in each of these areas, and the behavioral literature is replete with examples of contingency procedures applied to medical problems. Recent work on disorders such as seizures (13, 108), asthma (76), neuromuscular disorders (6, 13), sphincter control (27, 56), and blood pressure (24), combined with studies of adjunctive techniques such as medication compliance (28) and compliance with hemodialysis (61), strongly suggests the potential application of contingency-based procedures in health care.

Some Practical Considerations for Behavioral Medicine Approaches to Chronic Disorders

A great deal can be gained by approaching a chronic disorder, even with an exclusively behavioral treatment strategy, if one interfaces these specific procedures with current knowledge about the pathophysiology of the disorder in a way that facilitates the integration of the procedures into medical practice and ongoing health-care delivery programs, e.g., hospital services, clinics, health education programs, etc. From the perspective of the behaviorist working within a medical context, this implies some very specific practical considerations.

Medical Context

A behavioral medicine approach to chronic disorders must proceed on the assumption that the treatment of these disorders will be conducted on an appropriate medical service, for example, seizures by the neurologist, chronic renal failure by the nephrologist, and tetralogy of Fallot by the cardiologist. Chronic disorders are present in all subspecialties of medicine and in all age ranges—pediatrics, adults, and geriatrics. The behavioral medicine practitioner must be able to abstract common features from this wide range of pathologies to guide his inquiry and prescription.

A set of discriminative characteristics can be used to conceptualize the chronic disorders. A first consideration is that there be an existing, diagnosed, and documented pathological condition, such as asthma, functional heart disorders, or diabetes. Such an identifiable medical disorder is necessary to discriminate chronic medical disorders from hysterical reactions and other psychiatric conditions which may produce similar symptomatology. Information about disease status is important, since it is likely to produce differential control of the "course" of the disorder and suggest different methodologies for treatment.

This is by no means a trivial distinction. Treatment approaches aimed at behavioral symptomatology without consideration for etiology are at best irresponsible and possibly dangerous to the patient, as are behavioral programs that are not integrated into the patient's overall care plan. A recent case of a teenage girl with psychomotor seizures illustrates this dilemma. She presented with both a neurophysiological diagnosis by EEG and evidence of faked seizure episodes. When contingencies were placed on seizure rate, seizures decreased in number to meet the contingencies. As the "acceptable" number was lowered further, the girl still met the contingencies, and attempted suicide. The critical analysis, of course, was the consideration of circumstances under which the patient would fake a seizure. Her desperate needs for attention and control of the social context, at the expense of using socially unacceptable behaviors like seizures, were clearly not fulfilled by a simple contingency program for seizure rate. While faked seizures may have served as an operant, such a situation should indicate the need for psychiatric evaluation and training alternative compensatory behaviors.

Behavioral programs for patients with chronic disorders should be coordinated with an overall treatment plan. The risk of not interfacing with medical treatment can be disastrous. For example, a report has appeared concerning a diabetic patient who was trained to relax with EMG feedback, received a reduction in medication, and subsequently died (92). The insulin reduction was prescribed on the basis of the patient's estimated ability to relax and resist stress. Evidently the new regimen of reduced insulin and relaxation skills did not offer the degree of protection provided by the previous levels of insulin. Reliance on relaxation, or any behavioral treatment, to maintain an important therapeutic effect or take the place of traditional medical treatment methods in a chronic disorder is potentially dangerous and should be conducted with extreme caution under very close collaboration with the managing physician.

Course of the Disorder

An understanding of the course of chronic disorders is important to the treatment and especially critical for the outcome evaluation of behavioral medicine interventions. Chronic disorders are, by definition, long term. The state of the underlying disorder and the expression of symptoms are likely to vary, simultaneously or independently, based on both medical treatment and the influence of environmental factors such as family conflict and health habits. Usually the course of a chronic disorder is variable, with the variance in patient discomfort, response to treatment, and disease process controlled by a number of interacting variables. The natural course of these disorders often fluctuates from better to worse with and without behavioral and/or medical intervention.

Successful treatment of chronic disorders may be defined in two ways: Through intervention we may produce remediation of the disease itself, or through the combination of medical and behavioral intervention we may lessen the frequency, intensity, or duration of discomfort to the patient by minimizing the exacerbations of the disorder or by maximizing the patient's adjustment to and compensation for the disorder. The evaluation of treatments must be carefully conducted both medically and behaviorally to demonstrate therapeutic effectiveness and to rule out the possibility that symptom remission is unrelated to treatment.

The Importance of Patient Histories

Complete case records describing the course and treatment of a disorder can facilitate its management (50, 81, 102). Comprehensive medical histories allow the evaluation of current and previous treatment efforts. A complete account of previous medical tests and additional medical problems is very useful when a case is transferred to new physicians or a new treatment protocol is undertaken. A comprehensive medical history is also valuable to the behaviorist. By looking at the response of the disease to various treatments, the timing and events antecedent to exacerbations, and changes in factors such as weight or sleep habits, clues to the environmental determinants of the disorder may be obtained. Medical histories often do not provide enough information for a comprehensive behavioral evaluation (16, 86). A behavioral medicine treatment approach to chronic disorders should include a detailed review of the behavioral aspects of the history in addition to the standard medical history. This usually includes:

—Patient and family demographics, including age at onset of the disorder; number, age, and relationship of other persons in the family environment; presence of other disorders of a chronic or painful nature; and major events in the family history, e.g., death, divorce, etc.
—History of the disorder, with particular reference to exacerbations and remissions of symptoms.
—Frequency, duration, and intensity of symptoms.
—Antecedent events and maintenance reinforcers for symptoms, for example, situations that regularly precede or follow symptom presentation.
—Changes in symptoms, particularly those that can be related to environmental events, which may give clues about the behavioral determinants of the symptoms.
—Life-style change.

The Relationship Between Illness and Behavior

The duration, variability, and physical effects of chronic disorders generate situations in which changes in behavior are differentially influenced by the environment. Fordyce (35) has discussed this process in chronic pain patients and pointed out that patients learn new but sometimes inappropriate behaviors which are functional in the changed environment. This learning may be an overt attempt by the patient to obtain feedback from his environment, such as the exacerbation of symptoms to gain attention or "sympathy" from others, or more insidiously, the temporal pairing of behavioral states such as nonactivity with a reduction in symptoms. These states are likely to be maintained by the environment, and patients may develop a life style characterized by "learned helplessness" (29, 84). These patients are typically lethargic, and they have exaggerated symptomatic complaints.

Etiology and Treatment

Although many chronic disorders have underlying physical pathologies, or a physiological basis for acute exacerbations, treatment may also require attention to the antecedents and consequences of each symptom complex. Learning processes are often responsible for exacerbations of symptoms despite successful treatment of underlying pathology. Symptoms originally produced by pathological events, e.g., trauma, may be maintained by a different set of events. When considering an individual with a chronic disorder, one must be somewhat skeptical about the traditional beliefs in the difference between medical and psychosomatic illness (1). Physical pathology and learned responses must be considered jointly. This consideration is especially important in the case of chronic disorders because, from a learning perspective: 1) the patient has more opportunities to contact contingencies for learned or environmentally influenced exacerbations, and 2) the long learning history makes behavioral- and environment-based remediation strategies more difficult to effect.

Focus on Biobehavioral Measurement

Behavioral science focuses on observable behavioral events as the basis for inquiry. Statements about the effects of behavioral interventions in medicine should be in terms of changes in both behavioral and biological measures whenever possible. Under certain circumstances, the outcome measure may reflect symptomatic changes, for example, a decreased frequency of "seizurelike" behaviors or "asthmatic attacks." However, given the high probability of multiple causes for symptoms in chronic disease states, a reduction of symptom frequency should not be confused with treatment of underlying pathology unless correlated with biomedical measurement.

Role of the Physician and the Behaviorist

In most instances, the patient's overall course of treatment is the responsibility of a physician, with the behaviorist as a consultant or a provider of adjunctive treatments. This division of labor is appropriate considering the lengthy course of treatment, the need for coordination of many types of services, and the legal requirements for physician management and supervision.

Ethics

As a subspecialty, behavioral medicine must reflect not only the practice but also the ethical standards of both the behavioral and the medical communities. Since ethics represents a consensus of opinion, the ethical use of behavioral medicine procedures requires a firm grounding in the ethics of both professions and an evaluation of community opinion.

This has been neither an exhaustive nor a conceptually complete review of strategies in behavioral medicine. We have presented some of the considerations involved in developing behavioral treatments for chronic conditions. As the behavioral medicine specialty becomes defined, considerations of this type might serve as the basis for training of new practitioners in the behavioral and medical sciences. The next generation of behavioral medicine specialists, their research, and their innovations in treatment may provide at least a partial solution to the current crisis in health-care services for chronic disease.

DIRECT TREATMENT OF CHRONIC DISORDERS

There are many examples in the literature of the successful integration of behavioral and medical science. Cardiovascular disease is one area in which this synthesis has been well documented (26, 47, 64, 82, 93).

Another area showing the integration of behavioral and medical sciences is that of the chronic problems associated with neurological disorders. At the Kennedy Institute and Johns Hopkins Hospital, we have been able to apply behavioral techniques to these disorders in the areas of assessment, experimental analysis, and treatment strategies. A brief review of seizure and movement disorders will elaborate the unique approaches of behavioral medicine to these chronic problems, and the application of procedures that are ethical and effective from both a medical and a behavioral perspective. We wish to exemplify the contribution of experimental analysis of behavior to movement disorders, and the present need to study generalization or treatment transfer processes from both a behavioral and neurological standpoint.

Seizure Disorders

Background

Seizures are a diverse set of neurological symptoms which depend on CNS localization, age of the patient, basic neuropathophysiology, and topography of clinical responses for classification (72). The severity of seizure disorders varies from the common, very severe grand mal seizure, which includes complete loss of consciousness and postseizure coma, to milder forms of petit mal, which may produce brief disturbances of some aspects of consciousness or behavior (39).

Epilepsy refers to the chronic condition of recurrent seizures of any type. It is the most common chronic neurological disorder of childhood (80). Estimates of prevalence reported in the literature range from 6.25 per 1000 (45) to 18.6 per 1000 (77) in the general population. Although seizure disorders have been reported to seriously disrupt education (70), affect intelligence (55), produce behavioral disturbances (40), or render children at risk for behavior disorders (49) and for learning disabilities (80), little clinical research and few treatment programs have been directed at these problems (38).

Medical Management

Traditional medical management with pharmacological agents offers varying degrees of success, depending on the type of disorder and individual responsiveness to treatment (58, 72). Unfortunately, medication regimens have been reported to greatly affect cognitive, emotional, and behavioral variables, and may add to the risks of social and educational difficulties (38, 90). In addition to the effects of medication on seizures, behavioral variables have long been reported to influence the frequency of epileptic attacks (43, 72). The emotional reaction to the social consequences of a seizure disorder is a substantial problem for individuals with these disorders (70). Emotional difficulties have long been associated with exacerbation of epilepsy, and programs that reduce adverse emotional responses are already well accepted in clinical neurology (72). Indirect behavioral treatments that involve improving one or a variety of coping skills for emotional or social difficulties may be an important contribution to a comprehensive program for seizure patients.

Behavioral Approaches

Two types of behavioral treatments for seizure disorders have been reported in the literature: biofeedback training of EEG rhythms purported to be antagonistic to seizures, and behavioral conditioning of some aspects of seizure behavior.

The current literature on EEG biofeedback training for seizure disorders is controversial. Sterman (87, 88) and his colleagues have conducted basic research and a series of clinical research projects aimed at investigating the seizure-reducing effects of increasing an EEG rhythm of 12–14 Hz (called SMR, or sensorimotor rhythm) over the sensorimotor cortex. This rhythm has been reported to be a correlate of motor inhibition in cats and humans. After obtaining positive clinical findings, Sterman (87) and others (34, 59) have recently begun double-blind within-subject studies in which patients are trained to increase selected EEG frequencies to determine the effects on seizure rates. These studies should help resolve the conflicting evidence, which suggests that training any slow, synchronous, high-voltage EEG pattern (53) or training low-voltage, fast-frequency EEG arousal responses (106) may reduce seizure rates.

Two types of behavioral conditioning have been reported to reduce seizure rates. Efron (23) and Forster (37) have indicated that desensitization or counterconditioning is effective in reducing the rates of seizures which are "reflexively" triggered by very specific sensory stimuli. Utilizing an operant methodology, Zlutnick, Mayville, and Moffat (108) reported that applying aversive consequences, such as shaking the patient, to the initial components of stereotyped behavioral sequences of seizure activity (seen most frequently in Jacksonian seizures) not only disrupted the behavioral chain and prevented a grand mal seizure, but also reduced the future frequency of the entire seizure sequence. Although this finding is the clearest demonstration of an operant effect on seizure disorders, the report is somewhat weakened by a poor description of the neurological status of the patients and the nature of the seizures.

The following case study of a patient with a severe, chronic seizure disorder illustrates the importance of a thorough functional analysis leading to a successful behavioral intervention. It demonstrates the importance and ease of developing a treatment strategy which is ethical when judged by medical, behavioral, and lay standards.

Case Example

The patient was a 4½-year-old female who was admitted to be evaluated for uncontrollable myoclonic and grand mal seizures. All appropriate anticonvulsive medications, phenobarbital, dilantin, mysoline, zarontin, valium, clonazepam, tegretol, and a ketogenic diet had previously failed to reduce the frequency of myoclonic seizures below 50 to 400 per day, and grand mal seizures below 3 to 6 per week. Preliminary observation showed that the rate of seizures varied between days, and after several days of observation it became clear that certain activities were correlated with high rates of seizure activity. A behavioral analysis was undertaken to evaluate whether seizure rate might be systematically manipulated. The child was trained in a bar-pressing task under the discriminative control of a light placed above the reinforcement (M&M) dispenser. A combination reversal and multiple baseline design experiment was used to evaluate the patient. In this test situation, turning out the light signaled timeout or periods of nonreinforcement. Timeout was initially noncontingent, then contingent on the voluntary response of turning around, following which it was contingent or noncontingent on the occurrence of myoclonic seizures. There was a sharp reduction in the number of voluntary responses and a decrease in frequency of seizures in the contingent light-off condition.

The results of this operant analysis were transferred to the child's treatment program. When she had a high rate of seizures, she was asked to rest for a short period of time in a chair. This "contingent rest" corresponded to the termination of the discriminative stimulus for reinforcement (light off) in the laboratory when seizures occurred. Allowing the child to rest away from distracting events (and reinforcement) when she was having seizures proved effective, easy to implement, and ethical from any viewpoint. Partial results of this treatment are presented in Figure 2. A high rate of myoclonic seizures, followed by a grand mal seizure, was present during the baseline observation period. The contingent rest

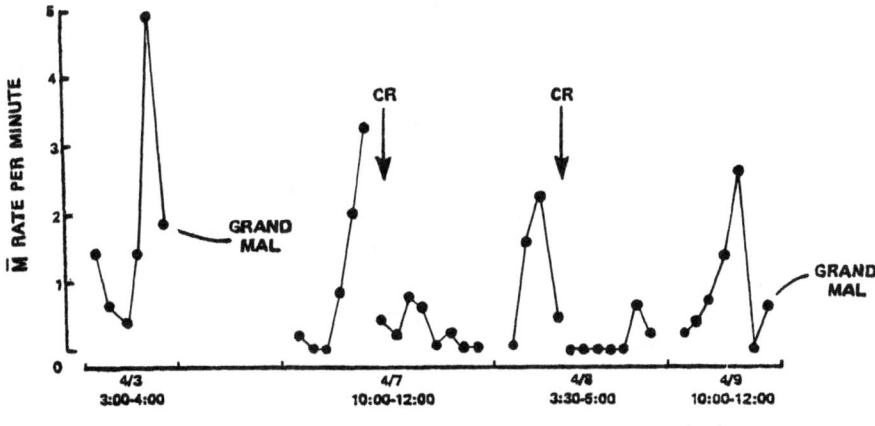

FIVE MINUTE OBSERVATIONS OF HIGH SEIZURE RATE

Fig. 2. Experimental analysis by reversal design of a "contingent rest" procedure to modify seizures. As can be seen, a grand mal seizure occurred after an increase in myoclonic seizures on 4/3. Contingent rest (CR) applied on 4/7 and 4/8, after a characteristic spike in myoclonic seizure rate, produced a decrease in myoclonic seizures and no subsequent grand mal. On 4/9, without CR intervention, a grand mal occurred after a spike.

procedure was introduced on the second and third days, and was followed by a reduction in the rate of myoclonic seizures, and the absence of grand mal seizures. On the fourth day, the removal of contingencies was followed by an abrupt increase in the number of myoclonic seizures followed by a grand mal seizure.

Although this procedure produced a decrease in the rate of behaviorally observable "seizures," it was unclear whether this represented a decrease in paroxysmal neurophysiological activity. Previous comparison of EEG records and behavioral observations had demonstrated a high correlation between the two, which suggests that the contingent rest procedure decreased the rate of neurophysiological seizures. Data collected after the child was discharged to home showed a decrease in average daily seizure rate of more than 50%.

Movement Disorders

Background

A variety of neurological movement and posture disorders produce chronic physical dysfunctions and have psychological sequelae. These include peripheral neuromuscular disorders—myelopathies and neuropathies; and central nervous system disorders—cerebral palsy, dystonia, posttraumatic spasticity, spasmodic torticollis, and Parkinsonism. Together, these disorders produce severe physical handicaps in a significant proportion of the population. For example, the prevalence of cerebral palsy has been estimated to be 1 in 1500 live births; approximately 700,000 persons were affected by cerebral palsy in the U.S. in 1974 (69). A large proportion of the cerebral palsy population is dependent on others for most care (73), and an equally large number is at risk for psychological difficulties (54). Over 500,000 strokes are estimated to occur in the U.S. each year, of which 40% require special rehabilitation services and physical therapy for hemiplegia (96). Less prevalent movement disorders such as dystonia and Parkinsonism severely disrupt motor functioning and often produce serious psychological problems.

Traditional Therapies

The pathophysiology of movement disorders is poorly understood (20, 25). Traditional medical treatments have included orthopedic bracing or surgery to correct muscular or bone deformities (79), physical therapies to teach patients maximum adaptive function within their neurological limitations (104), pharmacological treatments to correct biochemical abnormalities (31), and neurosurgical procedures to attempt to block or destroy dysfunctioning neural systems (18). Although these treatments have received widespread clinical acceptance, their effectiveness often lacks substantial documentation (32, 103). Of interest is the repeated finding that individual patients may respond dramatically to one or a few of those treatments, but not to all. Response often appears to be idiosyncratic, and general statements about treatment efficacy are not definitive (18, 31, 105). The medical management of a movement disorder is usually an individually tailored interdisciplinary treatment program (4, 101).

Behavioral Approaches

Behavioral programs for treating movement disorders offer three valuable additions to patient management: 1) objective assessment of treatment regimens of any type, 2) direct behavioral or biofeedback conditioning for improved motor control, and 3) behavior therapy programs for related behavioral problems.

Many studies in the literature and a number of respected clinics have reported clinical improvements in patients with movement disorders who received a comprehensive habilitation program of which biofeedback was a component, with evidence being particularly strong for effects in hemiplegia, spasmodic torticollis, and incomplete lesions of the spinal cord (33). However, despite encouraging reviews (9, 95), acceptable data are lacking on contributions of biofeedback to the efficacy of habilitation programs for movement disorders (6).

In our clinical research program, we have found that EMG biofeedback may be used to establish muscle control in the laboratory for patients with dystonia, cerebral palsy (athetoid and spastic types) and spastic hemiplegia. Using a single-subject experimental design, we have begun to identify and study variables that influence generalization and maintenance of laboratory biofeedback effects to produce clinical benefits. This approach suggests that EMG biofeedback is most useful when it is part of a total behavioral program which in turn may be complementary to physical therapy or medical treatment.

The patient's basic neurological substrate influences the rehabilitation and behavioral treatment program. Knowledge of the neurological causes of motor disorders, their relation to symptoms, and symptom topographies are critical to patient assessment and behavioral program design. For example, spastic paralysis of the lower limb may be produced by several neurological disorders which have different mechanisms, prognoses, and susceptibilities to medical and behavioral treatment. The natural history of these disorders varies; for example, hemiplegia due to stroke shows increasing return to normal function for a variable period after the vascular incident, while dystonia shows sporadic and progressive loss of function. The course of these disorders affects not only motor symptoms, but also the psychological and motivational status of the patient.

Motor dysfunction usually includes negative symptoms which are losses of normal function, and positive symptoms which are acquired abnormal reflexes, muscle tone disturbance, and unwanted muscular activity. The treatment literature does not adequately describe the effects of treating these types of symptoms or the differential outcome of sequential and simultaneous treatment programs (6, 57). Our approach has been to assess both positive and negative symptoms, but to focus on one or the other during treatment. For example, patients with disorders such as choreoathetoid cerebral palsy and dystonia have been effectively trained to inhibit involuntary tension or movement prior to shaping voluntary movements. In hemiplegics with spastic paralysis, training voluntary contraction in target muscles has been effective as an initial treatment strategy.

Case Example

The following case illustrates a behavioral approach that used biofeedback and adjunctive procedures to maximize clinical outcome. Our apparatus included three commercially available EMG biofeedback units which recorded surface EMG, feeding into a PDP-8E computer which provided moment-to-moment three-digit visual feedback and a teletype printout of EMG data every 20 seconds. EMG recording and analysis have been reviewed by Bird and Cataldo (6).

A 20-year-old male with a three-year history of dystonia and normal intelligence presented with severe involvement of facial, forearm, and lower leg muscles. His face was contorted by elevated tension into an exaggerated grimace during his waking hours. EMG relaxation training was begun with his mildly involved forehead muscles. His jaw and forearm muscles were selected for EMG recording and later EMG feedback training if necessary. For the first five days, no-feedback relaxation and no-feedback baseline conditions were alternated within sessions. The data indicated that no significant relaxation occurred. Feedback indicating forehead relaxation was added to the within-session reversals on the sixth day through the twenty-fifth day. Fifteen-minute videotapes of the patient's facial control while sitting and standing were made before and after training and were blindly scored using interval coding to measure facial muscle control.

The EMG feedback results during the first five sessions indicated relaxation in forehead muscles, which generalized to no-feedback relaxation conditions and to jaw and forearm muscles. Figure 3 depicts these changes over sessions, and Figure 4 depicts changes occurring within selected sessions, clearly demonstrating generalization effects. However, early in training, when a colleague entered the training room to observe the patient, his relaxation ceased. Also, the patient was unable to maintain relaxed forearm and facial muscles when he stood up. These problems were successfully overcome by generalization programs in which the patient was given EMG feedback training in the presence of other people and while sitting upright and standing. The behavioral raters indicated an increase in facial relaxation from 2% of the intervals before treatment to 100% after training. The patient was instructed to practice frequently and was reportedly able to produce relaxation in his home environment at three-month follow-up.

Using EMG biofeedback we have demonstrated successful relaxation training in other patients with dystonia and choreoathetoid cerebral palsy, and successful increases in voluntary muscle contraction in spastic hemiplegics. We have identified a number of variables that must be evaluated in order to assess the generalization of effects in the natural environment, and we have begun to develop programs for improving and maintaining these generalizations. A functional analysis of the patient's behavioral repertoire and its relationship to

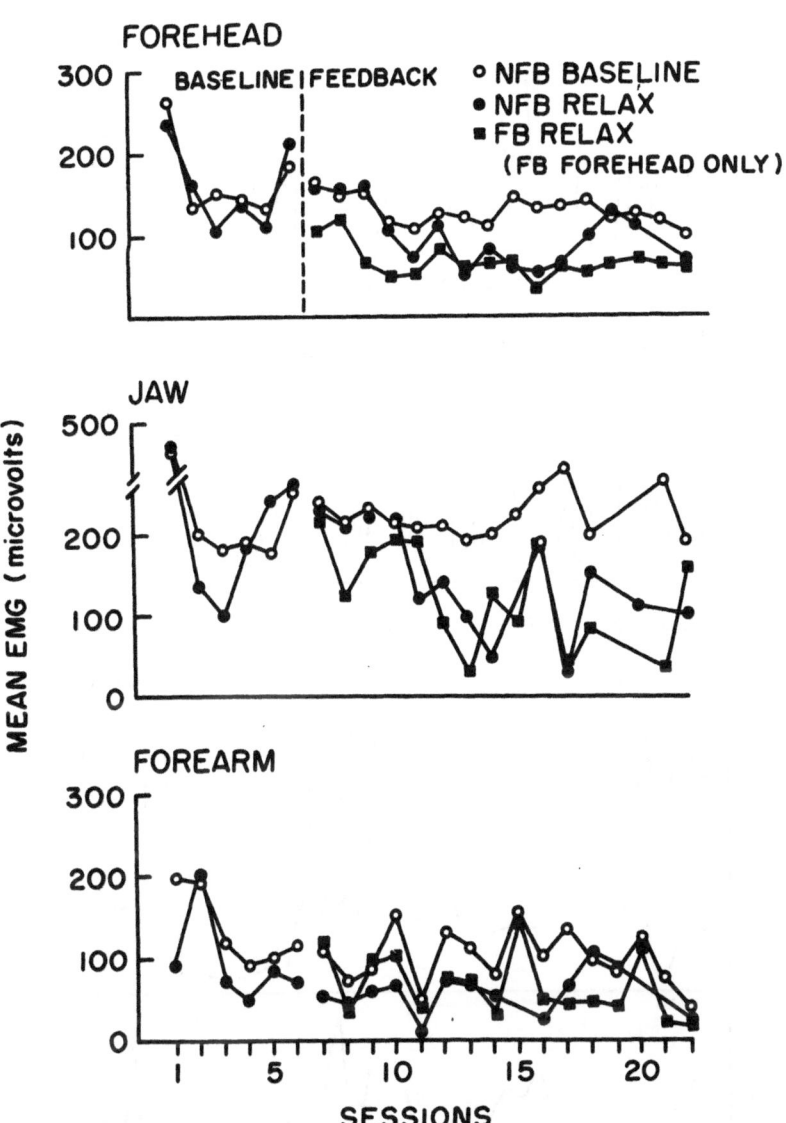

Fig. 3. Changes of average EMG voltages of forehead, jaw, and forearm muscles in no-feedback baseline (NFB Baseline), no-feedback relaxation (NFB Relax), and feedback plus relaxation (FB Relax) conditions over training sessions for forehead relaxation.
Source: Reprinted from *Annals of Neurology,* 1978, Vol. 3, page 312, by permission.

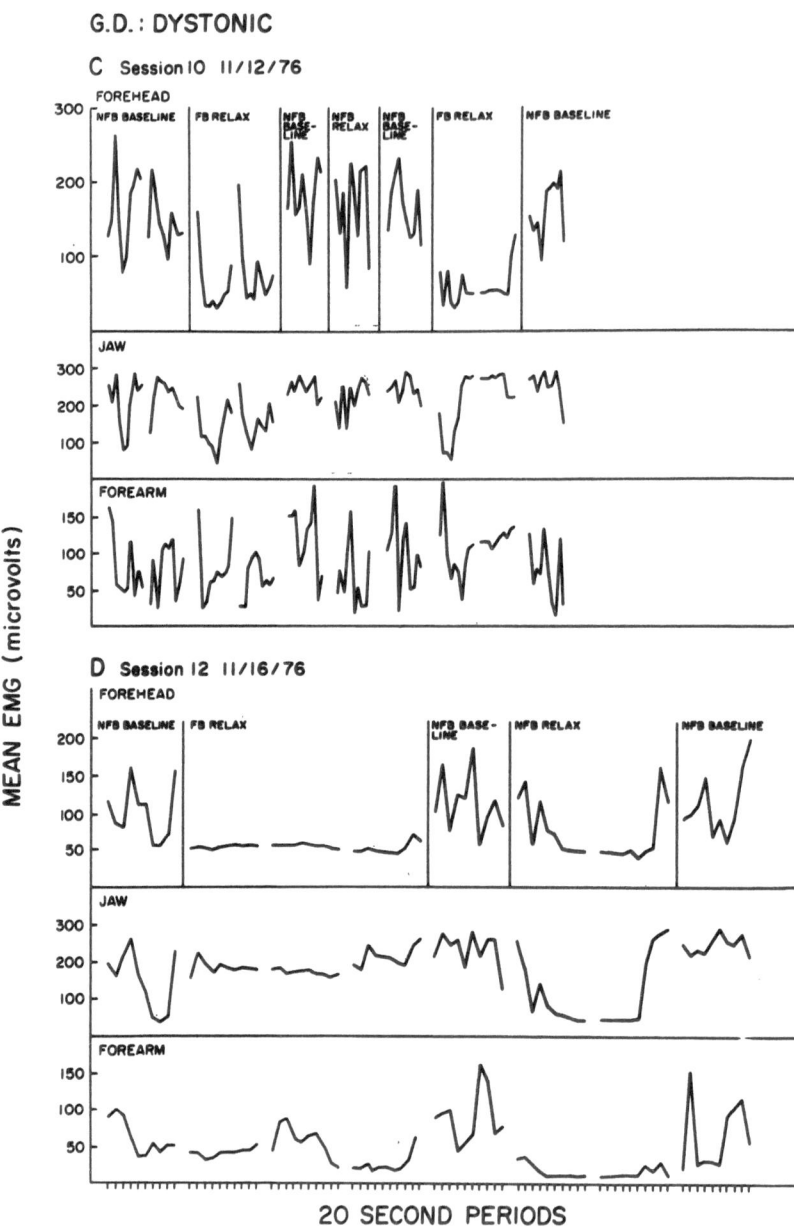

Fig. 4. Within-session changes in forehead, jaw, and forearm muscles during the third and fifth feedback sessions.
Source: Reprinted from *Annals of Neurology,* 1978, Vol. 3, page 313, by permission.

the environment is important in these cases. When necessary, additional behavior therapy programs can be used to maximize motor gains and rehabilitation. In our experience, these procedures are most helpful when they are part of a total behavioral program for managing the behavioral aspects of a chronic disorder.

TREATMENT CONSIDERATIONS
FOR THE PROBLEM OF CHRONICITY

Many similar behavioral problems are seen in a variety of chronic disorders—the problems which develop because the disorder is chronic. A patient must adjust to his disorder, find new sources of motivation, and develop new skills to compensate for those lost. When an illness is acute, the patient can "wait it out." When it is chronic, he must "learn to live with it." Behavioral therapies offer some hope for treating chronicity. Pediatric chronic pain is a symptom that illustrates the problem of chronicity and the contribution of behavioral treatments.

Pediatric Chronic Pain

Physical and psychological components appear to contribute to the intensity and character of perceived pain. The relative contribution of each varies between patients (51). Alternatively, pain perception can be seen to involve sensing painful stimuli and behaviorally or cognitively elaborating sensations of pain (67). Three categories of pain may be described: pain not linked to a disease state or identifiable source; pain linked to a disease state; and pain linked to a visible trauma, e.g., burns, fractures, and lacerations (30). While acute pain is clearly elicited by disease or injury (10), chronic pain is a sustained condition extending over a period of time, often without clear precipitating causes.

Children presenting with chronic pain often have a precipitating event with a history of surgery or physical injury (28). Merskey (68) cites evidence that patterns of pain behavior are learned through the interaction of the maturing organism and the social environment. In a study by Oster (74), 24% of the parents of children who had recurrent pain reported that they had experienced recurrent pains themselves in childhood or at the time of the investigation; 14% of the parents of children without pain reported a history of recurrent pain. It appears that pediatric chronic pain may be an interaction between an initial trauma or precipitating factor and multiple social-environmental influences (99).

The prevalence of pediatric chronic pain is unknown. Oster (74) conducted an eight-year longitudinal study of 18,162 children between 6 and 19 years of age to look for cases of recurrent pain. In this large nonselected population, the prevalence of recurrent abdominal pain was 14.4%, recurrent headache was 20.6%, and recurrent limb pain was 15.5%. For all three pain categories, the prevalence was higher in girls than in boys. These estimates, with estimates of the incidence of common problems in pediatric neurology (97), indicate that chronic pain is a significant problem in children.

The medical treatments available for chronic pain include medications (44), anesthetic nerve blocks (7), transcutaneous electrical stimulation (22), and surgical procedures (91). Unfortunately, the effectiveness of these procedures has been inconsistent (8, 94).

The behavioral assessment of chronic pain focuses on the external accompaniments of an assumed internal pain state (30). The external accompaniments are termed "pain behaviors" and the absence of "well behaviors" (35). Pain behaviors include verbal reports of pain, and such nonverbal signs as facial grimaces, compensatory posturing, restricted movement, limping, etc. Well-behavior deficits include decreased activity, depression, and decreased social contact. Assessment includes a description of actual and potential environmental influences on pain and well behaviors (35). Since Fordyce's original publication (36), an increasing amount of attention has been paid to the behavioral treatment of adult chronic pain (103). By contrast, the behavioral treatment approach for pediatric chronic pain has not been well investigated.

Case Example

In this example, we would like to present a treatment approach based on behavioral science principles and good clinical practice, which was designed to facilitate staff management of the patient. The treatment strategy is based on observations in other cases that attending to pain complaints in an attempt to comfort the child may not always be in the child's best interest, and that affection, concern, and comfort may be rescheduled to maximize rehabilitation, relieve pain, and improve the child's psychological functioning.

The patient was a three-year-old female who had been hospitalized for ten months at the Johns Hopkins Hospital for treatment of second- and third-degree burns to her buttocks, legs, and perineum which were caused by immersion in hot water. The circumstances of the burn incident indicated the possibility of child abuse. Scar contractures and subsequent decreased range of motion in both knees made it necessary for the patient to wear Jobst stockings and knee extension splints. At the time that behavioral treatment was begun, the patient was exhibiting many chronic pain behaviors that interfered significantly with her rehabilitation and interactions with the staff. Her pain behaviors increased in intensity and frequency during attention-seeking and demand situations. Data were obtained in three settings: the clinic room, where the patient wore knee extension splints in a contrived setting; her bedroom, where she wore her splints in her natural environment; and the physical therapy room, where the physical therapist focused on increased range of motion and independent ambulation.

Three categories of pain behaviors were defined: crying, which ranged in intensity from sobbing to screaming; verbal pain behaviors, which consisted of statements like "My stomach hurts," "Ouch," or "I can't stand up because of the pain"; and nonverbal pain behaviors, which were gestures expressing pain or discomfort, for example, facial grimaces, rubbing the legs or buttocks, or not following instructions because of pain. In the physical therapy setting, an additional measure was taken on activity—the number of steps the child descended when she was placed at the top of a short staircase. During baseline, the child's pain behaviors appeared to be a function of adult attention and demand situations. When no adults were present, chronic pain behaviors were significantly reduced in frequency. It was also noted that when the child engaged in interesting activities and received staff attention for these appropriate behaviors, pain complaints were infrequent.

Treatment consisted of rearranging existing contingencies and reinforcers. For example, in both the clinic and the bedroom, where the child wore her knee extension splints, attention and tangible reinforcers like ice cream were made contingent upon well behaviors such as helping to put on the splints, positive verbalizations, and smiling. After the procedure was successful in reducing pain behaviors in the clinic setting, the rationale for this type of treatment and a demonstration of the treatment techniques and data collection procedures were presented to other staff members. The nursing staff was taught how to apply the procedures in the bedroom setting. In physical therapy, the child was required to descend a number of steps as part of her therapeutic exercise program. During treatment, the therapist rewarded the child for descending the steps and ignored pain behaviors. Observations of pain and well behaviors were made throughout the baseline and treatment conditions, and they indicated a markedly positive change in both parameters. While it was not possible to determine whether the patient actually felt pain but learned not to display pain behaviors, these behaviors did not recur. Fordyce (35) suggested that patients may actually learn to experience pain in excess of its physiological basis or even in the absence of a physical cause. In these cases the pain behaviors serve patients' immediate needs but hinder rehabilitation. The behavioral approach is one of the ways of facilitating treatment in these cases. In the present case, the managing staff was successfully enlisted into the treatment program as a result of an explanation of the treatment rationale and a demonstration of changes in pain and well behaviors subsequent to changes in the social environment.

Adjunctive Behavioral Treatments

A variety of behavioral assessment and treatment procedures developed for other populations can be used with patients who have chronic medical disorders, for example, assertion and social skills training, contingency management, desensitization, graded activity exposure, life-style adjustment, medication compliance, relaxation, thought stopping/competing responses, verbalizations of sickness and health, and coping strategies. These therapies may be used to treat symptoms related to the chronic disorder or other concurrent behavior problems.

Assertiveness and Verbalization about Illness

Deficits in assertiveness and inappropriate verbalization about sickness instead of health are two common problems among the chronically ill (48). These patients often have few, if any, social behaviors other than those related to soliciting medical care, and their verbal behaviors are dominated by concerns about, solicitations of help for, or complaints about their disorder. Inappropriately assertive patients, who have experienced repeated failures of medical treatments for a chronic disorder, will often continue to seek and then agree to treatments about which they know little, despite having been informed of doubtful positive and possibly harmful outcomes (11).

Adherence to Medical Regimens

Adherence to medical prescription is a major problem in the practice of medicine (2, 21) and in medical research (85). With many chronic disorders, medical problems are made worse because patients do not adhere to treatment regimens. For example, a nine-year-old female diabetic patient was referred to us after it was discovered that she was periodically distorting her urine tests by substituting urine from her four-year-old brother. Though false, results within an appropriate range were immediately rewarded with a candy bar, and over a year, this behavior resulted in numerous emergency-room admissions. Patients with seizure disorders, hypertension, and many other chronic medical disorders are at risk if their treatment programs, including drugs, diet, and activity prescriptions, are not followed.

Adherence strategies for acute and chronic disorders may require two different technologies. Stokes and Baer (89) pointed out that, although there is a strong theoretical foundation for generalization and maintenance, little empirical research is available for applied problems. The behavioral literature applicable to chronic disorders such as pain (35), seizures (14, 108), and movement disorders (6) contains virtually no information about maintenance of treatment gains. Empirically, long-term maintenance programs must consider the treatment procedures as a part of the patient's life style, and identify and use existing reinforcers in the patient's environment. A structured schedule for assessment and follow-up is useful since some traditional assessments of treatment compliance, such as biochemical assays for drug levels, may not always be reliable (12) or available, and some form of behavioral assessment of treatment appears warranted (28).

Thought-Stopping and Competing Responses

Thought-stopping along with a competing-response strategy may be particularly useful for disorders in which recurrent thoughts or sensations are discriminative stimuli for early responses in a chain of maladaptive behaviors. For example, Cataldo, Varni, Russo, and Estes (15) studied a procedure in which a patient with a potent itch-scratch cycle from a severe dermatological condition was socially reinforced for folding his hands and imagining a particular competing scene instead of scratching. In addition to strictly behavioral interventions, Barber and others have conducted excellent studies using hypnosis to treat pain, a strategy which may have application in behavioral treatment programs for chronic disorders (3, 17).

Relaxation

Stress and extreme emotion adversely influence the symptoms of many chronic disorders, including some conditions not usually thought of as stress related, such as seizures and movement disorders. Relaxation training or one of its popular variants (5, 52, 60, 66) has been reported to have direct (75) and indirect benefits (63) for patients with chronic disorders. In addition, it has been suggested for its prophylactic benefits to general health (52) and against cardiovascular disorders (5).

Coping Strategies

Specific coping skills can be taught to patients to allow them to reduce their reactions to chronic conditions and modify or even prevent some of the adverse consequences of these disorders. Children with chronic illnesses may be deficient in social skills and assertiveness, and may have poor peer relationships and exaggerated reactions to adult authority (19). Epidemiological research has suggested that children with chronic illness and disability are at high risk for developing behavioral and emotional disorders (78). Behavioral procedures can be used to prevent the chronically disabled patient from developing further behavioral and personality disorders, or even to overcompensate by developing other areas of functioning (107). Patients with chronic disorders often feel depressed, partly as a result of not feeling in control of their lives. Self-management training often helps patients develop a sense of internal control and at least partial control of their environment (41, 100). For example, a patient might be taught school and learning skills, assertion training to help him deal more effectively with authority figures, and social-skills training to help him make and keep friends.

CONCLUSION

Any behavioral treatment for a chronic disorder relies on a behavioral conceptualization of the disorder and subsequently the generation of a set of procedural and methodological guidelines for evaluation and treatment. An empirical epistemology has been a primary determinant of the initial applicability and the dissemination of behavioral psychology. Empirically testable procedures have formed the basis for evaluating principles originally observed in animal and human laboratory settings. The excursion of the behaviorist into the assessment and management of chronic disorders is an attempt to interface with a well-developed and thoroughly researched technology which has procedures for identifying, managing, and following up these disorders. The behavioral inquiry into chronic disorders requires thorough behavioral analysis and systematic application of behavioral principles and, simultaneously, the evaluation of the medical environment, its technology, and its philosophy. Given the history and strength of both systems, what is likely to emerge is a unique field of inquiry governed by the outcome methodologies of both medical and behavioral sciences.

ACKNOWLEDGMENTS

This work was supported by Grants #917 and MC-R-240418 from the Maternal and Child Health Service, Grant #1RO3MH30346-01 from the National Institute of Mental Health, and Grant #R-294-78 from the United Cerebral Palsy Research and Education Foundation. The authors wish to thank Edith Stern and Margaret Weigel for their assistance. Research reported by the authors in this chapter was conducted at the Department of Behavioral

Psychology of the John F. Kennedy Institute and the Behavioral Medicine Center of the Johns Hopkins University School of Medicine.

REFERENCES

1. Anderson, D.E., and Brady, J.V. Experimental analysis of psychophysiological interactions: Behavioral influences in physiological regulations, in R. Davidson (ed.), *Experimental Analysis of Clinical Phenomena.* New York: Gardner Press, 1977.
2. Baile, W., and Engel, B.T. A behavioral strategy for promoting treatment compliance following myocardial infarction. *Psychosom. Med.,* in press.
3. Barber, T.X., Spanos, N.P., and Chaves, J.F. *Hypnosis, Imagination, and Human Potentialities.* Oxford: Pergamon, 1974.
4. Batshaw, M.L., and Haslam, R.H. Multidisciplinary management of dystonia misdiagnosed as hysteria, in R. Eldridge and S. Fahn (eds.), *Advances in Neurology, Vol. 14: Dystonia.* New York: Raven, 1976.
5. Benson, H. *The Relaxation Response.* New York: Avon Books, 1975.
6. Bird, B.L., and Cataldo, M.F. Experimental analysis of EMG feedback in treating dystonia. *Ann. Neurol.* 3:310-315, 1978.
7. Black, R.G. Management of pain with nerve blocks. *Minn. Med.* 57:189-194, 1974.
8. Black, R.G. The chronic pain syndrome. *Surg. Clin. North Am.* 55:999-1011, 1975.
9. Blanchard, E.B., and Young, L.D. Clinical applications of biofeedback training: A review of evidence. *Arch. Gen. Psychiatry* 30:573-589, 1974.
10. Bonica, J.J. (ed.). *International Symposium on Pain (Advances in Neurology, Vol. 4).* New York: Raven Press, 1974.
11. Brady, J.V., and Nauta, W.J.H. *Problems, Practices, and Positions in Neuropsychiatric Research.* London: Pergamon Press, 1972.
12. Brett, E. Implications of measuring anticonvulsant blood levels in epilepsy. *Dev. Med. Child Neurol.* 19:245-251, 1977.
13. Cataldo, M.F., and Russo, D.C. Developmentally disabled in the community: Behavioral/medical considerations, in L.A. Hamerlynck, P.O. Davidson, and F.W. Clark (eds.), *History and Future of Behavior Modification for the Developmentally Disabled: Programmatic and Methodological Issues.* New York: Brunner/Mazel, 1979.
14. Cataldo, M.F., Russo, D.C., and Freeman, J.M. A behavior analysis approach to high-rate myoclonic seizures. *Journal of Autism and Developmental Disorders,* 9:413-427, 1979.
15. Cataldo, M.F., Varni, J.W., Russo, D.C., and Estes, S. Behavior therapy techniques in the treatment of exfoliative dermatitis. *Archives of Dermatology,* in press.
16. Chamberlain, R.W. Early recognition and modification of vicious circle parent-child relationships. *Clin. Pediatr.* 6:469-479, 1967.
17. Chaves, J.F., and Barber, T.X. Hypnotism and surgical pain, in D. Mostofsky (ed.), *Behavior Control and Modification of Physiological Activity.* Englewood Cliffs, N.J.: Prentice-Hall, 1976.
18. Cooper, I.S. *Involuntary Movement Disorders.* New York: Harper & Row, 1969.
19. Creer, T.L., and Christian, W.F. *Chronically Ill and Handicapped Children.* Champaign, Ill.: Research Press, 1976.
20. Cruickshank, W.M. *Psychology of Exceptional Children and Youth.* Englewood Cliffs, N.J.: Prentice-Hall, 1971.
21. Dunbar, J., and Agras, W.S. A behavioral strategy for improving adherence to

medication. Paper presented at annual convention of the Association for Advancement of Behavior Therapy, Atlanta, Georgia, 1977.

22. Ebersold, M.J., Laws, E.R., Stonnington, H.H., and Stillwell, G.K. Transcutaneous electrical stimulation for treatment of chronic pain: A preliminary report. *Surg. Neurol.* 4:96-99, 1975.

23. Efron, R. The effect of olfactory stimuli in arresting uncinate fits. *Brain* 79:267-281, 1956.

24. Elder, S.T., Welsh, D.M., Longacre, A., and McAfee, R. Acquisition, discriminative stimulus control, and retention of increases/decreases in blood pressure of normotensive human subjects. *J. Appl. Behav. Anal.* 10:381-390, 1977.

25. Eldridge, R., and Fahn, S. (eds.). *Advances in Neurology, Vol. 14: Dystonia.* New York: Raven Press, 1976.

26. Enelow, A.J., and Henderson, J. *Applying Behavioral Science to Cardiovascular Risk.* New York: American Heart Association, 1975.

27. Engel, B.T., Nikoomanesh, P., and Schuster, M.M. Operant conditioning of recto-sphincteric responses in the treatment of fecal incontinence. *N. Engl. J. Med.* 290:646-649, 1974.

28. Epstein, L.H., and Masek, B.J. Behavioral control of medicine compliance. *J. Appl. Behav. Anal.* 11:1-9, 1978.

29. Epstein, M.H., and Harris, J. Children with chronic pain: Can they be helped? *Pediatr. Nurs.* 4:42-44, 1978.

30. Fabrega, H., and Tyma, S. Language and cultural influences in the description of pain. *Br. J. Med. Psychol.* 49:349-371, 1976.

31. Fahn, S. Medical treatment of movement disorders, in *Neurological Reviews.* Minneapolis: American Academy of Neurology, 1976.

32. Fahn, S., and Calne, D.B. Considerations in the management of Parkinsonism. *Neurology* 23:5-7, 1978.

33. Fernando, C.K. Report of the task force on applications of biofeedback in physical medicine and rehabilitation. Paper presented at Ninth Annual Meeting of the Biofeedback Society of America, Albuquerque, March 1978.

34. Finley, W.W. Effects of sham feedback following successful SMR training in an epileptic: Follow-up study. *Biofeedback Self Regul.* 1:227-236, 1976.

35. Fordyce, W.E. *Behavioral Methods for Chronic Pain and Illness.* St. Louis: C.V. Mosby, 1976.

36. Fordyce, W.E., Fowler, R., Lehmann, J., and Delateur, B. Some implications of learning problems of chronic pain. *J. Chronic Dis.* 21:179, 1968.

37. Forster, F.M. The classification and conditioning treatment of the reflex epilepsies. *Int. J. Neurol.* 9:73-83, 1972.

38. Freeman, J.M., Gayle, E.E., Hendler, L.M., and Pillas, D.J. *Epilepsy in Maryland: An Assessment of Services and Gaps in Service.* Baltimore: The Maryland Developmental Disability Council, 1975.

39. Gastaut, H. Clinical and electroencephalographical classification of epileptic seizures. *Epilepsia* 11:102-113, 1970.

40. Glaser, G.H. The problem of psychosis in temporal lobe epileptics. *Epilepsia* 5:271-278, 1964.

41. Goldiamond, I. Self-reinforcement. *J. Appl. Behav. Anal.* 9:509-514, 1976.

42. Goldiamond, I. President's message. *MABA Newsletter* 2:1-2, 1978.

43. Guey, J., Bureau, M., Dravet, C., and Roger, J. A Study of rhythm of petit mal absences in children in relation to prevailing situations. *Epilepsia* 10:441-451, 1969.

44. Halpern, L.M. Treating pain with drugs. *Minn. Med.* 57:176-184, 1974.

45. Hauser, W.A., and Kurland, L.T. The epidemiology of epilepsy in Rochester, Minnesota

1935-1967. *Epilepsia* 16:1-66, 1975.
46. Health Resources Administration. *Limitation of Activity and Mobility Due to Chronic Conditions: United States—1972.* Washington, D.C.: U.S. Government Printing Office, DHEW Publication No. HRA 75-1523, 1974.
47. Henderson, J.B., and Enelow, A.J. The coronary risk factor problem: A behavioral perspective. *Prev. Med.* 5:128-148, 1976.
48. Hersen, M., and Bellack, A.S. A multiple-baseline analysis of social skill training in chronic schizophrenics. *J. Appl. Behav. Anal.* 9:239-245, 1976.
49. Holdsworth, L., and Whitmore, K. A study of children with epilepsy attending ordinary schools. *Dev. Med. Child Neurol.* 16:746-758, 1974.
50. Hurst, J.W., and Walker, H.K. *The Problem-Oriented System.* Chicago: Modern Hospital Press, 1957.
51. Ince, L.P. *Behavior Modification in Rehabilitative Medicine.* Springfield, Ill.: Charles C Thomas, 1976.
52. Jacobsen, E. *Progressive Relaxation.* Chicago: University of Chicago Press, 1938.
53. Kaplan, B.J. Biofeedback in epileptics: Equivocal relationship of reinforced EEG frequency to seizure reduction. *Epilepsia* 16:477-485, 1975.
54. Keats, S. *Cerebral Palsy.* Springfield, Ill.: Charles C Thomas, 1965.
55. Klove, H., and Matthews, C.G. Psychometric and adaptive abilities in epilepsy with a different etiology. *Epilepsia* 7:330-338, 1966.
56. Kohlenberg, R.J. Operant conditioning of human anal sphincter pressure. *J. Appl. Behav. Anal.* 6:201-208, 1973.
57. Landau, W.M. Spasticity: The fable of a neurological demon and the emperor's new therapy. *Arch. Neurol.* 31:217-219, 1974.
58. Livingston, S. *Comprehensive Management of Epilepsy in Infancy, Childhood and Adolescence.* Springfield, Ill.: Charles C Thomas, 1971.
59. Lubar, J.F., and Bahler, W.W. Behavioral management of epileptic seizures following EEG biofeedback training of sensorimotor rhythm. *Biofeedback Self Regul.* 1:77-104, 1976.
60. Luthe, W. *Autogenic Therapy, Vols. 1-5.* New York: Grune and Stratton, 1969.
61. Magrab, P.R., and Papadopoulou, Z.L. The effect of a token economy on dietary compliance for children on hemodialysis. *J. Appl. Behav. Anal.* 10:573-578, 1977.
62. Mann, J. Uproar over medical bills. *U.S. News and World Report* (March 28, 1977), pp. 35-38.
63. Marshall, R.C., and Watts, M.T. Relaxation/Training: Effects on the communicative ability of aphasic adults. *Arch. Phys. Med. Rehabil.* 57:464-467, 1976.
64. McAlister, A.L., Farquhar, J.W., Thoreson, C.E., and Maccoby, N. Behavioral science applied to cardiovascular health: Progress and research needs in the modification of risk-taking habits in adult populations. *Health Educ. Monogr.* 4:45-73, 1976.
65. McClelland, D.C. Managing motivation to expand human freedom. *Am. Psychol.* 33:201-210, 1978.
66. Meichenbaum, D., and Turk, D. The cognitive-behavioral management of anxiety, anger, and pain, in P.O. Davidson (ed.), *The Behavioral Management of Anxiety, Depression, and Pain.* New York: Brunner/Mazel, 1976.
67. Melzack, R., and Wall, P.D. Pain mechanisms: A new theory. *Science* 150:971-979, 1965.
68. Merskey, H. On the development of pain. *Headache* 10:116-123, 1970.
69. Miller, N.E. Biofeedback and visceral learning. *Annual Review of Psychology.* 29:373-404, 1978.
70. Molnar, G.A., and Taft, L.T. Cerebral palsy, in J. Wortis (ed.), *Mental Retardation and Developmental Disabilities: An Annual Review.* New York: Brunner/Mazel, 1975.
71. Myklebust, H.R. *Educational Problems of the Child with Epilepsy.* Report to the Commission on the Control of Epilepsy and its Consequences, 1977.

72. National Health Education Committee. *Facts on Major Diseases in the United States Today.* New York: David McKay and Co., 1976.
73. Niedermeyer, E. *Compedium of the Epilepsies.* Springfield, Ill.: Charles C Thomas, 1974.
74. O'Reilly, D.E. Care of the cerebral palsied: Outcome of the past and needs for the future. *Dev. Med. Child. Neurol.* 17:141-149, 1975.
75. Oster, J. Recurrent abdominal pain, headache and limb pains in children and adolescents. *Pediatrics* 50:429-436, 1972.
76. Patel, C. Biofeedback-aided relaxation and meditation in the management of hypertension. *Biofeedback Self Regul.* 2:1-41, 1977.
77. Renne, C.M., and Creer, T.L. Training children with asthma to use inhalation equipment. *J. Appl. Behav. Anal.* 9:1-11, 1976.
78. Rose, S.W., Penry, J.K., Makush, R.E., Radloff, L.A., and Putnam, P.L. Prevalence of epilepsy in children. *Epilepsia* 14:133-152, 1973.
79. Rutter, M., Tizard, J., and Whitmore, K. (eds.). *Education, Health, and Behavior.* London: Longmens, 1970.
80. Samilson, R.I. *Orthopaedic Aspects of Cerebral Palsy.* Philadelphia: J.B. Lippincott, 1975.
81. Schain, R.J. *Neurology of Childhood Learning Disorders.* Baltimore: Williams and Wilkins, 1977.
82. Schmidt, B.D. The chronic disease flow sheet in ambulatory pediatrics. *Pediatrics* 51:722-730, 1973.
83. Schwartz, G.E. Self-regulation of response patterning: Implications for psychophysiological research and therapy. *Biofeedback and Self-Regulation.* 1:7-30, 1976.
84. Schwartz, G.E., and Shapiro, D. Biofeedback and essential hypertension: Current findings and theoretical concerns, in L. Birk (ed.), *Biofeedback, Behavioral Medicine.* New York: Grune and Stratton, 1974.
85. Schwartz, G.E., and Weiss, S.M. Yale Conference on Behavioral Medicine: A Proposed Definition and Statement of Goals. *J. Behav. Med.* 1:3-12, 1978.
86. Seligman, M.E. Submissive death: Giving up on life. *Psychol. Today* 7(12):80-85, 1974.
87. Soutter, B.R., and Kennedy, M.C. Patient compliance assessment in drug trials: Usage and methods. *Aust. NZ J. Med.* 4:360-364, 1974.
88. Starfield, B., and Barkowe, S. Physicians' recognition of complaints made by parents about their children's health. *Pediatrics* 43:168-172, 1969.
89. Sterman, M.B. Effects of sensorimotor EEG feedback training on sleep and clinical manifestations of epilepsy, in J. Beatty and H. Legewie (eds.), *Biofeedback and Behavior.* New York: Plenum, 1977.
90. Sterman, M.B., MacDonald, L.R., and Stone, R.K. Biofeedback training of the sensorimotor electroencephalogram rhythm in man: Effects on epilepsy. *Epilepsia* 15:395-416, 1974.
91. Stokes, T.F., and Baer, D.M. An implicit technology of generalization. *J. Appl. Behav. Anal.* 10:349-367, 1977.
92. Stores, G. Behavioral effects of anti-epileptic drugs. *Devel. Med. Child Neurol.* 17:647-658, 1975.
93. Stravino, V.D. The nature of pain. *Arch. Phys. Med. Rehabil.* 51:37-44, 1970.
94. Stroebel, C. Ethics and responsibilities of therapists in biofeedback and behavioral medicine. Symposium presented at the Eighth Annual Meeting of the Biofeedback Society of America, Orlando, Florida, 1977.
95. Stroebel, C. Report of study sections on clinical applications of biofeedback. Symposium at the Ninth Annual Meeting of the Biofeedback Society of America, Albuquerque, March 1978.
96. Swanson, D.W., Swenson, W.M., Manuta, T., and McPhee, M.C. Program for managing chronic pain 1: Program description and characteristics of patients. *Mayo Clin. Proc.*

51:401-408, 1976.

97. Taub, E. Introduction to invited addresses on biofeedback in neuromuscular re-education. Paper presented at Ninth Annual Meeting of the Biofeedback Society of America, Albuquerque, March, 1978.

98. Thompson, R.A., and Green, J.R. (eds.). *Advances in Neurology, Vol. 16: Stroke.* New York: Raven Press, 1977.

99. Tibbles, J.A.R. The functions and the training of a paediatric neurologist. *Dev. Med. Child. Neurol.* 18:167-172, 1976.

100. U.S. Department of Commerce, U.S. Bureau of the Census. *Statistical Abstract of the United States: 1977.* Washington, D.C.: U.S. Government Printing Office, 1977.

101. Varni, J.W., Bessman, C.A., Russo, D.C., and Cataldo, M.F. Behavioral management of pediatric chronic pain. *Archives of Physical Medicine and Rehabilitation,* in press.

1020. Varni, J.W., and Henker, B. A self regulation approach to the treatment of the hyperactive child. *Child Behavior Therapy,* 1:171-192, 1979.

103. Vining, E.P.G., Accardo, P.J., Rubenstein, J.E., Farrell, S.E., and Roizen, N.J. Cerebral palsy: A pediatric developmentalist's overview. *Arch. Am. J. Dis. Child.* 130:643-649, 1976.

104. Weed, L.L. *Medical Records, Medical Education, and Patient Care.* Cleveland: Case University Press, 1969.

105. Weisenberg, M. Pain and pain control. *Psychol. Bull.* 84:1008-1044, 1977.

106. Wolf, J.M. (ed.). *The Results of Treatment in Cerebral Palsy.* Springfield, Ill.: Charles C Thomas, 1969.

107. Wright, T., and Nicholson, J. Physiotherapy for the spastic child: An evaluation. *Dev. Med. Child Neurol.* 15:146-163, 1973.

108. Wyler, A.R., Lockard, J.S., Ward, A.A., and Finch, C.A. Conditioned EEG desynchronization and seizures. *Electroencephalogr. Clin. Neurophysiol.* 41:501-512, 1976.

109. Yule, W. The potential of behavioral treatment in preventing later childhood difficulties. *Behav. Anal. and Med.* 2:19-31, 1977.

110. Zlutnick, S., Mayville, W., and Moffat, S. Modification of seizure disorders: The interruption of behavioral chains. *J. Appl. Behav. Anal.* 8:1-12, 1975.

Cognitive
Treatment Strategies

Heide and Mahoney discuss the use of cognitive strategies for treating medical disorders. They point out that there are several extant cognitive therapies, included under the general categories of cognitive learning therapies, and covert conditioning therapies. The application of covert or cognitive techniques has been to headache, Type A behavior, alcoholism, and obesity. In each case there has been significant influence by these techniques, although like other behavioral techniques they do not offer a panacea. Clearly, cognitive processes play a significant role in human adjustment, human health, and human illness. These processes can be modified through the use of behavioral procedures. To date these procedures are relatively weak. Research in areas such as depression indicate that there may be ways to increase the effectiveness of these treatment strategies. The area of cognitive therapies is an exciting one and offers great potential for looking at thought processes and their influence on health-care behaviors.

CHAPTER 5

Cognitive Strategies for Medical Disorders

Frederick J. Heide
Michael J. Mahoney

Recent years have witnessed a trend within clinical psychology toward the integration of cognitive and behavioral approaches to therapy. The new perspective which has been emerging combines the behavioral emphasis on experimentation with the cognitive emphasis on the client's unique and influential interpretation of the world. A variety of intriguing therapies has sprung up both inside and outside the field of behavior modification, and they appear to offer some welcome conceptual breadth and clinical promise (28, 31, 37). Though only a few efforts have been made thus far to apply these therapies to medical disorders, preliminary results suggest that the cognitive-behavioral perspective may have considerable potential in this area. This chapter will discuss some of the available cognitive therapies, review the budding literature on their application to medical disorders, and finally consider some general strategies for applying them to selected medical problems.

THE COGNITIVE THERAPIES

First, it may be useful to consider what types of therapy are usually regarded as "cognitive" within the context of the recent cognitive-behavioral interface. Two broad categories of cognitive approaches can be distinguished: covert conditioning therapies and cognitive learning therapies (28).

Covert Conditioning Therapies

As the name implies, the covert conditioning therapies attempt to apply a conditioning model to private events. Thoughts, mental images, and memories are viewed as covert behaviors which conform to the same laws of learning that were developed through observation of overt behaviors. Thus, thoughts are considered to be stimuli, responses, or consequences, and principles such as reinforcement, punishment, and extinction are said to affect their frequency and intensity.

A good example of a covert conditioning therapy is Cautela's (8) technique of covert reinforcement. In this procedure, the client is instructed to imagine performing some difficult task (e.g., refraining from drinking alcohol) and then to reinforce himself by imagining some pleasant activity (e.g., skiing down a mountainside). A long involved task may be broken down into a series of discrete steps, each of which is covertly reinforced. A number of other covert conditioning techniques are available, including systematic desensitization and thought stopping (9, 10). By now most of the principles of learning which have been applied to overt behaviors have been incorporated into some covert technique.

A sizable literature has accumulated examining the conceptual foundations and therapeutic efficacy of these procedures. Unfortunately, with the exception of systematic desensitization, the effectiveness of these procedures has generally been meager (28, 31). Most of the better-controlled studies have found these techniques to be little better than attention-placebo controls. Even when clinical effectiveness has been clearly established, as in systematic desensitization, serious questions have arisen about the adequacy of traditional conditioning principles to explain this success (1, 24, 57). However, a blanket pronouncement on the effectiveness of these procedures or their underlying mechanisms is premature. Better-controlled research is needed to determine which of these techniques offer clear promise to the practitioner.

Cognitive Learning Therapies

The second class of cognitive approaches are those which have been labeled "the cognitive learning therapies" (29). They are a much more heterogeneous set of strategies, sharing a few assumptions but differing widely in their derivation and procedure. Though a precise model unifying these approaches has yet to be developed, one or more of the following principles appear to be fundamental to most of them:

1. that human beings respond not to environments per se but to their cognitive representations of those environments;

2. that thinking, emotion and behavior are all causally interrelated;
3. that human learning involves the active acquisition of complex rules and skills ("deep structural changes") rather than the passive conditioning of simple habits or responses ("surface structural manifestations");
4. that the task of the clinician is to teach skills and offer experiences which replace maladaptive cognitive representations with more adaptive cognitive systems.

A further feature of several of the cognitive learning therapies included in this chapter is that they attempt to modify cognitive representations in a more or less direct fashion, by making the client's beliefs and attitudes an explicit part of therapeutic discussion. In this way they can be contrasted with a number of other approaches such as participant modeling (1), which presume cognitive change mechanisms but which have not focused on cognitive compoents per se.

Deciding whether or not a particular procedure is cognitive is obviously somewhat arbitrary. Indeed, it appears that this decision is often influenced more the terminology and theoretical orientation of the procedure's inventor than any intrinsic characteristic of the procedure itself. Ultimately, most therapeutic techniques will probably be found to engage complex interacting systems of cognition, affect, and behavior, rendering the cognitive-noncognitive distinction less meaningful. In the meantime, however, we will continue to use the term "cognitive" to refer to those procedures which conform fairly closely to the principles presented above.

Mahoney and Arnkoff (31) have classified the cognitive learning therapies into three major categories: cognitive restructuring, coping skills therapies, and problem-solving therapies. The first category includes Beck's (4) cognitive therapy, Ellis's (13) rational-emotive therapy, and Meichenbaum's (37) self-instructional training. Though differing in a number of subtle ways, these three approaches share a common emphasis on training clients to identify their maladaptive thought patterns, become aware of their negative consequences, and substitute more adaptive thoughts in their place. The second category, coping skills therapies, includes Suinn and Richardson's (54) anxiety management training, Meichenbaum's (35) stress inoculation training, and covert modeling (9, 23). These approaches are similar in their common attempt to train clients in one or more skills which can be applied in a variety of stressful situations. These skills may include relaxation training, cognitive restructuring, imagery manipulation, and preperformance rehearsal. Many programs which train clients in biofeedback, assertiveness, and the like can also be considered coping skills therapies.

The final category, which overlaps with the other two, is problem-solving therapies. Included under this heading are behavioral problem-solving (12), problem-solving therapy (48), and personal science (30). These approaches train clients to identify personal problems and their causes, to generate alternative ways of dealing with these problems, and to evaluate the success of whatever alternative is chosen. It can be seen that these approaches constitute a broad conceptual scheme into which the other cognitive therapies as well as many behavior therapies can fit.

A number of controlled outcome studies of the various cognitive learning therapies have been conducted, particularly with anxious and depressed clients. A recent summary of this literature concluded that the data thus far were "promising but preliminary" (31). The results appear sufficiently encouraging to warrant more elaborate outcome studies using general clinical populations as well as persons manifesting medical problems.

APPLICATIONS TO MEDICAL DISORDERS

Having skimmed over the variety of cognitive strategies available, let us briefly review studies in which they have been applied to medical disorders. Work in this area is just beginning. Only a few studies have been conducted, and these have varied widely in their methodological adequacy. Though results of these early studies seem promising, the lack of adequate controls and attention-placebo groups in most studies requires that an attitude of healthy skepticism be retained. Since a review of the application of covert conditioning procedures in behavioral medicine has recently been presented elsewhere (14), this review will be confined to applications of cognitive learning strategies.

Cognitive learning approaches have been principally applied to five types of medical problems: pain, headache, Type A behavior, obesity, and alcoholism.

Pain

Probably the most common problem thus far addressed by cognitive techniques is the control of pain. This is probably due to the ease with which pain can be studied in a laboratory setting, the clearly defined dependent variable, and the usefulness of using pain as an analog for a variety of stressful stimuli. A great variety of different strategies has been examined, including attention diversion (2, 21), relaxation and attentional focus (6, 49), imaginative transformation of pain (3, 5), verbal/symbolic activity (11, 18), and calming self-talk (26). As Stevens and Heide (49) have pointed out, the relationship between these strategies is complex and perhaps interactive. Though a number of comparative studies of techniques have been conducted, no one strategy has emerged as being clearly superior to others in all situations or with all types of pain.

Several recent attempts have been made to develop and test package programs which combine a number of pain control techniques. One of the most comprehensive of these package programs is stress inoculation training, developed by Meichenbaum and his colleagues (35, 38, 55). When this procedure is applied to pain, clients are presented a rationale derived from Melzack and Wall's (39) gate control theory of pain. They are told that the pain experience consists of three components, each of which can be controlled by a different set of techniques. The *sensory-discriminative* component, or raw sensory input of pain, is dealt with through physical and mental relaxation and deep breathing. The *motivational-affective* component, which includes feelings of helplessness and lack of control, is dealt with by attention diversion (focusing attention on some external object), somatization (focusing attention on physical sensations in the body, including the pain), and imagery manipulations (e.g., imagining that you are a spy who has been shot in the arm and are now escaping from enemy agents). Finally, the *cognitive-evaluative* component of pain is dealt with by teaching clients a variety of self-statements or calming things to say to themselves while coping with the pain (e.g., "Just relax, breathe deeply, and use one of the strategies").

It is noteworthy that this approach differs from many of the pain studies cited above in providing clients with a choice of many coping strategies rather than requiring them to use one or two selected by the experimenter. This emphasis on self-control rather than passive responding may be a significant factor in the effectiveness of the package in view of evidence favoring self-control strategies for pain (22). It also appears to incorporate elements of all three categories of the cognitive learning therapies discussed above.

Laboratory research on this program using ischemic pain produced by a blood pressure cuff indicated that subjects could almost double their pain tolerance after undergoing training. This was in marked contrast to an attention-placebo group given psuedo-training without specific coping procedures (38). Further work is underway applying this approach to clinical populations. A component analysis of the package has recently been presented (20).

Headache

Two reports on the application of cognitive learning strategies to headache are available. In a case study of tension headache, Reeves (40) trained a subject to identify negative self-statements and thoughts, substitute coping self-instructions (e.g., "Don't worry, worry won't help anything"), and then rehearse these coping self-instructions while imagining stressful situations. Following this, the subject was also trained in EMG biofeedback. This combined procedure resulted in a 66% reduction of headache activity, maintained at a six-month follow-up.

A more elaborate study of tension headache compared a cognitively oriented stress-coping program with biofeedback and a waiting-list control group (19).

Clients in the stress-coping group were trained to identify thoughts associated with tension and headaches and to interrupt them with each of three types of covert coping techniques: cognitive reappraisal, attention deployment, and fantasy. Only the stress-coping group displayed substantial reduction in number of recorded headaches. Though this study is an improvement over previous work, its interpretation is hampered by absence of a placebo group and by use of the two senior authors as therapists in the stress-coping group but not the biofeedback group. Further work is clearly called for.

Type A Behavior

Suinn and his colleagues (51, 52, 53) have conducted several studies applying a type of coping skills therapy to persons displaying the coronary-prone (Type A) behavior pattern. This pattern is characterized by self-imposed deadlines, eagerness to compete, sense of time urgency, strong desires for achievement, and impatience. Suinn's Cardiac Stress Management Program places major emphasis on a procedure called Anxiety Management Training (AMT). This procedure trains subjects in relaxation and then deliberately arouses anxiety through imagery. Subjects are asked to attend to the subjective cues associated with anxiety and to practice relaxation as a coping response.

The best-controlled study of this approach (53) compared AMT and a waiting-list control group in treating healthy subjects manifesting the Type A behavior pattern. The experimental group showed significant reductions in some Type A behaviors and self-reported anxiety, but differences in blood pressure, cholesterol, and triglyceride levels were not significant. These results may be interpreted as encouraging, but more definitive conclusions must await replications with larger sample sizes, adequate placebo groups, and comparisons with other behavioral interventions. Suinn is also exploring applications of other cognitive techniques, such as refocusing thoughts to something other than worry or engaging in stressful thoughts only in certain places or at certain times of day (52).

Obesity

Although cognitive factors in obesity have long been recognized (7), very few behavioral interventions have incorporated cognitive strategies (50). This is somewhat surprising in that a client's expectancies and perceptions may dramatically influence weight-relevant patterns. Wooley (58), for example, has shown that a person's food consumption may be affected more by their *perception* of calorie content than by actual calorie content. Likewise, it would appear that a person's expectancies may influence their responsiveness to a treatment strategy (28).

At the present time, very few behavioral weight control programs have focused on the alteration of weight-relevant thought patterns. One of these (32) was an exploratory two-year study involving a combination of cognitive and non-cognitive strategies (33). A subsequent group study involving 86 obese adults who were studied for two years suggested that the package was variable in its effectiveness with a wide range of weight loss and changes in cardiovascular health. Interestingly, one of the best predictors of successful treatment was cognitive—i.e., self-reported attitudes and beliefs about obesity and personal ability to lose weight (27). The most effective methods for changing these cognitive patterns and for measuring their impact remain an issue for continuing research.

Alcoholism

A comprehensive approach to treating alcohol problems has been developed by Sobell and Sobell (44, 47). Their training package, called Problem Solving Skills Training, can be viewed as a cognitive learning approach because of its coping-skills orientation and its attempt to teach problem-solving, which is usually considered a cognitive skill. The Sobells' program consists of four stages: 1) *Problem Identification,* in which clients are trained to identify specific circumstances under which they drink inappropriately; 2) *Delineation of Behavioral Options,* in which clients generate a series of alternative behaviors that they might engage in when facing problem situations; 3) *Evaluation of Behavioral Options,* in which clients identify the short-term and long-term consequences of using each of the behavioral options generated previously; and 4) *Employing the Option(s) Evaluated to Have the Best Probable Total Outcome,* in which clients learn and practice the option(s) anticipated to have the best total consequences. At this stage, clients may be trained in relaxation, biofeedback, assertiveness, self-monitoring, contingency management, behavioral contracting, or a variety of other skills.

It is interesting to note the similarity of this program to the stress-inoculation and coping-skills programs discussed previously. All of these programs employ a broad-spectrum approach in which clients are offered a wide array of techniques from which to choose. In this way, clients become active participants in their own growth process and are free to develop strategies uniquely suited to them. Rather than being tied to the success or failure of any one technique, these programs also offer built-in flexibility by emphasizing the overall problem-solving *attitude* more than the specific alternatives that may be selected.

The Sobells have undertaken a substantial research project to test the efficacy of this approach (44, 45, 46). Seventy male alcoholics at a state hospital were selectively assigned to a treatment goal of either controlled drinking or complete abstinence. Subjects in each group were then randomly assigned to either an experimental group receiving 17 behavioral treatment sessions or a control group receiving conventional state hospital treatment. The experimental treatment was a combination of problem-solving skills training, videotape feedback on drunken behavior, and electrical shock to punish inappropriate drinking. Differences between experimental and control groups on drinking and general adjustment measures were significant at six-month and one-year follow-ups. However, only the experimental group given the goal of controlled drinking was significantly different from the respective control group at the two-year follow-up.

These results are encouraging and indicate that this approach is worth pursuing. Unfortunately, selective assignment of subjects to controlled and abstinent conditions hampers interpretation of this study. It is difficult to know whether the sustained success of the controlled drinking group is due to their more lenient treatment goal, to some interaction between the treatment package and their treatment goal, or simply to factors such as motivation and presence of outside social support which were used in determining assignment to treatment goals. For clearer interpretation, future studies will need to employ random assignment to conditions and more isolation of treatment components.

ISSUES AND IMPLICATIONS

Clinical Implications

Space limitations make it impossible to do justice to the complexity of the many cognitive-learning therapies available or to provide detailed suggestions for their application. Practical guidelines are available in several other sources (4, 30, 37). However, it may be helpful to suggest several ways in which cognition might be taken into account in dealing with general medical problems.

In his discussion of cognitive factors in biofeedback therapy, Meichenbaum (36) has presented one possible way of applying a cognitive perspective to treatment of somatic disorders. He argues that biofeedback therapy can be broken down into three fairly distinct phases: 1) a conceptualization phase, in which diagnosis takes place and attempts are made to foster the client's motivation; 2) a training phase, in which the client acquires and rehearses a set of cognitive, behavioral, and physiological coping skills; and 3) a transfer of treatment phase, in which the client applies these new skills outside the treatment setting.

Meichenbaum argues that cognitions or thoughts should be taken into account during each of these three phases in order to enhance effectiveness of treatment. During the conceptualization phase, he suggests that the therapist attend to the personal meaning that the client has given his or her problem. In many cases, the client feels helpless and incapable of controlling the problem. By assessing the client's internal dialogue (e.g., asking what he is saying to himself in stressful situations), the therapist may tap a source of inner stimulation which is perpetuating the physiological disorder. During the treatment phase, the therapist might attempt to modify this internal dialogue by providing the client with coping self-statements or by suggesting the use of relaxing self-instructions and imagery during biofeedback. Finally, in order to foster transfer of treatment to real-life settings, the therapist might use an imagery rehearsal technique such as Suinn's (51) anxiety management training or a covert modeling procedure (23).

Meichenbaum's recommendation to use cognitive strategies during the training phase gains some support from discussion of cognitions in the biofeedback literature. For example, Schwartz (42) reports that clients will spontaneously employ aggressive and sexual fantasies to raise their heart rate and that they often report using quiet, relaxing fantasies to lower it. He also reports the case of a patient treated for Raynaud's disease who used "hot thoughts" about warm, sunny beaches to raise the temperature of his feet (41). A similar use of thought patterns to control heart rate has been reported by Weiss and Engel (56).

Another way in which a cognitive perspective might be applied to medical disorders is through use of the problem-solving approach discussed earlier. In this approach, clients are taught the skills relevant to identifying problems and their causes, generating options for dealing with these problems, anticipating the outcome of employing these options, and finally putting the selected options into practice and evaluating their effectiveness. As in Meichenbaum's model of biofeedback, cognitions enter during each phase of this training. In identifying causes of problems, clients are encouraged to recognize maladaptive beliefs and attitudes which contribute to their tendency to overreact or to lose control. The generation of options can be aided by the use of helpful self-statements (e.g., "Just relax and let the possibilities present themselves"). Several of the options selected might involve cognitive strategies (e.g., positive self-statements, cognitive restructuring, etc.). Anticipation of outcomes is clearly a cognitive process, which can be aided by realistic feedback from the therapist and practice in means-ends thinking. Finally, implementation and maintenance of a given option can be assisted by making clients aware of their inner dialogues about the option they have chosen and by helping them to modify these dialogues if they are counterproductive.

Psychosomatic Cognitions

A fairly sizable literature is now available documenting the impact of thought processes on physiological reactions (34, 42). This literature is often cited in support of one of the assumptions of the cognitive learning model presented earlier, i.e., that thinking, emotion, and behavior are all interrelated. In addition, several other lines of research have suggested that certain patterns of beliefs may be associated with particular physiological disorders. Such links have been postulated in disorders as diverse as asthma (25) and cancer (43). If this is indeed the case, cognitive therapy may be a logical intervention to modify these maladaptive belief patterns.

Perhaps the most extensive work in this area has been conducted by Graham and his colleagues (15, 16, 17). In a series of studies, these researchers have identified a number of "mental attitudes" which they believe to be associated with specific psychosomatic disorders. An example is the mental attitude associated with uticaria (hives), in which subjects felt that they were taking a beating and were helpless to do anything about it. In one elaborate study (16), hypnotized subjects were given the attitude suggestions associated with hives and essential hypertension in counterbalanced order. The authors predicted that the rise in skin temperature in response to the hives suggestion would be greater than the rise, if any, in response to the hypertension suggestion (skin temperature is elevated by hives). Similarly, they predicted a rise in blood pressure in response to the hypertension suggestion that would be greater than the rise, if any, in response to the hives suggestions. Both predictions were corroborated and no differences were found in other physiological variables for which no differential effect was predicted.

This hypothesis of mental attitudes specific to various psychosomatic disorders is similar to Beck's (4) postulation of thought patterns associated with clinical syndromes such as depression, anxiety, paranoia, and obsession. In both cases, the intriguing possibility arises of developing therapies to modify the particular cognitive set associated with a distinct syndrome. Just as Beck's therapy with depressives subtly challenges their belief that they are worthless or hopeless, cognitive therapy with hives patients might challenge their mistaken belief that the world is picking on them. In both cases, clients would learn to be aware of these faulty beliefs, to substitute accurate beliefs, and to engage in active behavioral performance to demonstrate to themselves that their former beliefs were wrong.

A FINAL NOTE

We have reviewed several attempts to apply a cognitive learning perspective to medical disorders. Some encouraging results have been obtained thus far, but this work is far from definitive. As more outcome studies are conducted, some of these techniques will undoubtedly prove more useful than others. Nevertheless, it is important to emphasize that one can endorse the cognitive learning perspective without necessarily endorsing the use of currently available cognitive therapies. It is entirely possible that cognitive *processes* play a significant role in human adjustment, but that these processes are best modified through the use of behavioral or affective *procedures*. Whether the techniques presented here will prove more powerful than other techniques is ultimately an empirical issue. The preliminary promise of cognitive techniques in treating anxiety and depression gives us reason to be optimistic about their usefulness in treating medical disorders. However, the best strategy at this early stage of inquiry is to adopt an attitude of critical evaluation and open-minded empiricism in regard to these approaches.

REFERENCES

1. Bandura, A. *Principles of Behavior Modification.* New York: Holt, Rinehart and Winston, 1969.
2. Barber, T.X., and Cooper, B.J. Effects on pain of experimentally induced and spontaneous distraction. *Psychol. Rep.* 31:647-651, 1972.
3. Barber, T.X., and Hahn, K.W. Physiological and subjective responses to pain producing stimulation under hypnotically-suggested and waking-imagined "analgesia." *J. Abnorm. Soc. Psychol.* 65:411-418, 1962.
4. Beck, A.T. *Cognitive Therapy and the Emotional Disorders.* New York: International Universities Press, 1976.
5. Blitz, B., and Dinnerstein, A.J. Role of attentional focus in pain perception: manipulation of response to noxious stimulation. *J. Abnorm. Psychol.* 77:42-45, 1971.
6. Bobey, M.J., and Davidson, P.O. Psychological factors affecting pain tolerance. *J. Psychsom. Res.* 14:371-376, 1970.
7. Bruch, H. *Eating Disorders.* New York: Basic Books, 1973.
8. Cautela, J.R. Covert reinforcement. *Behav. Ther.* 1:33-50, 1970.
9. Cautela, J.R. Covert conditioning, in A. Jacobs and L.B. Sachs (eds.), *The Psychology of Private Events: Perspectives on Covert Response Systems.* New York: Academic Press, 1971, pp. 109-130.
10. Cautela, J.R. Rationale and procedures for covert conditioning, in R.D. Rubin, H. Fonsterheim, J.D. Henderson and L.P. Ullmann (eds.), *Advances in Behavior Therapy.* New York: Academic Press, 1972, pp. 85-96.
11. Chaves, J., and Barber, T.X. Cognitive strategies, experimenter modeling, and expectation in the attenuation of pain. *J. Abnorm. Psychol.* 83:356-363, 1974.
12. D'Zurilla, T.J., and Goldfried, M.R. Problem solving and behavior modification. *J. Abnorm. Psychol.* 78:107-126, 1971.
13. Ellis, A. *Reason and Emotion in Psychotherapy.* New York: Lyle Stuart, 1962.
14. Gentry, W.D. Cognitive treatment of somatic disorders, in J.P. Foreyt and D.P. Rathjen (eds.), *Cognitive Behavior Therapy: Research and Application.* New York: Plenum, 1978.
15. Graham, D.T. Psychosomatic medicine, in N.S. Greenfield and R.A. Sternbach (eds.), *Handbook of Psychophysiology.* New York: Holt, Rinehart and Winston, 1972, pp. 839-924.

16. Graham, D.T., Kabler, J.D., and Graham, F.K. Physiological response to the suggestion of attitudes specific for hives and hypertension. *Psychosom. Med.* 24:159-169, 1962.

17. Graham, D.T., Stern, J.A., and Winokur, B. Experimental investigation of the specificity of attitude hypothesis in psychosomatic disease. *Psychosom. Med.* 20:446-457, 1958.

18. Grimm, L. and Kanfer, F.H. Tolerance of aversive stimulation. *Behav. Ther.* 7:593-601, 1976.

19. Holroyd, K.A., Andrasik, F., and Westbrook, T. Cognitive control of tension headache. *Cog. Ther. Res.* 1:131-133, 1977.

20. Horan, J.J., Hackett, G., Buchanan, J.D., Stone, C.I., and Demchik-Stone, D. Coping with pain: A component analysis of stress modulation. *Cog. Ther. Res.* 1:211-232, 1977.

21. Kanfer, F.H. and Goldfoot, D.A. Self-control and tolerance of noxious stimulation. *Psychol. Rep.* 18:79-85, 1966.

22. Kanfer, F.H. and Seidner, M.L. Self-control factors enhancing tolerance of aversive stimulation. *J. Pers. Soc. Psychol.* 20:55-64, 1973.

23. Kazdin, A.E. Covert modeling and the reduction of avoidance behavior. *J. Abnorm. Psychol.* 81:87-95, 1973.

24. Kazdin, A.E., and Wilcoxon, L. Systematic desensitization and nonspecific treatment effects: A methodological evaluation. *Psychol. Bull.* 83:729-758, 1976.

25. Kinsman, R.A., Dahlem, N.W., Spector, S., and Staudenmeyer, H. Observations on subjective symptomatology, coping behavior, and medical decisions on asthma. *Psychosom. Med.* 39:102-119, 1977.

26. Langer, E., Janis, I., and Wolfer, J. Reduction of psychological stress in surgical patients. *J. Exper. Soc. Psychol.* 11:155-165, 1975.

27. Mahoney, B.K., Rogers, T., Straw, M.K., and Mahoney, MJ. *Human Obesity: Assessment and Treatment.* Englewood Cliffs, N.J.: Prentice-Hall, in press.

28. Mahoney, M.J. *Cognition and Behavior Modification.* Cambridge, Mass.: Ballinger, 1974.

29. Mahoney, M.J. Reflections on the cognitive-learning trend in psychotherapy. *Am. Psychol.* 32:5-13, 1977.

30. Mahoney, M.J. *Self-Change.* New York: W.W. Norton, 1979.

31. Mahoney, M.J., and Arnkoff, D. Cognitive and self-control therapies, in S.L. Garfield and A.E. Bergin (eds.), *Handbook of Psychotherapy and Behavior Change,* vol. 2. New York: Wiley, 1978.

32. Mahoney, M.J., and Mahoney, K. Treatment of obesity: A clinical exploration, in B.J. Williams, S. Martin, and J.P. Foreyt (eds.), *Obesity: Behavioral Approaches to Dietary Management.* New York: Brunner/Mazel, 1976.

33. Mahoney, M.J., and Mahoney, K. *Permanent Weight Control.* New York: W.W. Norton, 1976.

34. McGuigan, F.J. and Schoonover, R.A. (eds.). *The Psychophysiology of Thinking.* New York: Academic Press, 1973.

35. Meichenbaum, D. A self-instructional approach to stress management: A proposal for stress inoculation training, in I. Sarason and C.D. Spielberger (eds.), *Stress and Anxiety,* vol. 2. New York: Wiley, 1975, pp. 227-263.

36. Meichenbaum, D. Cognitive factors in biofeedback therapy. *Biofeedback and Self-regulation* 1:201-216, 1976.

37. Meichenbaum, D. *Cognitive-Behavior Modification: An Integrative Approach.* New York: Plenum, 1977.

38. Meichenbaum, D., and Turk, D. The cognitive-behavioral management of anxiety, anger and pain, in P.O. Davidson (ed.), *The Behavioral Management of Anxiety, Depression,*

and Pain. New York: Brunner/Mazel, 1976.

39. Melzack, R. and Wall, P. Pain mechanisms: A new theory. *Science* 150:971, 1965.

40. Reeves, J.L. EMG-biofeedback reduction of tension headache: A cognitive skills-training approach. *Biofeedback and Self-Regulation* 1:217-225, 1976.

41. Schwartz, G.E. Biofeedback as therapy: Some theoretical and practical issues. *Am. Psychol.* 28:666-673, 1973.

42. Schwartz, G.E. Biofeedback, self-regulation, and the patterning of physiological processes. *Am. Scientist* 63:314-324, 1975.

43. Simonton,, O.C., and Simonton, S.S. Belief systems and management of the emotional aspects of malignancy. *J. Transper. Psychol.* 7:29-47, 1975.

44. Sobel, M.B., and Sobell, L.C. Individualized behavior therapy for alcoholics. *Behav. Ther.* 4:49-72, 1973.

45. Sobell, M.B., and Sobell, L.C. Alcoholics treated by individualized behavior therapy: One year treatment outcome. *Behav. Res. and Ther.* 11:599-618, 1973.

46. Sobell, M.B., and Sobell, L.C. Second year treatment outcome of alcoholics treated by individualized behavior therapy: Results. *Behav. Res. and Ther.* 14:195-215, 1976.

47. Sobell, C.C., and Sobell, M.B. Alcohol problems, in R.B. Williams and W.D. Gentry (eds.), *Behavioral Approaches to Medical Treatment.* Cambridge, Mass.: Ballinger, 1977.

48. Spivack, G., and Shure, M.B. *Social Adjustment of Young Children: A Cognitive Approach to Solving Real-Life Problems.* San Francisco: Jossey-Bass, 1974.

49. Stevens, R.J., and Heide, F.J. Analgesic characteristics of prepared childbirth techniques: Attention focusing and systematic relaxation. *J. ·Psychosom. Res.,* 21:429-438, 1977.

50. Stunkard, A.J., and Mahoney, M.J. Behavioral treatment of the eating disorders, in H. Leitenberg (ed.), *Handbook of Behavior Therapy and Behavior Modification.* Englewood Cliffs, N.J.: Prentice-Hall, 1976.

51. Suinn, R.M. Behavior therapy for cardiac patients. *Behav. Ther.* 5:569-571, 1974.

52. Suinn, R.M. Type A behavior pattern, in R.B. Williams and W.D. Gentry (eds.), *Behavioral Approaches to Medical Treatment.* Cambridge, Mass.: Ballinger, 1977.

53. Suinn, R.M., and Bloom, L.J. Anxiety management training for Type A persons. *J. Behav. Med.,* 1:25-36, 1978.

54. Suinn, R.M., and Richardson, F. Anxiety management training: A nonspecific behavior therapy program for anxiety control. *Behav. Ther.* 4:498-510, 1971.

55. Turk, D.C. Cognitive-behavioral techniques in the management of pain, in J.P. Foreyt and D.P. Rathjen (eds.), *Cognitive Behavior Therapy: Research and Application.* New York: Plenum, 1978.

56. Weiss, T., and Engel, B.T. Operant conditioning of heart rate in patients with premature ventricular contractions. *Psychosom. Med.* 33:301-322, 1971.

57. Wilkins, W. Desensitization: Social and cognitive factors underlying the effectiveness of Wolpe's procedure. *Psychol. Bull.* 76:311-317, 1971.

58. Wooley, S.C. Physiologic versus cognitive factors in short-term food regulations in the obese and non-obese. *Psychosom. Med.* 34:62-68, 1972.

Compliance

Once prescriptions have been written or advice given, a patient's compliance may become the determining factor in successful outcome of therapy. In this chapter, Dunbar and Agras provide an extensive review of the problem of compliance with medical instructions. The problem of poor adherence to medical regimens has been well documented, and in some cases the percentage of noncompliant patients is extremely high. With the individual patient, the failure to receive maximum benefit from health programs is apparent. From a larger viewpoint, it becomes impossible to monitor treatment efficacy, safety, and side effects without knowing the rate of compliance to drug prescription or other therapeutic instructions. Dunbar and Agras point out that much is known about the broad phenomenon of adherence, but much needs to be learned about the details. Studies in this area are too young to know long-term outcome for various intervention strategies. Nonetheless, the technology has been developed which stresses factors such as the organization of a clinic, the method of administering medication, the quality of the interaction between patient and physician, and other staff members, and the effect of altering patient reception of health-care benefits. Although it is still not clear why patients fail to follow treatment advice, answers are beginning to emerge, and the technology is beginning to be developed to change the course of poor adherence.

CHAPTER 6

Compliance with Medical Instructions

Jacqueline M. Dunbar
W. Stewart Agras

Interest in adherence to health regimen has proliferated in recent years. Most of this interest has been directed to medication taking, where reports indicate that 33% (15) to 82% (119) of patients do not follow or err in following their regimens. More recent reports suggest that other health regimens fare as poorly. Dropout rates in weight-loss programs reach as high as 70% within two years (48), with some suggestions that dietary adherence itself may average 50% (39). About 50% of appointments are kept if the provider makes the appointment; 80% are kept if the patient makes the appointment (108). Forty-nine percent of postmyocardial infarction patients drop out of exercise programs within the first year (108). And, reportedly, just 16% to 59% of persons use seat belts (101, 102).

Thus, a substantial portion of individuals fail to receive maximum benefit from health regimens. The problem is further compounded when one realizes that good adherence is necessary and that knowledge of the degree of patient adherence is required to monitor treatment efficacy, safety, and side effects. This is not only crucial to the evaluation of treatment for the individual patient, but also to the interpretation of clinical research involving self-administered regimen. Indeed, Joyce (69) has aptly demonstrated that drug intervention studies may arrive at different conclusions, depending on whether or not patient adherence is accounted for in the evaluation of the data.

FACTORS CONTRIBUTING TO POOR ADHERENCE

Exactly why patients fail to follow treatment advice is not entirely clear, although considerable research has examined this question. The temptation is to ascribe nonadherence to a lack of motivation, to certain socioeconomic factors, or to personality characteristics. None of these has held up well as reasons. Indeed, no personality traits or socioeconomic indicators have been associated with adherence (83). Neither age, educational level, occupation, religion, nor any other demographic features make independent contributions. In studies where a relationship has been demonstrated, a second contributing factor can often be found, e.g., comprehension of the regimen, ability to financially afford the regimen, or continuance in care.

Motivation

Motivation is a difficult construct to measure and evaluate. But it does not appear to be a primary factor in most adherence problems. In one study, for example, only 15% of patients reported having no intention of following their physician's advice and did not do so, and yet the proportion of patients adhering was considerably lower than 85% (33). More often patients do feel willing to adhere, but other factors interfere with their *ability* to do so.

Education and Information

Lack of knowledge may be one of the factors interfering with the patient's ability to adhere. But it should be noted that this is lack of knowledge about the *regimen,* not the disease. Information about the disease itself is of limited value (109). But knowledge of the regimen, such as how many pills to take and at what time, is crucial. Indeed, in one study, medication scheduling errors decreased from 17% to 3% when the patient's understanding of the regimen was taken into account (59).

A major contribution to patients' understanding is made by their recall of their clinicians' advice. Indeed, patients can be expected to do no more than they remember, and yet accurate recall of advice cannot be taken for granted (20, 58, 65, 72). For example, Joyce et al. (68) questioned patients about what the physician had told them in an office visit. One group was interviewed immediately after the visit, while a second group was interviewed at home two weeks after the visit. Both groups had forgotten two-thirds of the diagnoses and treatment explanation and one-half of the instructional statements. There was no relationship between the passage of time and loss of information. However, forgetting increased in direct proportion to the amount of information given by the physician, suggesting that recall should be improved if information is dispensed in discrete quantities over time.

The problems inherent in overloading the patient with information were further demonstrated in a study of the effect of consent forms of varying complexity upon patient recall (41). Three forms were used containing similar information presented in brief, in an intermediate format, and finally with every complexity exposed. Volunteers for an experiment were randomly allocated to one of the three groups, each receiving one version of the consent form, and were than tested for recall of the salient points. The group receiving the short form demonstrated the best recall, while those receiving the long form showed the poorest, remembering only about half as much as those receiving information in its simplest form. Moreover, those with higher recalls in all groups tended to volunteer to take part in the study more often than those who recalled less. Nineteen of 22 subjects exposed to the short form volunteered, while only 11 of 22 subjects exposed to the long form decided to participate.

In addition to the quantity of information relayed at any one time, the way the information is presented influences recall. For example, the manner in which the material is organized is important. Ley et al. (72) found that patients were more likely to remember information when it was organized according to specific categories. Thus, the clinician might discuss diagnoses, then move on to diagnostic tests, then to each prescribed treatment, then to what the patient must do, rather than shifting among categories. Recall has been raised between 25 and 50% with just this modification alone (72).

Using visual aids in patient instruction also increase retention. For example, Boyd et al. (20) reported that over a three-day period patients retained 10% of the verbally transmitted information, 20% of that presented visually, and 65% of that presented by both modalities. Clinite and Kabat (28) also reported that combining presentation modalities was superior to either modality alone. However, in this case, written materials were poorer than an oral presentation if each was done alone. Both Dickey et al. (35) and Linkewich et al. (75) have confirmed the greater efficacy of combining verbal and written instructions.

Even a well-organized instruction presented through oral and written modalities, however, must be at a level which the patient can comprehend. We might expect that simple rather than complex information would be associated with better comprehension and adherence. Ley, Jain, and Skilbeck (73) tested this notion with 160 patients being treated either with antianxiety agents or with antidepressants. Patients were randomly assigned either to usual care or to receive a leaflet containing brief information including the name of the medication, what to do if a tablet was forgotten, and an explanation that the medicine would take some time to be effective. In addition, patients received this information at three different levels of comprehension, ranging from easy, in which 90% of all persons would be expected to understand, to difficult, in which less than 10% would understand. Adherence measured by a clinic pill count demonstrated a distinct advantage for those receiving the simplest form of information. Complexly written information was no better than usual care.

In a very similar study, patients taking a short course of oral penicillin were randomly allocated to two groups receiving either medication labeled in the usual way, or medication with an auxiliary label and a simple instruction sheet (112). A surreptitious pill count at home showed that simple augmentation of information was associated with 85% consumption of pills as against 63% in the usual practice group. Finally, a slightly more complex form of information provision within a predischarge conference with a pharmacist led to marked augmentation of adherence two weeks later—to 92% versus 24% for the group not receiving the counseling session (29).

Thus, the instructional strategies used by the clinician can have a substantial impact on adherence by improving the patient's memory and comprehension of the advice given. However, these findings have been with patients on short-term regimen for acute illnesses. The picture in chronic disease is not as encouraging. For example, Sackett and his colleagues (109) tested the effects of a "mastery learning" program versus usual care. Mastery learning consisted of a slide-tape show, a booklet, and a follow-up to determine recall and to remind participants about salient facts. Items covered included the facts about hypertension and its effects on life expectancy, the benefits of treatment, the need for compliance, and some simple reminders about pill taking. After six months of treatment, no effects of this program on either adherence as measured by a surreptitious home pill count or blood pressure were found. Even more remarkable was that in the group treated at work, education seemed to have a detrimental effect, with adherence rates of 48% vs. 62% for the usual-care group.

In another study with hypertensive patients, two different methods of conveying information were compared with routine care (24). One group of patients received a series of lectures about the disease, its treatment, and adherence problems. Another group received and discussed similar information in small groups aimed at providing a maximum of social support. A number of measures, such as self-report of adherence, knowledge of the disease, and social support, suggested that the lecture and group method were equally beneficial and that both were better than usual care. But no differences were found between the three groups when blood pressure was measured, suggesting that education had no practical effect on adherence.

Thus, the role of education and information in patient adherence is somewhat bewildering. There does appear to be ample evidence to support the importance of instructional strategies in improving patient recall and understanding of the regimen. Since this is basic to any patient's ability to adhere, instructional methods ought to be attended to. However, once recall and comprehension have been accounted for, it is not clear that the method of advising the patient has any independent bearing on adherence, particularly in long-term care. In looking at the content of education programs, there does seem to be some consistency in the finding that those concerned with the disease and its effects, the medication and its complications, and adherence problems have not been worthwhile, and, indeed, under some circumstances may be counterproductive. On the other hand, short, simple information about the regimen presented both orally and in writing has been useful in short-term treatment. Its impact in longer-term care remains to be seen. It would appear, at any rate, that well-designed instruction about the regimen would be more useful than programs dealing with the disease and, most likely, should form a basis for setting the conditions for good adherence. Even if patients know what to do, however, a number of other factors contribute to their ability to follow through.

Social Support

The positive role of the family in the good adherence of its members has been reported in a number of studies (5, 14, 93). This has been the case particularly in dietary regimens. The Anti-Coronary Club, for example, reported that married men more often participated actively in the dietary program than the unmarried (2, 5). Greater weight loss has also been reported in patients with supportive spouses (22, 120).

The influence of the family has not been limited to the dietary area, however. Oakes et al. (93) noted the importance of family expectation on the wearing of an arthritis splint. A positive association between the wife's attitude toward a physical fitness program and the husband's adherence patterns has been demonstrated with dental visits (4) and alcoholism treatment (60).

The family can affect adherence in a variety of ways (14). As noted, the expectations held for the patient's behavior as well as the attitudes toward the regimen itself may play a significant role, perhaps by influencing the level of encouragement, reminding, and reinforcement offered the patient. The family may also exert some control over the patient's environment, making adherence easier. For example, smoking may be prohibited in certain areas of the home or only diet-appropriate foods purchased for the home. And, of course, members of the family may actually assume full or partial responsibility for carrying out the regimen, e.g., reminding the patient, administering a medication, preparing diet-appropriate foods. All of these might be considered methods of supervising the patient, a factor which itself has been associated with adherence (61, 63, 113).

A note of caution should be injected here. Although social support may encourage the patient to adhere, at least one instance has been reported where support was stressful for certain patients (24). Presumably, the level of support given threatened the patients' perceptions of their self-sufficiency. It would seem advisable, then, to build in just that quantity of support which the patient needs and can tolerate.

Clinician Characteristics

The clinician also affects the patient's adherence. The ability to instruct the patient as to how to follow a regimen will contribute to the patient's comprehension and recall. Of equal importance is the style of interacting. In a review of 35 studies, Baekeland and Lundwall (7) reported that 100% of the studies indicated that the clinician's relationship with his patients influenced their subsequent adherence.

A number of behaviors characterize the more successful clinician. Of particular importance is a warm and empathic manner (26, 47, 70). The successful clinician also actively interacts with the patient (70). Thus, patients participate in planning their regimen, with the clinician supplying both feedback and individualized instruction. Social conversation also becomes a part of the interaction (70).

For the relationship between the clinician and the patient to be effective, however, requires some ongoing contact. Indeed, one of the most consistent findings in the literature is that adherence is better if the patient sees the same clinician over time (2, 11, 12, 15, 23).

Environmental Factors

The notion that the provision of health care at the work site might enhance adherence is extremely plausible. In one such model, a screening and treatment program for hypertension was offered for employees at a New York department store (1). For those selecting treatment the dropout rate at the end of one year was remarkably low (3%), and 66% had blood pressures lower than 160/95. However, in a randomized controlled clinical trial involving 230 hypertensive Canadian steel workers, no advantage was found at the end of six months for those treated at work as compared with those treated by their personal physicians (109). The dropout rate was 7% in each group, and 54% were designated compliant (taking 80% of medication by pill count) in the factory-treated group versus 51% in the office-treated group. One striking difference, however, was that 76% of the group treated by the company physician were placed on medication as against 49% treated by their own physicians. Thus, the effects of treatment at work site are equivocal. It may be that specific, but yet unidentified features of work-site treatment contribute to its success or lack thereof.

Specific characteristics of the clinic setting have been demonstrated to be important. Alpert (2) suggests that good participation in care may be related to a positive identification with the clinic. This is fostered by the same warm, personalized approach that characterizes the successful clinician being carried out by the entire office staff (23, 44, 50, 114).

The clinic setting is particularly important in minimizing appointment failures and dropouts from treatment. A consistent finding is that waiting time is associated with missed appointments (8, 57). An aspect of clinic care affecting waiting time and appointment keeping appears to be the type of scheduling system used. Two dimensions seem important: whether or not a block of patients is scheduled at the same time, and whether or not an appointment is made with a particular physician. In one nonexperimental comparison of these parameters, 22% of patients scheduled in block fashion did not attend compared with 13% of patients given individual appointments (103). Perhaps equally interesting was the behavior of physicians. In a block system when patients were not assigned to a particular doctor, physicians came to the clinic 35 minutes late, compared with 9 minutes late for patients given individual appointment times, and 2 minutes early when appointments were given with a specific physician. Under the latter system, patients outdid their physicians by arriving 14 minutes early. Thus, the physicians were able to spend more time with their patients, and patients spent less time waiting when an individualized system was used.

While it is to be hoped that enhancing appointment keeping will reduce the number of dropouts from treatment, this problem has received less attention in the experimental literature. When Finnerty et al. (44) reorganized a clinic to reduce waiting time and provide a consistent health caretaker for each patient, dropout was reduced from 42% to 8%. In a better-controlled study, a group receiving extra counseling as to side effects and problems encountered with taking medication showed better clinic attendance (90%) than a usual-practice group (60%) (98).

Attendance is also related to the use of an appointment reminder system. The simplest system is to telephone or send a reminder letter to patients before each appointment. This system has been documented in several studies, for the most part within clinics serving low-income populations. In one such study, patients were assigned sequentially to groups either receiving or not receiving a reminder card mailed one week before the appointment (90). Those receiving a card kept 64% of their appointments while those in the control group kept only 48%, a clear and significant difference. Other studies using random assignments have made similar findings (122). Naturally, the question then arises as to which system is better, card reminders or telephone calls. To answer this question patients attending a comprehensive health-care clinic were randomly assigned to one of the three groups, a usual-practice control, and either a telephoned or written reminder (49). No differences were found between these methods, although both reduced unkept appointments to about 9% compared with 38% for the control group.

One might expect that such a system would be costly. However, the cost effectiveness of prompting appointment keeping was dramtically illustrated in one study (122). One thousand telephone prompts using a standard message delivered by an appointment clerk cost $162, an amount recovered when just six appointments were kept, when the time wasted by idle staff was taken into account.

We can conclude then that appointment keeping is beneficially influenced by several relatively simple methods in the clinic, including individualized appointments made for a specific physician at a particular time, which in turn is likely to reduce waiting time; choosing the most convenient time for the patient; using a simple prompting system either by telephone or by mail; and finally, enhancing the relationship between health-care provider and patient. It seems possible that by using these techniques early in the treatment of the disorder, dropping out of treatment might also be beneficially influenced.

Medication Regimen

The patient himself, his support system, his relationship with the clinician, and his experience with the clinic itself all contribute to his ability and willingness to follow a medical regimen. But perhaps the single most important determinant of compliance is the regimen itself.

One striking feature of the regimen which is related to adherence is its degree of complexity. The probability of poor adherence rises as complexity increases (19). Perhaps the most strongly associated factor is the number of daily medications prescribed (126), with three or more drugs significantly lowering adherence (47). Frequent doses also contribute to an increase in scheduling misconceptions, which in turn are related to adherence errors (58).

In a retrospective study of this issue with hypertensives, the effect of one–tablet equivalent of three separate tablets was studied (27). It was found that patients who were shifted from the separate to combined dosage schedule showed an average drop of 19 mm Hg diastolic blood pressure, the mean time on the combination being 10 months. Retrospective studies, of course, are fraught with error, particularly in the possibility of differential assignment of poor–risk patients to one or another group, and differential retrieval of data from the record. One prospective study corrected for this difficulty but used a sequential design, in which hypertensive patients were placed on placebo, followed by separate tablets, followed by combination tablets, with two weeks spent in each phase (31). Both separate and combination tablets were found superior to placebo, but no differences were found between the two regimens. However, the very short time periods used might well have obscured the longer–term benefit of the simpler medication regimen.

Thus, a controlled study in which 50 hypertensives were randomly allocated to either separate or combined tablets and in which blood pressure was measured at the end of some 16 weeks provides one of the best tests of the effect of a simple medication regimen (110). Sitting blood pressures were not significantly different before randomization (P = .63 systolic; P = .69 diastolic). However, when the raw data presented in the original paper were reanalyzed, it was found that after treatment both systolic (P = .04) and diastolic pressure (P = .02) were different, although this difference was not found in standing blood pressures.

Thus, while the evidence for an advantage of a simple dosage regimen over a complex regimen is somewhat questionable as regards efficacy in terms of therapeutic effect such as blood pressure, at least some evidence of superiority has been presented. Moreover, a simple regimen has never been found less effective than a complex one of equal pharmacologic effect. Unfortunately, no data as to the effect of the simple dosage schedule on adherence behavior such as pill count exists.

Combining a medication with another treatment has also been found to decrease adherence to as little as 25% in one study (47). Combining three behavior changes (changes in diet, work, and personal habits) leads to even more profound adherence problems. One study (34) reported that only 9% of patients complied with three, and 42% with two of three prescribed behaviors. Individuals may only be able to cope with a limited number of changes and intrusions in their lives at any given time.

These findings certainly suggest that the regimen should be kept as simple and nonintrusive as possible. And, if there is no pressing health reason to begin a complex regimen at once, adherence may be enhanced by a gradual introduction to its various components.

In addition to its complexity, the length of time the regimen must be enacted is also important. Adherence tends to decrease over time with long–term regimen. There is some suggestion that complacency, boredom, tedium, and forgetfulness are involved in this decline (19).

Side effects of the regimen have also been discussed as contributors to adherence. However, their impact is not as strong as one might assume (46). Blackwell (19) suggests that alarming or unexpected side effects are often among the reasons patients give for stopping treatment. Weintraub, Au, and Lasagna (124), for example, found that 8% of patients on digitalis reported side effects as a reason for noncompliance, whereas a total of 34% of patients were non-compliant. On the other hand, a more extensive number of persons may complain of side effects. For example, 92% of patients on niacin complained of one symptom alone in the Coronary Drug Project (30). Such complaints, however, may not always be drug induced. Reidenberg and Lowenthal (99) were able to elicit a history of symptoms commonly thought of as drug side effects from healthy persons not on medication.

The management of such complaints may be a factor in how they affect adherence. Blackwell (18) suggests that reassurance and inquiry about improvement may yield fewer complaints than probes for side effects and less optimism about improvement. Interestingly, forewarning patients of the potential occurrence of side effects has not been demonstrated to affect either the incidence of reported side effects or the patient's continuance with medication (87, 88).

Summary

A number of factors have been found to be associated with adherence. With regard to the patient, demographic factors, personality characteristics, and motivation are not related to adherence, although comprehension and recall of the prescribed regimen, and supervision in the conduct of the regimen are. The clinician is important in fostering good adherence. Interest, involvement with patients, as well as warmth, degree of empathy, and skill in instructing patients all appear relevant, as does the continuous relationship between clinician and patient. The treatment setting, which minimizes waiting through scheduling and reminder systems and offers a personalized approach, supports adherence, particularly to appointment keeping. Perhaps the most important factor, however, is the nature of the regimen itself. The complexity of the regimen, the incidence of side effects and their management, as well as the length of time the regimen is to be carried out all have an impact on patient adherence.

PREDICTION OF ADHERENCE

Although a variety of factors have been shown to be associated with adherence, none will allow the clinician to predict reliably a given patient's subsequent adherence. A few studies have related a patient's beliefs regarding susceptibility to the illness (12) and the efficacy of the prescribed treatment (13, 37, 40) to adherence. However, the nature of the regimen itself is more likely to predict adherence than are these beliefs.

Other associated factors have also been poor predictors. Davis (32) reported finding no single factor which predicted adherence and, further, a combination of nine variables yielded a correlation of just .44 with outcome. In this combination of factors, education and health insurance accounted for most of the variance.

As one might assume, if the factors associated with adherence do not allow for predictability of adherence, it is difficult for clinicians to assess whether or not their patients will follow advice. And, indeed, studies have shown just that (19, 25). Patients appear to do a better job of predicting their own performance if interaction with the clinician is such that they do not feel threatened. At least one report has suggested that some 70% of patients can predict their future health behavior accurately (33). Interestingly, patients made errors in both directions— i.e., stating they would adhere and did not, as well as stating they would not adhere but did.

Thus, there do not appear to be any reliable methods of predicting patient behaivor. To have such a method would, of course, allow clinicians to place their prevention and remediation efforts specifically where they would be needed. Until future research efforts identify such methodologies, clinicians are advised to consider all patients as potential nonadherers and to periodically assess the adherence of their patients.

ASSESSMENT OF ADHERENCE

Adherence can be measured by a number of methods, e.g., interview, clinician rating, pill count, biochemical indicators, and self-report. Unfortunately, no single measure appears to be highly reliable, with perhaps the least effective method being the clinician's judgment or rating of the patient's behavior. Clinicians tend to identify poor/nonadherence at no better than chance levels (19, 25). Indeed, Caron and Roth (25) reported a median correlation of .01 between an objective measure of adherence and physician estimates. More than 80% of the physicians overestimated the patients' medication consumption. Similarly, correlations of .10 and .23 have been reported between nutritionists' estimates of dietary adherence and serum cholesterol responses (89). Thus, it would seem advisable for the clinician to utilize other methods of evaluating adherence, and, given the limited reliability of these other methods, to combine two or more modes of assessment.

Biochemical Assessment

Biochemical measures of adherence generally include the assessment of the metabolic byproducts of a drug or diet, the detection of a marker placed in the medication, or the detection of the therapeutic agent itself in urine or blood. Thus, some estimation can be made about whether or not the patient made some effort to follow the regimen. Unfortunately, this process is subject to problems (89, 116). First, it provides no information on adherence over time, and, if the substance or marker is rapidly excreted, provides information only on very recent behavior. Second, the variability among individuals in the absorption, metabolism, and clearance of therapeutic substances limits the reliability of the assessment. As a single determination of adherence, biochemical assessments may be of limited utility. Additional information can be gained, however, by combining them with other measures.

Pill Count

The pill count is simply a determination of the percentage of the prescribed regimen which was followed. This requires knowledge of the quantity of medication dispensed as well as the quantity which should have been ingested within some specific time period. The pill count does give an estimate of the patient's adherence over time, but does not detect patterns of errors. Correlations with urine markers tend to be low (64, 77, 106), with the pill count tending to overestimate adherence. Reliability seems to be increased if the patient is unaware that the count will be done (97). Although the pill count is fraught with these problems, it is a relatively simple and inexpensive measure which is more reliable than a verbal report.

Verbal Report

Reliance on patients' reports of their adherence to the prescribed regimen is probably the most commonly used method of evaluating adherence in the clinic. The validity of patients' reports, however, depends upon their memory, their ability to observe and evaluate their behavior, and willingness to report accurately to the clinician, as well as upon the clinician's skill in interviewing the patient. If the patient is willing and able to report accurately, specific adherence problems can be reviewed in depth. However, there is substantial evidence that patients tend to underreport low or nonadherence (38, 51, 56, 95, 100). Haynes et al. (56) did find they could identify one-half of poor adherers with an interview procedure. There is some suggestion that among the poor adherers, less-adherent patients are more likely to report accurately, perhaps because they are more aware of deviations from the prescription (100).

Self-Monitoring

A fourth method of assessing adherence is through patient self-monitoring. With this method patients observe and record their regimen-related behavior. These records then supply the adherence data. This procedure relies on patients' willingness to comply with the record-procedures, which is closely related to the manner in which self–monitoring is introduced by the clinician. Records may be kept on either a continuous basis or at periodic intervals throughout treatment. This process of assessing adherence has a long history in the diet and weight–loss areas and is more recently being introduced to smoking and medication regimens.

The advantages of self–monitoring include the collection of continuous data on the conduct of the regimen, which can help the clinician identify adherence patterns as well as specific problems in carrying out the regimen. As with other measures, problems with reliability are well known (66, 76, 91, 105, 115). One of the major problems in obtaining good reliability is that self–monitoring may have reactive or therapeutic effects (68, 78, 79, 92, 104). Accuracy can be improved, however, if certain guidelines are followed, as demonstrated by a correlation of .90 between self–monitoring and packet (pill) count in one medication adherence study (38). The guidelines include: 1) asking the patient to observe positively valued behaviors, e.g., recording medication taken rather than medication missed; 2) using readily accessible, easy–to–use records; 3) asking the patient to assess readily observable behaviors, e.g., recording the quantity of meats eaten rather than the amount of saturated fat; 4) training the patient in self–monitoring; 5) reinforcing the patient's *accuracy* rather than any improvements or changes in regimen–related behavior; 6) letting patients be aware that their records will be checked for accuracy; 7) asking patients to record at the time that behavior occurs, rather than at the end of the day or end of the week (10).

Summary

The clinician (or researcher) has a variety of methods available for assessing adherence, each with its own advantages. Biochemical procedures provide a direct measure of whether or not the regimen has been carried out but provide no knowledge of the degree of adherence, and they tend to assess adherence within a very short time of the assessment itself. The pill count offers information on the degree of adherence over time, but little on the specific patterns or problems. It is confounded by the patient's memory, ability to assess behavior, and willingness to report to the clinician. Self–monitoring can provide a continuous record of adherence as well as patterns and problems specific to regimen conduct, but may have reactive effects, thus diminishing its accuracy. Because of the problems inherent in each single measure's reliability, the clinician or researcher is advised to use more than one of the assessment procedures.

The clinician or researcher is also advised to avoid using physiological outcome (e.g., weight loss, reduced blood pressure, etc.) as an indicator of adherence. Individual variability in response to treatment allows some patients to achieve a therapeutic goal with poor adherence rates, while others may not have a therapeutic response despite excellent adherence. This was clearly demonstrated by Haynes and his colleagues (56) in a study of a group of 100 hypertensives. While 57% were adherent, just 35% had attained good blood pressure control (121). On closer examination, it was found that of the 35 patients who achieved blood pressure control, 12 (34%) were *poor* adherers. And, similarly, of the 65 who failed to achieve blood pressure control, 34 (52%) were *good* adherers. While outcome is related to adherence, there is not a one-to-one correspondence. Thus, outcome should not be used as an adherence measure but as a criterion for deciding whether or not adherence needs to be improved in the poorly adhering patient.

INTERVENTION STRATEGIES

Clinicians can anticipate that, on the average, 50% of their patients (20% to 80%) will have adherence problems. If Taylor et al.'s (121) data are representative, about 70% of that poorly adhering group will not demonstrate a therapeutic response, suggesting the need for improvement in the conduct of the regimen. Fortunately, a number of strategies can be employed to minimize the extent of adherence problems in practice. With good assessment techniques, those problems which do arise can be identified and, efforts made to remediate them.

It should be noted, however, that the mammoth literature documenting the extent of the adherence problem is in sharp contrast to the small number of studies on what to do about the problem. Indeed, the contrast is so great that it is likely to lead to the perception that nothing can be done, or worse still that the problem has been over-emphasized. Luckily, much is known about the process of behavior change, and this knowledge can be combined with the growing research literature on adherence intervention to develop a rational approach to improving adherence. As the research findings accumulate, the approach will become increasingly certain and effective, but for the present, extrapolations from uncontrolled studies and from studies in other areas will be necessary to flesh out our skeletal knowledge.

Preventive Strategies

As noted in the discussion of factors contributing to adherence—1) the method of instructing the patient to improve his knowledge and recall of the regimen, 2) the extent of the family's involvement in supporting and carrying out the regimen itself, 3) the level or warmth, empathy, and concern evidenced by the clinician, 4) the type of scheduling system used to minimize waiting, 5) the use of appointment reminders, as well as 6) the degree of warmth and personalized attention offered by the clinic staff—effect the patient's willingness to remain in treatment and his ability to adhere to the prescribed regimen. Each of these factors is modifiable to some degree and should be attended to.

Positive Environment

A basic step in preventing adherence problems, particularly dropping out of treatment, is to provide a positive, organized environment. Staff should be warm and friendly individuals who make the clinic a pleasant place for the patient. The clinician, too, should give adequate time, attention, and empathy to his patients. Waiting time should be minimized through careful attention to patient scheduling. And reminders, either telephone or mailed, should be given to patients preceding their scheduled appointments.

Stamler et al. (117), for example, report the first two years' experience with a hypertensive clinic, one of 14 centers involved in the hypertension detection and follow-up program. Emphasis was placed on making the treatment center one of high quality, with an atmosphere encouraging participation. All visits are by appointment, with little or no waiting. In almost all cases the same physician sees the patient at all phyician consultations. The center is physically attractive, and the staff aims to be receptive and sympathetic, with enough time per visit to permit ample staff–patient communication. Intervals between visits vary from two weeks to three months, the longer intervals being for patients with normal blood pressure after a period of accommodation to the medication with no important side effects. The greater frequency in early visits was designed to permit better titration of the effects of therapy, as to both efficacy and possible unwanted effects.

The clinic makes use of paramedical personnel for blood pressure measurement and for monitoring possible side effects and problems of adherence to therapy. The paramedical personnel underwent an intensive period of training, both locally and nationally, aimed at understanding the effects and side effects of drugs. Physician supervision at the training level and physician monitoring of paramedical personnel performance are accomplished through daily chart review as well as general staff case review. Patients responding well to medication (i.e., with pressures reduced below 90 mm Hg diastolic and with no important side or toxid effects) are transferred to paramedical personnel for care between semiannual physician visits.

The dropout rate in this clinic was 20% for the first year, in line with the high initial dropout observed in other clinical trials; however, this was reduced to 3% annually thereafter. Moreover, 82% of patients remaining in the program had diastolic blood pressures below 90 mm Hg after two years' treatment as compared with 67% of patients in a control group who had been referred to and treated by their own physicians.

Thus, an attractive clinic environment with short waiting time and adequate opportunity to communicate with health–care personnel, who in turn are well trained and closely supervised, would seem to be necessary factors in improving adherence. Similar well–organized clinics have been successful in helping patients to lower cholesterol levels by diet and to maintain those levels for several years (3, 71).

Minimizing Regimen Complexity

A regimen should then be prescribed for the patient in a manner that minimizes its complexity. As noted earlier, one method of doing this is to prescribe the fewest number of medications the least number of times per day possible. A regimen which must be complex might be introduced gradually in its component parts. One way to do this is to use a graduated regimen implementation, which borrows from the principles of behavior shaping.

In using a graduated approach to introduce a therapeutic regimen, the clinician is proceeding in an essentially stepwise fashion to introduce components of the regimen until the patient has attained full performance of the prescribed behavior. For example, in the dietary area, a patient who is advised to lose weight might begin with modification of breakfast habits. When that is successfully achieved, then the diet is extended to lunch, and so on. Similarly, with a therapeutic diet, e.g., a low cholesterol diet, a patient might first be advised to learn to identify foods high in cholesterol, then to make dietary modifications at home, then to learn to make diet–appropriate restaurant selections. In the medication area, this would be comparable to a graduated–dose approach to medication administration, a procedure which has been used to minimize the occurrence of side effects (21, 111). The medication, if there is no urgency about rapid attainment of the full dosage, might first be introduced once a day. When adherence has been achieved, a second medication is added at a second time per day, and so on.

In using such an approach, the regimen is divided into a series of behaviors in order of difficulty. The patient is then started on the simplest step which can reasonably be expected. As the patient achieves good adherence, components are gradually added, building successful performance. Although a systematic investigation has not been carried out to test the efficacy of this approach in minimizing adherence problems, it has intuitive appeal as well as demonstrated efficacy in the shaping of other types of behaviors (9, 67).

Individualizing Treatment

Individualizing the patient's regimen also has intuitive appeal for enhancing adherence. One process by which this can be accomplished is by tailoring the regimen to specific patient characteristics. This can be done in two ways. The first is to select a treatment which is more likely to be followed by a successful outcome for a given patient. For example, the obese hypertensive patient who refuses to follow an initial weight–loss program might initially be prescribed medication treatment alone. Or obese patients who live alone might be advised to join a group weight–loss program which could offer social support and reinforcement, rather than be given a specific diet to follow on their own. A second way to tailor the regimen is to adapt it to features of the patient's life style. For example, once–a–day medication might be recommended to be taken at morning tooth–brushing time or at the time of some other daily habit, to enhance adherence.

Limited research has been carried out on the efficacy of this approach. However, the results have been encouraging, though not conclusive, in the studies which have been undertaken (16, 54). For example, Hallburg (54) reported that medication errors were reduced in elderly ambulatory patients using a procedure which tailored the prescribed medication regimens to the patients' routines. One example she cited was that of developing a pill–an–hour regimen, which was compatible with the prescriptions for a patient on multiple medications who felt that he could only take one pill at a time. Although Hallburg did not demonstrate statistical significance, she did report that serious errors were made by 23.5% of a control group as compared with 11.5% of the tailoring group. Best (16) also demonstrated an advantage to a tailoring procedure with smoking cessation, although statistically significant differences were not found.

Support and Reinforcement

Support and reinforcement for regimen adherence are important factors in the patient's conduct of prescribed tasks, as noted earlier. Thus, it becomes imprtant to include the family in the instruction of the patient—both regarding what the patient is to do and why it is to be done (43). If the family or other significant persons can be involved in the regimen in any way, this should further enhance adherence.

One way to increase the probability of support and reinforcement for adherence is through the use of contracts. Contracting refers to formalized process of specifying the rules and consequences of adhering/nonadhering to the regimen. In this case, the consequences would not be the long–term health benefits of adherence, but rather more immediate rewards and punishments (or witholding rewards). For example, a patient prescribed a daily medication might receive a "point" from his wife, a certain number of which would be exchanged for a meal at a restaurant of his choice. Failure to take the medication might result in a point being subtracted from the total accumulated.

Contracts have been used successfully to improve blood pressure control (118). In this case, the patients did have a choice of treatment modalities—medication, wight loss, stress management. Contracts have also been used successfully in maintaining appointment keeping for disulfiram administration among alcoholics (17). And modest success has been reported in the treatment of obesity using contracting procedures (36, 55, 81). Several advantages are offered by this procedure. The regimen can be individualized by enlisting the patient's cooperation in the design of the contract. Then, by agreeing to and signing the contract, the patient makes a public commitment to adhere. Further, by enlisting the cooperation of another person, support and reinforcement can be fostered.

Building in Reminders

Attention to building reminders into the patient's environment should also enhance adherence by minimizing the periodic forgetting which patients report (38, 62). A number of investigations have reported success in achieving better adherence when reminders are utilized (6, 74, 82, 84, 86). The reminders ranged from stickers on the refrigerator door (74) to medication calendars (86), to dispensers providing feedback on dosages taken and missed (82).

Packaging medication to provide feedback on missed doses should also enhance adherence, both by allowing missed doses to be taken (if this is feasible) and by promoting more accurate behavior. In one clinical trial with 100 hypertensive patients, pills were dispensed either in the usual bottle or in a specially designed compliance PAK which displayed the pills to be taken by date (42). Urinalysis to detect chlorthalidone revealed that this display resulted in a compliance rate of 93% against 69% for the bottle prescription. No data for blood pressure were given.

In a very similar study, two methods of medication display proved superior to both the usual bottled prescription and a bottle together with a calendar which allowed patients to check off each dose of antibiotic as it was taken (75). In this case the measure was a pill count at an unannounced home visit. The two methods of display were the compliance PAK, previously described, and a strip package in which each strip contained one day's dosage of medication; compliance was 92.5% and 97.3%, respectively, as against 83.9% and 73.3% for the calendar and bottled prescription, the last two percentages not being significantly different from the first two. Finally, however, another randomized trial with hypertensive subjects, a display device quite similar to those previously described did not lead to more effective lowering of blood pressure than the usual bottled prescription (98). However, when this device was used in conjunction with pharmacist's counseling, diastolic blood pressure was significantly reduced (−10 m Hg) when compared with counseling alone.

These data may suggest that enhanced packaging works better with short-term prescriptions, and that a counseling relationship might increase the efficacy of the packaging. Other forms of display, such as containers or pill calendars to be mounted on a wall in the kitchen or bathroom—serving both as reminders and providing feedback as to doses taken—have been developed but have not yet been tested.

Adherence Counseling

The studies so far considered have suggested that appointment keeping can be enhanced by the systematic use of reminders; that specific information concerning the dosage regimen can be helpful; as can the simplest possible dosage schedule, reminders, and packaging which provides feedback as to doses taken. Moreover, there has been a strong hint that enhancing the relationship between health–care providers and their patients by establishing a counseling relationship will also prove helpful, as we have seen in appointment keeping and perhaps dropout prevention; as a method of providing information concerning the medication and scheduling; and even enhancing the effect of other adherence strategies. The question now arises, what would be the effect of early and extended counseling upon adherence?

Luckily, the effect of what appears to have been a model treatment program from the viewpoint of adherence has been published (85). Hypertensive patients were randomized into two groups, one receiving usual care from their physician, while the other received extra counseling from a pharmacist at regular visits over a five–month period. During visits patients were first informed about the nature and treatment of hypertension, using pamphlets followed by a discussion. At subsequent visits, lasting an average of six minutes each, the pharmacist "evaluated the patients' therapeutic responses to the drug and dietary management; identified and managed additional complications, reactions, and problems; evaluated the patient's understanding of the educational material; provided additional educational material; identified and managed some adverse reactions to drug therapy; referred patients to health–center personnel for specialized care; and recommended therapy changes to the physician based on the patient's therapeutic responses and compliance with prescribed therapy..." partly assessed by a pill count. A substantial proportion of counseling time was devoted to the early identification and management of medication side effects. During five months of counseling, 50 suspected adverse drug reactions were identified and promptly dealt with in 24 patients. The compliant patients (those taking more than 90% of their medication) experienced a mean of 2.0 adverse reactions each, while noncompliant patients had a mean of 4.4 side effects or drug reactions.

By the end of the five–month study, the counseled group showed superior knowledge of hypertension and its treatment compared with the control group, and 78% of patients were showing excellent (above 90%) adherence as measured by pill count, compared with 16% of the control group. Blood pressure for the counseled group was 146/90 compared with 166/101 for the control group. Despite these excellent results, over a relatively lengthy time, one disappointing finding was reported. When counseling was stopped, the advantage shown by the counseled group vanished, as their blood pressures rose to baseline levels. Adherence counseling, it seems, must be a continuous process if optimum results are to be achieved. Nonetheless, this study does suggest that the development of an excellent therapeutic relationship, provision of information, early attention to side effects, and presumably social reinforcement of successful adherence, substantially contributes to the management of the hypertensive patients. Moreover, such a program could well be carried out by a physician, a pharmacist, or a nurse, making it easy to fit within a routine clinic visit.

Adherence Remediation

Unfortunately, even with the systematic use of the various procedures so far described, it is probable that adherence problems will occur. Thus the question arises that, given a method of identifying poor adherence within a clinical setting, perhaps by a combination of pill counts and interview, can anything be done? Three investigations have examined this problem, two in hypertensive patients and the other with participants in the Coronary Primary Prevention Trial taking cholestyramine.

The first experiment was a follow–up to the study of Canadian steel workers described earlier (56). Thirty–nine hypertensives who had not reached a diastolic blood pressure of 90 mm Hg or less after six months of treatment were allocated to one of two groups, usual care or a multicomponent intervention. In the latter condition, patients were seen every two weeks by a high school graduate counselor, were taught to measure their own blood pressure, and asked to record both blood pressure and the amount of medication taken each day. In addition, the pattern of adherence and their life schedule were examined to identify regularly occurring events to which pill taking could be tailored. Finally, patients were praised for improvement in adherence behavior, and for each 4 mm Hg improvement in diastolic pressure given a $4 credit toward purchase of their sphygmomanometer. This combination of self–monitoring, stimulus control, and reinforcement over six months of counseling led to an increase in medication adherence, as measured by a surreptitious home pill count, in 80% of the counseled patients compared with 39% of the usual–care patients. The pill count in the former group averaged 65.8% at the end of the study as compared with 44.7% in the latter group. Diastolic blood pressure fell by 5.4 mm Hg in the counseled group compared with 1.9 mm Hg in the usual–care group. The blood pressure changes compared between groups were not significantly different (p=0.12), although the counseled group showed a significant change (p=.001) from the beginning to the end of the study. Obviously these are modest gains, perhaps even of dubious clinical significance; nonetheless they provide a point of departure for other studies. Moreover, were the counseling to be continued, as it should be in a clinical setting, larger differences between the groups might be seen over time. The specific contribution of each of the components of the intervention package, including simply the added attention, was not assessed.

In a second remedial study, the contributions of home blood pressure monitoring and home visits by the health aide were evaluated by the same group of investigators (62). Using a 2 × 2 factorial design, 140 uncontrolled hypertensive patients who had been on antihypertensive medication for a year or more were randomly assigned to either a 1) self–monitoring group, 2) home visit group, 3) combined self–monitoring and home visit group, or 4) control group. Subjects who self–monitored their blood pressure did so daily, taking their records to their physicians at usual appointments. Home visits were made on a monthly basis, for those receiving them, at which time the blood pressure was taken by a lay health worker. This was reported to both the subject and his physician. During the six–month intervention period, subjects remained in the care of their own physician. Adherence measures included both the interview and the pill count.

The authors reported that diastolic blood pressure was reduced by approximately 8 mm Hg in all groups after change scores were adjusted for initial diastolic values. Nor were significant differences found between groups in adherence, with adherence averaging approximately 66.5%. Gains in adherence, however, tended to be larger in the subjects who self–monitored blood pressures. These gains were accounted for by those subjects who had reported difficulty in remembering to take their medication. Thus, the added attention given through the home visits and the self–monitoring of blood pressure were not demonstrated to effect adherence, with the exception of the subgroup of patients who had remembering problems.

In the third remedial study (38), 60 poor adherers from three participating Lipid Research Clinics were randomly allocated to one of three groups: a multicomponent procedure; an attention–control group which received the same amount of therapist contacts and self–monitoring; and a usual–care group. The men entering the study were all poor adherers taking between 5% and 50% of a prescribed dose of six packets daily. Counseling, largely conducted by scheduled telephone calls and by nonmedical clinic personnel who had been trained in a workshop setting, consisted first of determining the average dosage taken and the time of day at which most success was obtained, using self–monitoring records kept by the patients. A prescription to take one packet less than the average taken, at the most successful time of day—usually morning—was then given. If the patient took 75% of this prescription, then one extra package was added using a graduated regimen implementation procedure. Other elements included social reinforcement and emphasis on the motivations that led the patient to enter the study in the first place.

The multicomponent package was more effective in bringing a significantly greater proportion of patients above a preestablished 75% adherence criterion than either of the other groups (p=0.006). Modest differences were also found in the mean packet counts between groups (p=0.057). Changes in adherence were supported by significant differences in the percent reduction in serum cholesterol (p=0.048) at the end of treatment. The reduction was maintained in two of the clinics in the experimental group, but the third clinic experienced a rebound to entry levels. Interestingly, this clinic lost the adherence counselor who was administering treatment during the follow–up period, again emphasizing the need for continuity of care. It was also of interest that over a six–month follow–up period the therapist contact with self–monitoring group made continuous and significant gains, exceeding the multicomponent intervention group by the sixth follow–up month. Generally the subjects who were most responsive to this particular strategy were those who were more variable in their daily habits and overestimated the quantity of medication they took over time.

These three studies are similar on a variety of dimensions. First, they have each shown the utility of lay health workers or allied health professionals as adherence counselors for the poorly adhering patient on medication. The effectiveness of nonphysicians as adherence educators and counselors with patients at the outset of care has been well documented (23, 44, 69, 118). These three studies suggest that with training and supervision, the role of the nonphysician can be expanded to include remediation of the poor adherer.

These three studies have also demonstrated that improvement in both adherence and physiological outcome can be made in the poorly adhering patient. The multicomponent package programs seemed to fare better for a larger group of patients, perhaps because one or more of the components affected various problems in regimen conduct. Considerable work remains to identify specific adherence problems and the strategies affecting them.

Taking these studies as models for a clinically useful adherence remediation program, however, the major elements of remedial counseling can be outlined as in Table 1. Having calculated the average dose taken by the patient and identified the time of day at which medication is most frequently taken (or other adherent

Table 1. Elements of Adherence Counseling

1. Self-monitoring
2. Shape medication dosage (or other regimen behavior, e.g., diet, exercise, etc.)
   (a) start at average or below average taken/performed
   (b) at the most frequently taken time of day
   (c) build up dose/behaviors slowly
3. Help patient identify reminders
4. Reinforce adherence behaviors
5. Identify and reinforce patient's initial reasons for starting treatment

behavior is most frequently performed), the counselor can start the process of shaping the regimen. The prescription should be at or slightly below the average taken and at the time of day most likely to lead to success. In this way failure is turned into success. Patients should be helped to increase stimulus control by identifying reminders, for example by attaching pill taking to regularly occurring events, such as brushing teeth and eating meals. Pills should be stored so that engaging in the one behavior reminds patients of the other, i.e., pill taking. Thus, a toothbrush and pills can be stored together or pills can be stored with the utensils or food used at every meal. In addition, recording the number of pills taken or other adherent behaviors performed each day should continue to provide feedback on progress and help to identify areas of difficulty.

The counselor should arrange to call the patient about one week after the initial session and at that time inquire about regimen conduct by having patients read their daily logs. If the patient has successfully (75% or better) adhered to the regime as prescribed, the regimen should be increased by one pill or one unit of behavior. In the case of multiple daily dosages of medication, it is better to keep to one time until the original fully prescribed dose is being taken, and then move to the next time. Each adherence success can easily be commented on and praised during the phone conversation and the patient reminded of the reasons for originally seeking treatment. In this way regimen can be increased to as near optimal levels as possible over the course of a few weeks.

Some other less well specified remediation procedures have been used which might prove useful with some individual or subpopulations of a clinic. Wilber and Barrow (125) found that 88 of 220 individuals (40%) were willing to participate in a program involving regular home visits by a public-health nurse. During these visits the nurse checked the patient's blood pressure, reemphasized the importance of taking medication, and made sure that patients were seeing a physician and had a supply of medication. Before the visiting-nurse program began, only 15% of the patients were well controlled (diastolic blood pressure at 95 mm Hg or less). After participating for two years, 80% of patients showed good control compared with 34% of the nonvolunteer group, an excellent record.

Once more, however, two years after the program was stopped only 29% of patients showed good control, again emphasizing the need for continued attention to the problem of adherence. The successful elements in this program were presumably continual prompting by the nurse, reinforcement of adherence behavior, and probably increasing the importance of blood pressure treatment for the whole family by making adherence to the regime more public. Increased public attention to behavior has been shown in several studies to enhance performance, particularly if combined with reinforcement (94, 96).

Maintenance

The problem of maintaining adherence behavior once it has been attained by the patient is a dilemma in health care. Not only does there tend to be a persistent decline in adherence over time (52, 106, 123), but the adherence interventions that have been tested have not shown continuation of effects when the intervention is withdrawn (38, 55, 56, 81, 85).

Two strategies, however, do show some promise for obtaining more enduring changes. The first is involvement of the spouse in the regimen, although caution is indicated, as noted earlier. Brownell et al. (22) reported that included spouses in a weight-loss program with their obese partner resulted in greater weight loss than treating the obese patient alone—whether or not spouses were cooperative. Indeed, after a six-month follow-up, the cooperative participating spouse group averaged a 29.6-pound weight loss, compared with 19.4 pounds in the cooperative nonparticipating spouse group and 15.1 pounds in the noncooperative spouse group. Interestingly, group differences were not apparent at the end of treatment but were evidenced, as noted, at the six-month follow-up period.

Similarly, Dunbar (38) reported finding no immediate posttreatment benefits to self-monitoring of medication taking. Yet after a six-month follow-up period, the group of patients who had self monitored were outperforming other groups. This would suggest that self-monitoring might also have delayed but more enduring effects, at least with the patients who are variable in their regimen habits and who overestimate their performance.

The problems of maintenance of adherence are far from being solved. At least two strategies show some promise of obtaining more enduring change. It is likely, however, that periodic attention to the patient will be necessary even though maintenance strategies are developed and utilized (80).

Overview

The problem of poor adherence to the medical regimen has been well documented in recent years, and the findings have been echoed in the problem of poor maintenance in relation to weight reduction, smoking cessation, and other life-style behavior changes. Indeed, from an even broader viewpoint, the problem may be divided into two components: achieving initial behavior change and maintaining that change over time. Less is known about maintaining behavior than about achieving acute behavior change, particularly about behavior such as medication taking, which occurs at a relatively low frequency in the patients' own environment and is not amenable to direct supervision.

While much is known about the broad phenomenon of adherence, more needs to be learned about the details. Relatively little information is available about the fate of adherence in selected cohorts of patients followed for several years. Can patients be classed as good or poor adherers or, as seems more likely, do good adherers become poor and vice versa? And, if this is so, what events are associated with such changes? Similarly, little is known about daily variation in medication taking or about the implications of such variability for remediation and maintenance. Finally, the relationship between adherence and therapeutic outcome needs further study, for, as we have seen, there is not an exact correspondence between these two aspects of patient care.

Nonetheless, the elements of an adherence technology have emerged, and a number of strategies have shown some promise in improving and maintaining patient adherence. The continuing study of adherence will inevitably lead to an examination of the process of health-care delivery. For it is evident that factors such as the organization of a clinic or the mode of administering a medication have an effect upon adherence, and that not only are the patient and physician involved, but clinic administrators, a variety of health-care personnel, and the pharmaceutical industry as well. Ultimately the longer-term consequences of improving adherence to the medical regimen should be examined, including the effect on the perception of well-being and the costs and benefits of such an approach. Finally, since adherence remediation, which necessarily involves counseling, is likely to be relatively costly, research into the prevention of poor adherence should be given a high priority.

This relatively new field of research has made an excellent start and has begun to generate information of interest to both the clinician and the research worker. It is unlikely that any major breakthrough will occur in this complex field. Instead, we can look forward to steady progress in our understanding of the phenomenon of adherence and in our efforts to enhance adherence to the medical regimen.

ACKNOWLEDGMENTS

Preparation of this article was partially supported by Contract No. WIH NHLI 71-2161 from the National Heart, Lung, and Blood Institute.

REFERENCES

1. Alderman, M.H., and Schoenbaum, E.E. Detection and treatment of hypertension at the work site. *N. Eng. J. Med.* 293:65-68, 1975.
2. Alpert, J.J. Broken appointments. *Pediatrics* 53:127-132, 1964.
3. American Heart Association. The national diet-heart study final report. *Circulation* 37:Supplement No. 1, 1968.
4. Antonovsky, A., and Kats, R. The model dental patient: An empirical study of preventive health behavior. *Soc. Sci. Med.* 4:367-380, 1970.
5. Archer, M., Ringler, S., and Christakis, G. Social factors affecting participation in a study of diet and coronary heart disease. *J. Health Soc. Behav.* 8:22-31, 1967.
6. Azrin, N.H., and Powell, J. Behavioral engineering: The use of response priming to improve prescribed self-medication. *J. Appl. Behav. Anal.* 2:39-42, 1969.
7. Baekeland, F., and Lundwall, L. Dropping out of treatment: A critical review. *Psychol. Bull.* 82:738-783, 1975.
8. Badgley, R.F., and Furnal, M.A. Appointment breaking in a pediatric clinic. *Yale J. Biol. Med.* 34:117-123, 1961.
9. Bandura, A. *Principles of Behavior Modification.* New York: Holt, Rinehart and Winston, 1969.
10. Barlow, D. Self-report measures. Paper presented at the High Blood Pressure Education Research Program meeting. New Orleans, 1976.
11. Becker, M.H. Sociobehavioral determinant of compliance, in D.L. Sackett and R.B. Haynes (eds.), *Compliance with Therapeutic Regimens.* Baltimore: The Johns Hopkins University Press, 1976, pp. 40-50.
12. Becker, M.H., Drachman, R.H., and Kirscht, J.P. Predicting mothers' compliance with pediatric medical regimens. *J. Pediatr.* 81:843-845, 1972.
13. Becker, M.H., Drachman, R.H., and Kirscht, J.P. A new approach to explaining sick-role behavior in low-income populations. *Am. J. Public Health* 64:205-212, 1974.
14. Becker, M.H., and Green, L.W. A family approach to compliance with medical treatment: A selective review of the literature. *Int. J. Health Educ.* 18:2-11, 1975.
15. Becker, M.H., and Morman, L.A. Sociobehavioral determinants of compliance with health and medical care recommendations. *Med. Care* 13:10-24, 1975.
16. Best, J.A. Tailoring smoking withdrawal procedures to personality and motivational differences. *J. Consult. Psychol.* 43:1-8, 1976.
17. Bigelow, G., Strickler, D., Leibson, I., and Griffiths, R. Maintaining disulfram ingestion among outpatient alcoholics: A security-deposit contingency contracting procedure. *Behav. and Res. Ther.* 14:378-381, 1976.
18. Blackwell, B. Commentary: The drug defaulter. *Clin. Pharmacol. Ther.* 13:841-848, 1972.
19. Blackwell, B. Drug therapy: Patient compliance. *N. Engl. J. Med.* 289:249-252, 1973.
20. Boyd, J.R., Covington, T.R., Stanaszck, W.F., and Coussons, R.T. Drug defaulting—Part I: Determinants of compliance. *Am. J. Hosp. Pharm.* 31:362-364, 1974.
21. Brosens, I.A., Robertson, W.B., and Van Assche, F.A. Assessment of incremental dosage regimen of combined oestrogen-progestogen oral contraceptive. *Br. Med. J.* 4:643-645, 1974.
22. Brownell, K.D. The effect of spouse training and partner cooperativeness in the behavioral treatment of obesity. Doctoral Dissertation, Rutgers University, 1977.
23. Caldwell, J.R., Cobb, S., Dowling, M.D., and de Jonga, D. The drop out problem in antihypertensive treatment. *J. Chron. Dis.* 22:579-592, 1970.
24. Caplan, R.D., Robinson, E.A.R., French, J.R.P., Caldwell, J.R., and Shinn, M. *Adhering to Medical Regimens: Pilot Experiments in Patient Education and Social*

Support. Ann Arbor: University of Michigan, 1976.
25. Caron, H.S., and Roth, H.P. Patients' cooperation with a medical regimen: Difficulties in identifying the noncooperator. *JAMA* 203:120-124, 1968.
26. Charney, E. Patient-doctor communication: Implications for the clinician. *Pediatr. Clin. North Am.* 19:263-279, 1972.
27. Clark, G.M., and Troop, R. One table combination drug therapy in the treatment of hypertension. *J. Chron. Dis.* 25:57-64, 1972.
28. Clinite, J.C., and Kabat, H.F. Improving patient compliance. *J. Am. Pharm. Assoc.* 16:74-76, 1976.
29. Cole, P., and Emmanuel, Sr. Drug consultation: Its significance to the discharged hospital patient. *Am. J. Hosp. Pharm.* 28:954-960, 1971.
30. Coronary Drug Project Research Group. Clofibrate and niacin in coronary heart disease. *JAMA* 231:360-381, 1975.
31. David, N.A., Welborn, W.S., and Pierce, H.I. Comparison of multiple and combination tablet drug therapy in hypertension. *Curr. Ther. Res.* 18:741-754, 1975.
32. Davis, M.S. Predicting non-compliant behavior. *J. Health Soc. Behav.* 8:265-271, 1967.
33. Davis, M.S. Physiologic, psychological and demographic factors in patient compliance with doctor's orders. *Med. Care* 6:115-122, 1968.
34. Davis, M.S., and Eichhorn, R.L. Compliance with medical regimens: A panel study. *J. Health Hum. Behav.* 4:240-249, 1963.
35. Dickey, F.F., Mattar, M.E., and Chudzek, G.M. Pharmacist counseling increases drug regimen compliance. *Hospitals* 49:85-88, 1975.
36. Dinoff, M., Rickard, N.C., and Colurck, J. Weight reduction through successive contracts. *Am. J. Orthopsychiatry* 42:110-113, 1972.
37. Donabedian, A., and Rosenfeld, L.S. Follow-up study of chronically ill patients discharged from hospitals. *J. Chron. Dis.* 17:847-856, 1964.
38. Dunbar, J. Adherence to medication: An intervention study with poor adherers. Doctoral Thesis, Stanford University, 1977.
39. Dunbar, J., and Stunkard, A. Adherence to diet and drug regimen, in R. Levy, B. Rifkind, B. Dennis, and N. Ernst (eds.), *Nutrition, Lipids, and Coronary Heart Disease*. New York: Raven Press, in press.
40. Elling, R., Whittemore, R., and Green, M. Patient participation in a pediatric program. *J. Health Hum. Behav.* 1:183, 1960.
41. Epstein, L.C., and Lasagna, L. Obtaining informed consent: Form or substance. *Arch. Intern. Med.* 123:682-688, 1969.
42. Eshelman, F.N., and Fitzloff, J. Effect of packaging on patient compliance with an antihypertensive medication. *Ther. Res.* 20:215-219, 1976.
43. Fass, M.F., Green, L.W., and Deeds, S.G. The effect of family education on patient adherence to antihypertensive regimens. Paper presented at the National Conference on High Blood Pressure Control, Washington, D.C., 1977.
44. Finnerty, F. Jr. New techniques for improving patient compliance, in *The Hypertension Handbook*. West Point, Pa.: Merck, Sharp, and Dohme, 1974, pp. 117-124.
45. Finnerty, F.A., Mattie, E.C., and Finnerty, F.A. Hypertension in the inner city. 1. Analysis of clinic drop-outs. *Circulation* 47:73-75, 1973.
46. Fitzgerald, J. Desmond. The influence of the medication on compliance with therapeutic regimens, in D.L. Sackett and R.B. Haynes (eds.), *Compliance with Medical Regimen*. Baltimore: The Johns Hopkins University Press, 1976, pp. 119-128.
47. Francis, V., Korsch, B.M., and Morris, M.J. Gaps in doctor-patient communication: Patient's responses to medical advice. *New Engl. J. Med.* 280:535-540, 1969.
48. Garb, J.R., Garb, J.L., and Stunkard, A.J. Effectiveness of a self-help group in obesity

control. *Arch. Int. Med.* 134:716-720, 1974.

49. Gates, S.J., and Colborn, D.K. Lowering appointment failures in a neighborhood health center. *Med. Care* 14:263-267, 1976.

50. Glogow, E. Effects of health education methods on appointment breaking. *Public Health Rep.* 85:441-450, 1970.

51. Gordis, L. Methodologic issues in the measurement of patient compliance, in D.L. Sackett and R.B. Haynes (eds.), *Compliance with Therapeutic Regimens.* Baltimore: The Johns Hopkins University Press, 1976, pp. 51-66.

52. Gordis, L., Markowitz, M., and Lilienfeld, A.M. Why patients dont't follow medical advice: A study of children on long-term antistreptococcal prophylaxis. *J. Pediatr.* 75:957-968, 1969.

53. Haefner, D.P., and Kirscht, J.P. Motivational and behavioral effects of modifying health beliefs. *Public Health Rep.* 85:478-484, 1970.

54. Hallburg, J.C. Teaching patients self-care. *Nurs. Clin. North Am.* 5:223-231, 1970.

55. Harris, M.B., and Bruner, C.G. A comparison of a self-control and a contract procedure for weight control. *Behav. Res. and Ther.* 9:347-354, 1971.

56. Haynes, R.B., Sackett, D.L., Gibson, E.S., Taylor, D.W., Hackett, B.C., Roberts, R.S., and Johnson, A.L. Improvement of medication compliance in uncontrolled hypertension. *Lancet* 1:1265-1268, 1976.

57. Hieb, E., and Wang, R.I.H. Compliance: The patient's role in drug therapy. *Wis. Med. J.* 73:152-153, 1974.

58. Huika, B.S., Cassel, J.C., and Kupper, L.L. Disparities between medications prescribed and consumed among chronic disease patients, in L. Lasagna (ed.), *Patient Compliance.* Mount Kisco, N.Y.: Futura Publishing Co., 1976, pp. 123-152.

59. Hulka, B.S., Cassel, J.C., Kupper, L.L., and Burdette, J.A. Communication, compliance, and concordance between physicians and patients with prescribed medications. *Am. J. Public Health* 66:847-853, 1976.

60. Hunt, G.M., and Azrin, N.H. A community-reinforcement approach to alcoholism. *Behav. Res. and Ther.* 11:91-104, 1973.

61. Irwin, D.S., Weitzel, W.D., and Morgan, D.W. Phenothiazine intake and staff attitudes. *Am. J. Psychiatry* 127:67-71, 1971.

62. Johnson, A.L., Taylor, D.W., Sackett, D.L., Dunnett, C.W., and Shimizu, A.G. Self blood pressure recording: An aid to blood pressure control? *Ann. R. Coll. Phys. Sur. Can.* 10:32-36, 1977.

63. Johnson, D.A.W. Drug defaulting by patients on long-acting phenothiazines. *Psychol. Med.* 3:115-119, 1973.

64. Joyce, C.R.B. Patient co-operation and the sensitivity of clinical trials. *J. Chron. Dis.* 15:1025-1036, 1962.

65. Joyce, C.R.B., Capla, G., Mason, M., Reynolds, E., and Mathews, J.A. Quantitative study of doctor-patient communication. *Q. J. Med.* 38:183-194, 1969.

66. Kanfer, F.K. Self-monitoring: Methodological limitations and clinical applications. *J. Consult. Clin. Psychol.* 35:148-152, 1970.

67. Kanfer, F.K., and Phillips, J.S. *Learning Foundations of Behavior Therapy.* New York: John Wiley and Sons, 1970.

68. Kazdin, A.E. Self-monitoring and behavior change, in M.J. Mahoney and C.E. Thoresen (eds.), *Self-control, Power to the Person.* Monterey, Cal.: Brooks/Cole, 1974.

69. Kersh, E. Prospective comparison of a paramedical clinic to a university medical clinic in the evaluation and treatment of high blood pressure. Paper presented at the National Conference on High Blood Pressure Control, Washington, D.C., 1977.

70. Korsch, B.M., and Negrete, V.F. Doctor-patient communication. *Sci. Am.* 227:66-74, 1972.

71. Leren, P. The effects of plasma cholesterol lowering diet in male survivors of myocardial infarction. *Acta Med. Scand. Supplement* 466, 1966.
72. Ley, P., Bradshaw, P.W., Eaves, D., and Walker, C.M. A method for increasing patients' recall of information presented by doctors. *Psychol. Med.* 3:217-220, 1973.
73. Ley, P., Jain, V.K., and Skilbeck, C.E. A method for decreasing patients' medication errors. *Psychol. Med.* 6:599-601, 1976.
74. Lima, J., Nazarian, L., Charney, E., and Lahti, C. Compliance with short-term antimicrobialtherapy: Some techniques that help. *Pediatrics* 57:383-386, 1976.
75. Linkewich, J.A., Catielano, R.B., and Flack, H.L. The effect of packaging and instruction on outpatient compliance with medication regimes. *Drug Intell. Clin. Pharm.* 8:10-15, 1974.
76. Lipinsky, D., and Nelson, R. The reactivity and unreliability of self-recording. *J. Consult. Clin. Psychol.* 42:118-123, 1974.
77. Maddock, R.K. Jr. Patient cooperation in taking medicines. *JAMA* 199:137-172, 1967.
78. Mahoney, M.J. Self-reward and self-monitoring techniques for weight control. *Behav. Ther.* 5:48-57, 1974.
79. Mahoney, M.J., Moura, N.G.M., and Wade, T.C. The relative efficacy of self-awards, self-punishment and self-monitoring techniques for weight loss. *J. Consult. Clin. Psychol.* 40:404-407, 1973.
80. Maletzky, B.M. Behavior recording as treatment: A brief note. *Behav. Ther.* 5:107-111, 1974.
81. Mann, R.A. The behavior-therapeutic use of contingency contracting to control an adult-behavior problem: Weight control. *J. Appl. Behav. Anal.* 5:99-109, 1972.
82. Marshall, G.D., Agras, W.S., and Rotchstein, N. The use of medication dispensers in improving adherence. Unpublished manuscript. Stanford University Laboratory for the Study of Behavioral Medicine, 1978.
83. Marston, M. Compliance with medical regimens: A review of the literature. *Nurs. Res.* 19:312-323, 1970.
84. Mattar, M.E., Markello, J., and Yaffe, S.J. Pharmaceutic factors affecting pediatric compliance. *Pediatrics* 55(1):101-108, 1975.
85. McKenney, J.M., Slining, J.M., Henderson, H.R., Devins, D., and Barr, M. The effect of clinical pharmacy services on patients with essential hypertension. *Circulation* 48:1104-1111, 1973.
86. Moulding, T. Preliminary study of the pill calendar as a method of improving the self-administration of drugs. *Am. Rev. Respir. Dis.* 84:284-287, 1961.
87. Myers, E.D., and Calvert, E.J. The effect of forewarning on the occurrence of side effects and discontinuance of medication in patients on amytriptylene. *Br. J. Psychiatry* 122:461-472, 1973.
88. Myers, E.D., and Calbert, E.J. The effect of forewarning on the occurrence of side-effects and discontinuance of medication in patients on dothiepen. *J. Int. Med. Res.* 4:237-240, 1976.
89. National diet—heart study: Final report. *Circulation,* Supplement Number One. Volume 37, March 1968.
90. Nazarian, L.F., Michalier, J., Charney, E., and Coulter, M.P. Effect of a mailed appointment reminder on appointment keeping. *Pediatrics* 53:349-352,m 1974.
91. Nelson, R.O. Methodological issues in assessment via self-monitoring, in J.D. Cone and R.P. Hawkins (eds.), *Behavioral Assessment.* New York: Brunner/Mazel, 1977, pp. 217-240.
92. Nelson, R.O., Lipinsky, D.P., and Black, J.L. The relative reactivity of external observations and self-monitoring. *Behav. Ther.* 7:314-321, 1976.
93. Oakes, T.W., Ward, J.R., Gray, R.M., Klauber, M.R., and Moody, P.M. Family

expectations and arthritis patient compliance to a hand resting splint regimen. *J. Chron. Dis.* 22:757-764, 1970.

94. Panyon, M., Boozer, H., and Morris, N. Feedback to attendants as a reinforcer for applying operant techniques. *J. Appl. Behav. Anal.* 8:1-19, 1975.

95. Park, L.C., and Lipman, R.S. A comparison of patient dosage deviation reports with pill counts. *Psychopharmacologie* 6:299-302, 1964.

96. Pomerleua, O., Bobrove, R.H., and Smith, R.H. Recording psychiatric aids performance for the behavioral improvement of assigned patients. *J. Appl. Behav. Anal.* 6:383-395, 1973.

97. Porter, A.M.W. Drug defaulting in a general practice. *Br. Med. J.* 1:218-222, 1969.

98. Rehder, T.L., McCoy, L.K., Blackwell, B., Whitehead, W., and Robinson, A. Improving compliance by counseling and pill container. Unpublished manuscript, 1977.

99. Reidenberg, M.M., and Lowenthal, D.T. Adverse nondrug reactions. *N. Engl. J. Med.* 279:678-679, 1968.

100. Rickels, K., and Briscol, E. Assessment of dosage deviation in outpatient drug research. *J. Clin. Pharmacol.* 10:153-160, 1970.

101. Robertson, L. Safety belt use in automobiles with starter-interlock and buzzer-light reminder systems. *Am. J. Public Health* 65:1319-1325, 1975.

102. Robertson, L., and Haddon, W. The buzzer-light reminder system and safety-belt use. *Am. J. Public Health* 64:814-815, 1974.

103. Rockart, J.F., and Hofmann, P.B. Physician and patient behavior under different scheduling systems in a hospital outpatient department. *Med. Care* 7:463-470, 1969.

104. Romanczyk, R.G. Self-monitoring in the treatment of obesity: parameters of reactivity. *Behav. Ther.* 5:531-540, 1974.

105. Romanczyk, R.G., Tracey, D.A., Wilson, G.T., and Thorpe, G.L. Behavioral techniques in the treatment of obesity: A comparative analysis. *Behav. Res. and Ther.* 11:629-640, 1973.

106. Roth, H.P., Caron, H.S., and Hsi, B.P. Measuring intakes of a prescribed medication: A bottle count and a tracer technique compared. *Clin. Pharmacol. Ther.* 11:228-237, 1970.

107. Roth, H., Caron, H.S., and Hsi, B.P. Estimating a patient's cooperation with his regimen. *Am. J. Med. Sci.* 262:269-273, 1971.

108. Sackett, D.L. The magnitude and distribution of compliance. Paper presented at the Second McMaster Workshop/Symposium on Compliance. Hamilton, Ontario, May 25-27, 1977.

109. Sackett, D.L., Gibson, E.S., Taylor, D.W., Haynes, R.B., Hockett, B.C., Roberts, R.R., and Johnson, A.L. Randomized clinical trial of strategies for improving medication compliance in primary hypertension. *Lancet* 1205-1207, 1975.

110. Schultz, F.B. The evaluation of hypertensive drugs. *J. Med. Assoc. State Ala.* 32:105-111, 1962.

111. Seybold, M.E., and Drachman, D.B. Gradually increasing doses of prednisone in myasthenia gravis: Reducing the hazards of treatment. *N. Engl. J. Med.* 290:81-84, 1974.

112. Sharpe, T.R., and Mikeal, R. Patient compliance with antibiotic regimens. *Am. J. Hosp. Pharm.* 31:479-484, 1974.

113. Shaw, S.M., and Opit, L.J. Need for supervision in the elderly receiving long-term prescribed medication. *Br. Med. J.* 1:505-507, 1976.

114. Shmerak, K.L. Reduce your broken appointment rate: How one children and youth project reduced its broken appointment rate. *Am. J. Public Health* 61:2400-2404, 1971.

115. Simkins, L. The reliability of self-recorded behaviors. *Behav. Ther.* 2:83-87, 1971.

116. Soutter, B.R., and Kennedy, M.B. Patient compliance assessment in drug trials: Usage and methods. *Aust. N. Z. J. Med.* 4:360-364, 1974.

117. Stamler, R., Stamler, J., Civinelli, J., Pritchard, D., Gosch, F.C., Ticho, S., Restivo, B., and Fine, D. Adherence and blood pressure response to hypertension treatment. *Lancet* 1227-1230, 1975.

118. Steckel, S.B., and Swain, M.A. Written contracts to improve adherence to hypertensive patients. Paper presented at the National Conference on High Blood Pressure Control, Washington, D.C., 1977.

119. Stewart, R.B., and Cluff, L.E. Commentary: A review of medication errors and compliance in ambulant patients. *Clin. Pharmacol. Ther.* 13:463-468, 1972.

120. Stuart, R.B., and Davis, B. *Slim Chance in a Fat World: Behavioral Control of Obesity.* Champaign, Ill.: Research Press, 1972.

121. Taylor, D.W., Sackett, D.L., Haynes, R.B., Johnson, A.L., Gibson, E.S., and Roberts, A.S. Compliance with antihypertensive drugs in food and nutrition in health and disease. *Ann. N.Y. Acad. Sci.,* in press.

122. Turner, A.J., and Vernon, J.C. Prompts to increase attendance in a community mental health center. *J. Appl. Behav. Anal.* 9:141-145, 1976.

123. Vincent, P. Factors influencing patient noncompliance: A theoretical approach. *Nurs. Res.* 20:509-516, 1971.

124. Weintraub, M., Au, W.Y.W., and Lasagna, L. Compliance as a determinant of serum digoxin concentration. *JAMA* 224:481-485, 1973.

125. Wilber, J.A., and Barrow, T.G. Reducing elevated blood pressure: experience found in a community. *Minn. Med.* 52:1303-1306, 1969.

126. Wilson, J.T. Compliance with instructions in the evaluation of therapeutic efficacy. *Clin. Pediatr.* 12:333-340, 1973.

Maintenance
of Behavioral Changes

In the field of behavioral medicine, no problem is more urgently in need of attention than that of maintenance. A variety of long–term studies on obesity, relaxation, and smoking have shown that, although behavioral techniques may have more effective short–term effects, the long–term effects, those of six months or longer, are less certain. Strategies to improve maintenance are desperately needed. Unfortunately, these studies must extend over a many–year time course, which is often impossible within our current university structure. A comparison of maintenance strategies requires a study that is at least one year long, with up to five years of follow–up data. In our mobile society, few subjects stay in one area for this length of time and fewer experimenters, who often must be evaluated more frequently by their university for promotion and tenure.

Hall and Hall examine some of the issues of maintenance from a behavioral standpoint. Relapse, for example in the case of an alcoholic, can relate to stimulus conditions—like having friends that continue to be alcoholics and no nonalcoholic friends, or biological pressures in the case of a childhood obese individual who manages to lose weight but retains an excessive number of fat cells, or from external reinforcement as in the case of a child who finds the only way to gain attention within the family is to starve himself. Hall and Hall review the literature of maintenance and point out that some technology is available currently which appears to increase the probability of maintaining change. This includes booster sessions, which need not be either frequent or extensive, follow–up visits which are as much like treatment sessions as possible, and continued concern on the part of the therapist. The simplicity of these recommendations, they point out, reflects the state of the art.

CHAPTER 7

Maintaining Change

Sharon M. Hall
Robert G. Hall

This chapter deals with maintenance once therapeutic change has been achieved. Much of the relevant research on maintenance of behavior change is in the area of addictive disorders—obesity, smoking, and alcoholism—where relapse is a serious problem. Because of this emphasis, much of our discussion will be organized around research in these problem areas. However, the strategies and concepts discussed presumably also apply to other health–related disorders.

Interest in maintenance strategies has greatly increased in the last decade. The source for much of this interest has been the application of behavioral self-management treatments to obesity and other recalcitrant, self-destructive disorders. In these treatments the client is taught to modify problem behaviors in his natural environment. Ideally, the client becomes his own therapist, and change is maintained even after "treatment" terminates. Investigation into the efficacy of these self–management treatments has naturally led to evaluation of long-term success and maintenance of change. A second source of interest has been the creative and clinically encouraging application of aversive control to cigarette smoking and alcoholism; since these disorders are prone to relapse, treatment goals have emphasized permanence of change, and techniques leading to long–term success are considered essential.

THEORIES OF RELAPSE AND MAINTENANCE

Early behavioral theorists hoped that once change was achieved, adaptive responses would automatically be reinforced by the environment and maintained without continued therapeutic contact. This may be the case for behaviors which have immediate social impact and for which easy alternative behaviors are readily available, for example increased assertiveness, improvements in aberrant behaviors in psychotics, and decreased avoidance in phobics. However, adaptive health–related behaviors often evoke no social response, do not produce observable change immediately, and may be limited in complex ways by physiological factors. The immediate satisfaction of a craving tends to encourage relapse; the relaxing effect of alcohol, the stimulating effect of cigarettes, and the satisfaction of food are all immediate results that reinforce the problem behavior. When we also consider the social reinforcement that accompanies the misuse of these substances, the influence of the advertising media in selling them, and our national ambivalence about drinking, smoking, and overeating, we can understand the ease of relapse and the need to program therapies to deal specifically with the posttreatment periods.

Recently, writers have suggested strategies for maintaining therapeutic change. Most of these are limited adaptations of more comprehensive theories (8) or deal with very specific segments of behavior (14). Among these is Kopel and Arkowitz's (16) application of an attribution analysis to maintenance. They noted that self–attributed behavior change is maintained to a greater extent than behavior change attributed to an external agent. On the basis of this principle, they suggested several strategies for enhancing maintenance, including the following: using the least powerful reward or punishment effective so that the saliency of the external agent is reduced; fading therapist involvement over time to shift perceptions from therapist–attributed to client–attributed change; teaching clients self–control skills, which emphasize self–generated reward and punishment; allowing the client to play an active role in treatment; and decreasing the use of external aids to which change can be attributed.

The most comprehensive models dealing specifically with the posttreatment period are those attempting to explain relapse in alcoholism and drug abuse. Wikler (30) proposed a classical conditioning model of opiate use and relapse which has been adopted by Ludwig (20) and his colleagues to deal with relapse from alcohol abstinence. The model proposes that both withdrawal symptoms and other drug–related cues become classically conditioned to the environment in which they occur. In the presence of these environmental stimuli, a "craving" for alcohol or opiates occurs. This craving is labeled a "conditional withdrawal" syndrome. Craving is a necessary, but not a sufficient condition for relapse; other factors, such as the availability of the substances, influence whether the abstainer will in fact relapse. The initial instance of substance use by the abstainer serves as an "appetizer" (or conditioned stimulus for further use), which results in the loss of control as seen with alcohol or narcotic relapse. Suggested treatment strategies emphasize extinction of the conditioned response, for example with antagonists in the case of narcotics.

Marlatt (22) proposed a theory of relapse to alcohol use in which certain high–probability situations present a decision point for the "abstainer". If the abstainer has an appropriate coping response available, he will use it, continue to perceive himself in control, and continue abstaining. If no appropriate response is available, the client will engage in his "forbidden" behavior. This will result in a phenomenon called the Abstinence Violation Effect (AVE), which is composed of two cognitive elements: cognitive dissonance (e.g., drinking behavior is dissonant with the conception of self as abstinent) and the personal attribution effect (e.g., attribution of the break in abstention to personal weakness). Both of these effects increase the probability that continued abuse will occur. According to this formulation, maintenance strategies should include direct training in handling high–risk situations and methods which increase one's sense of control cross situationally, such as meditation.

None of the above formulations has been subjected to extensive examination. Data on causes of relapse gathered from a behavioral perspective are lacking, as are studies on behavioral differences between relapsers and nonrelapsers. At this point, an analysis of actual outcome studies of therapeutic maintenance provides the most information about factors of importance in maintenance. Further theory development is needed, both to tie together our observations and to generate new experiments and hypotheses.

RESEARCH ON MAINTENANCE STRATEGIES

Several strategies designed to produce maintenance of changed behaviors have been evaluated. These can be divided into treatment and posttreatment interventions. Most work has been done on posttreatment strategies, and we will consider these first.

Posttreatment Strategies to Maintain Change

Perhaps the most obvious maintenance strategy is continuation of the treatment itself—usually in an attenuated form. Several studies indicate that booster sessions help maintain change. These are usually brief versions of treatment sessions designed to provide support but not introduce new treatment techniques.

Stuart's (25) pioneering work in obesity included booster sessions over a one-year period. Treatment techniques included weight and food monitoring, stimulus control, weakening the chain leading to eating, and the development of an alternative response repertory. Treatment extended over a four- to five-week period with subsequent sessions as needed, and follow–up meetings on a monthly basis. Eight of twelve subjects lost 24 to 41 pounds over a 12–month period. Data after termination of follow–up contacts were not reported.

In the excitement over these impressive results, most investigators ignored the possibility that Stuart's follow–up sessions were partly responsible for the weight losses he reported. Early controlled experiments with behavioral treatment packages for obesity provided treatment techniques in brief periods of time (11, 31) and generally used short–term follow–up evaluation. In most of these studies, weight changes were not well maintained (7, 26).

In an effort to discover techniques that would help maintain changed behaviors, Hall, Hall, Borden, and Hanson (9) provided subjects who had received a self-management treatment for obesity with either booster sessions, instruction to continue monitoring but no further contact, or no posttreatment support or instruction. Booster sessions consisted of hourly meetings bimonthly to provide support for continued adherence to self–management strategies and to discuss difficulties experienced in applying these techniques. Although interpretation of the results of this study is difficult due to methodological problems, the data appear to indicate that both self–monitoring and booster sessions produced at least some maintenance of weight changes. This seemed to be true, however, only if the booster subjects continued with the therapist that they had seen during active treatment.

Two studies without the methodological problems experienced by Hall et al. provide limited support for the value of booster sessions in obesity treatment. Kingsley and Wilson (14) compared group and individual behavior therapy with a social pressure placebo control. Following an eight–week treatment period, a limited booster condition (four meetings irregularly spaced over a 16–week period) was compared with no booster for all three treatment conditions. They found significant differences between the behavioral groups and social pressure control group at the end of treatment, but not at any of the follow–up sessions. The booster condition was more effective than the no–booster condition, and both groups showed increases in weight after booster sessions were terminated.

Hall, Bass, and Monroe (6) extended the earlier Hall et al. study. Subjects who completed a 10–week course of behavioral self–management were assigned to one of three conditions: minimal contact, monitoring with minimal contact, and continued contact in bimonthly groups. At two and six months after treatment termination, the continued–contact subjects had lost significantly more weight than minimal–contact subjects. Follow–up support terminated six months after treatment termination. At one year from the start of the study, differences between treatments were no longer significant. Thus, continued contact did differ from minimal contact and did produce small losses. When contact was terminated subjects began to regain lost weight. Monitoring alone did not at any period differ from either continued or minimal contact.

Brightwell (2), in a series of case studies, found a similar effect. He treated six patients with food and weight monitoring, stimulus control, and a self-reward program. Following two weeks of instruction, subjects were followed in brief (15–30 minutes) monthly meetings for one year. At the end of that year, all subjects had lost weight (from 48.8 to 9.0 pounds). During the second year, when contact with the therapist ceased, four of the six subjects showed weight gain and two weight loss.

These data appear to indicate that booster sessions are of value in the treatment of obesity. Even contacts as brief as 15 minutes occurring as infrequently as once per month may be helpful. However, in most cases weight losses during treatment are moderately slow and losses during booster periods slower still, and subjects rarely reach goal weight. Booster sessions appear to maintain the weight loss *process*; we cannot specify what this process is or which elements are active during the posttreatment period. The function of booster sessions when goal weight has been attained has not been determined.

What is being maintained is clearer when one considers the disorders for which abstinence is traditionally considered the ideal outcome of treatment—alcohol abuse and cigarette smoking. Voegtlin et al. (27) reported results from an uncontrolled trial with 285 alcoholic patients. All patients who completed a course of aversion conditioning were asked to return between 30 and 60 days after the original treatment and thereafter at 90–day intervals for one year. At each return, the patient was given a single aversion trial. Among the patients who elected to continue on boosters, there was a 19% increase in abstinence over patients receiving no boosters. Similarly, Stojiljkovi'c (24) reported clinical data suggesting booster sessions were of value in the maintenance abstinence in alcoholics. Nearly 51% of his clients who had repeatedly failed at other treatments underwent monthly "stabilization" sessions and were abstinent at 18 months (136 of 264 subjects). At these follow-up sessions held 60 to 150 days after termination, he reduced the amount of the emetic or used none at all if the conditional response was elicited in the presence of alcohol.

Vogler et al. (28) compared a variety of aversive conditions: booster, conditioning only, pseudo–conditioning, sham conditioning, and no aversion–treatment control, and monitored the number of days to relapse. By far the most effective treatment included booster sessions, with a median of 66 days to relapse. Conditioning only was the next most effective condition, with a median relapse of 19.5 days. In all three studies the authors comment on the high dropout rate for persons who were scheduled for booster sessions. Clearly, a self–selection factor was operating, and the differences seen could be explained by higher motivation of subjects attending the booster sessions.

Despite the high relapse rates noted in some treatments for cigarette smoking (6, 18, 19), few studies of posttreatment maintenance strategies have been reported. Kopel (15) failed to find increased maintenance with booster sessions following rapid smoking therapy. However, he suggested this failure was due to less than optimal treatment and to introduction of maintenance strategies *after* smoking had been resumed. More recently, Colleti and Kopel (5) have obtained preliminary evidence that the type of booster condition is closely related to maintenance. They suggest that maintenance strategies that lead to self–attribution for change are more successful than those which do not.

The clinical data indicate that booster sessions should be further studied; for example, if the findings of Voegtlin et al. (27) and of Stojiljkovi'c (24) could be replicated, we might be able to offer effective follow–up strategies to aversion treatments that include only a single aversion session, monitoring of the conditioned response, or even support alone. The support for booster sessions in abstinence–oriented treatments is less clear than in the case of obesity. This is due in part to a paucity of data and in part to methodological problems in existing studies.

When a limited number of clients are involved, booster sessions are moderately economical. However, for a busy practitioner with a large caseload, they may be too time consuming to be practical, especially if professional leaders are employed.

Less time–consuming posttreatment strategies have been studied. One possibility is the use of self–help groups for maintenance of change. Levitz and Stunkard (17) introduced behavioral procedures in TOPS (Take Off Pounds Sensibly) chapters. These groups were either provided with instructions in behavioral techniques by a professional leader or by a TOPS leader who had been trained in behavior modification. The two control groups were given nutrition instruction or given no special treatment. At posttreatment, the behavioral groups were superior to both control groups. At one–year follow–up, professionally led groups continued to lose weight, while groups led by TOPS leaders returned to baseline, and the two control groups faired even more poorly, both gaining weight.

Preexisting self–help groups often have ideologies that are not compatible with change strategies. Since changing the beliefs of an organization may be more difficult than changing the behavior of individuals, it may be more effective to form groups that receive professional assistance initially and gradually prepare such groups to become self–sustaining self–help units.

Janis and Hoffman (12) built a self–help social support network for smokers. Subjects wishing to quit smoking were assigned to high–contact companion therapy, low–contact companion therapy, and a no–treatment control condition. Although there were no differences immediately at posttreatment, at one–year follow–up high–contact partners smoked significantly less than control subjects and low–contact partners.

Strategies Provided During Active Treatment

Once behavioral change has occurred, reinforcement for change must be faded and replaced by reinforcement for maintenance. There are at least two strategies for this transition: provision of durable treatments without posttreatment support and incorporation of natural reinforcers to help maintain change. The family unit is a system with a relatively long duration of existence which usually does not have an official policy about behavioral change and does not have to rely on arranged treatment sessions for its reinforcing properties and support. Two studies indicate that including family members in a change program may help create an environment conducive to maintenance. Mahoney and Mahoney (21) report a clinical obesity treatment program with 13 subjects where family members were invited to all sessions. One treatment session was devoted to the family's role in the program. The family members were asked to avoid teasing and criticizing, offering food for any reason, and to change their own eating patterns. The subjects were taught how to be socially reinforcing to their spouses. The authors computed an index based on family attendance and reports of social support. The index was found to correlate with posttreatment change and change at six months and one year. Brownell et al. (3) noted the importance in a weight loss program of a family member with bilateral power, and they were able to demonstrate both maintenance and continuing change over an 8½-month period. This change was especially striking when the couple was treated as a unit. The investigators demonstrated that the effectiveness was due to active spouse involvement rather than passive cooperation or lack of interference.

Self–management training was originally proposed as a brief, cost–effective therapy. Much of the early work teaching self–management skills to clients proposed transforming clients into their own therapists with an assumption that this would produce better maintenance of change than externally imposed treatments. Studies tested this proposition by comparing self–managed treatments with treatments that produced change by the use of external reinforcers, such as money. Jeffrey (13) compared a self–control condition with an external–control condition in the treatment of weight reduction. The self–control group used self–reinforcement and was told explicitly that they alone were responsible for their weight. In the external–control condition the experimenter provided reinforcement, and subjects were told that the therapist was responsible for weight loss. The self–control subjects did as well as the external–control subjects during treatment and surpassed the external control at the brief (six–week) follow–up.

Bellack and Rozensky (1) compared self– and external control in a weight reduction program, along with the responses of high and low self–reinforcers to each condition. They assessed subjects at seven (posttreatment) and 14 weeks (follow–up). They found that self–control was more effective at both assessments, and they found especially poor results for subjects who were high self–reinforcers in the external–control condition. Differential effects during maintenance were not noted.

Hall et al. (9) compared self–management, external management, and self– and external management combined with two control conditions. They hypothesized that combining the two would result in early weight loss, which should reinforce further efforts, while self–management training would provide the skills needed for long–term treatment. This hypothesis was not supported. The three groups did not differ at posttreatment, or at three– and six–month follow–up evaluations.

Thus, experiments that have directly evaluated the role of self–control training in maintenance of change are not conclusive. The data do not support the asumption that self–control training leads to better maintenance. This failure may be due to a variety of factors, including use of techniques that were not optimally effective or high levels of variability that occurred because of changes in life situations during follow–up.

Research on pragmatic issues related to treatment durability is rare. However, the available studies do indicate some direction for further study. Maintenance of change may be enhanced when treatments emphasize relatively simple procedures. For example, in obesity research there is some evidence that relatively simple techniques, such as stimulus control procedures, may be more effective than complex self–management packages. These procedures are practical and easy for the client to maintain after treatment has been terminated, and they are easy for the client to understand and recall when necessary.

An important example is a study by McReynolds et al. (23), who evaluated two groups of overweight women treated for obesity by doctoral and master's level nutritionists. The first group received the standard complex self–management program including shaping, stimulus control, manipulation of satiation and deprivation, self–reward, response chaining, aversive control, and response substitution. The second group received a limited stimulus control treatment including special dishes, which were the only dishes from which they ate, and received instruction in environmental control for eating at all stages in the eating process, beginning with buying food and ending with clearing the serving table and cleaning up the kitchen. They found no difference at termination in weight between the two treatment groups. However, at three and six months, the stimulus control group was superior. Most impressively, this group continued to lose weight until a three–month follow–up, after which weight losses were maintained.

Weiss (29) also used stimulus control procedures to treat obese adolescents. He compared five conditions: a no–treatment control group, a diet–only control group, and a diet with points for diet adherence which could be exchanged for a variety of reinforcers, a group which received stimulus control instructions along with the diet, and a group which received the stimulus control condition without a diet. At posttreatment and at one–year follow–up, both stimulus control groups were superior to the other treatments. In addition, these two groups showed a 9.77% decrease in percent overweight at the one–year follow–up visit. These two studies suggest that focused procedures hold some promise for maintenance of change which may be lacking in more diffuse, complicated techniques.

The role of the therapist in treatment has not been thoroughly explored from a behavioral standpoint. Data from studies completed with other objectives in mind have indicated that the patterning and intensity of the therapeutic relationship should be further explored as a factor in behavior maintenance.

Carter et al. (4) found that when the therapist was faded from treatment (he met with subjects during weeks 1, 3, 6, and 10 of a 10–week treatment), subjects were able to maintain weight change over a six–month follow–up period, which was not the case when therapeutic contact was abruptly terminated after weekly meetings. Unfortunately in this experiment, the subjects with therapist fading also lost more weight at the end of treatment, suggesting they may have been more motivated initially. Kingsley and Wilson (14) found that subjects given individual behavioral therapy were more likely to regain lost weight than those seen in groups, even when boosters were provided. They hypothesized that group sessions were more motivating than individual sessions. After new behaviors are learned, motivation to use therapeutic techniques should be the primary factor in determining weight loss, hence the difference. This admittedly post hoc analysis does not explain *why* a group should be more motivating than individual therapy.

Another explanation for these findings might lie in the differences in dependency which developed in the two treatments. The more intensive contact may have produced dependency on the therapist which did not occur in the group situation. This dependency may not have been appropriately decreased by gradual fading of the therapist during the booster sessions. Additional evidence for the need to minimize dependence on the therapist was found by Hanson et al. (10). They reported that if subjects were given a programmed text and little contact during treatment, the subjects lost moderate amounts of weight during treatment and continued to lose weight after treatment termination. Subjects given the same text and additional therapeutic support during treatment did not continue to lose weight. Unfortunately, the crucial one–year follow–up in this study was obtained by telephone rather than direct weighing. The results of these three studies, taken together, are suggestive. They indicate that high levels of therapist contact during treatment and follow–up may be deleterious to maintenance of behavioral change. They also suggest that gradual changes in the amount of therapist contact may produce better maintenance than sharp changes. It is possible that attributional processes mediate these results and provide a better explanation for the finding. Subjects with high therapist contact may attribute losses during treatment to the therapist rather than their own efforts. When contact is reduced or removed, therapeutic changes are not maintained because the source to which they have been attributed has been lost. An alternate explanation is that high therapist contact may promote a high level of dependency, and when this dependent relationship is terminated the client is unable to continue these behaviors.

IMPLICATIONS

Theory and Research

Fitting the data available to the theoretical conceptions presented earlier would be a difficult undertaking. Most of the research reviewed does not stem from a particular conception of successful maintenance, and the data available and kinds of questions asked are limited. At best, we can summarize the findings and tentatively explore their relationship to conceptual schemes.

Booster sessions seem to be a promising strategy for maintenance. Comparisons of different kinds of booster sessions have not been reported, and detailed descriptions of what occurs within these sessions are rare. We do not know how they maintain change. It is possible that they continue to reinforce values learned in treatment; they may serve as motivators for continued practice of treatment techniques, provide cues for subjects about the appropriateness of their behaviors, or maintain newly learned aversions to previously reinforcing events; they may gradually decrease dependency on treatment contacts and shift attribution of change from the therapist to themselves.

The evidence supporting the efficacy of booster sessions does not directly contradict any model of maintenance, nor is it specific enough to lend strong support to any of them. Many questions about booster sessions remain to be answered. Optimal content needs to be determined; for example, in aversive conditioning, does monitoring for conditioned response work as well as continued conditioning? Is continued support or continued conditioning the important factor? There is evidence (4, 15) that timing may be important both in terms of introduction of boosters and their termination.

The data indicate that posttreatment support from others, especially the family, is important. Replication of early work describing family support (3, 21) is needed along with studies describing the acceptability of such treatments to families. The effect of treatment on other behavioral subsystems in the family needs to be determined. Other aspects of treatment procedures deserving further study are the comparison of different sorts of techniques and the durability of changes they produce, and further research into this issue of therapist–client relationship and its effect on maintenance of behavioral change. The feasibility of introducing behavioral strategies into existing self–help groups and their effectiveness in this situation needs examination, as does the acceptability of professionally formed posttreatment support groups.

Very little work has been designed to test various theoretical formulations of behavior maintenance. The area most studied has been change produced by self–control training. Unfortunately, this research has added little support for the concept that "self–management" skills are more likely to persist than skills taught in other ways.

Treatment Implications

What are the implications for the practitioner? The seemingly simplistic statement, "make follow–up as much like treatment as possible," seem to be the best summary of the available data. Treatment procedures should be easily duplicated during posttreatment periods; for example, simple stimulus control procedures with low–frequency therapist contact in self–help groups. Posttreatment support should include the important parts of the treatment as much as possible; for example, booster sessions should certainly provide support for those aspects of the treatment the clinician considers essential. This recommendation is somewhat clouded by a lack of agreement on *what* is essential for change. Lacking objective data, the clinician might well choose to rely on the client's report, his own careful analysis of the problem behaviors unique to the client, and such basic "commonsense" principles as the cost–benefit ratio of the procedure, particularly the subjective aspects of the ratio.

ACKNOWLEDGMENTS

Preparation of this manuscript was supported in part by Demonstration Grant H81 DA 01978 and in part by Program Project Grant DA 4RG012, both from the National Institute on Drug Abuse.

REFERENCES

1. Bellack, A.S., and Rozensky, R. Subjects' self–reinforcement tendencies and their responses to behavioral weight reduction programs. Paper presented at the European Association for Behavioral Therapy Conference, 1974.
2. Brightwell, D.R. One year follow–up of obese subjects treated with behavior therapy. *Dis. of the Nerv. Sys.* 37:593–594, 1976.
3. Brownell, K., Heckesman, C.L., Westlake, R.J., Hayes, S.C., and Monti, P.M. The effect of couples training and partner cooperation—new in the behavioral treatment of obesity. Paper presented at the Eleventh Annual Association for the Advancement of Behavior

Therapy Conference, Atlanta, Georgia 1977.

4. Carter, E.N., Rice, A.P. and de Julio, S. Role of the therapist in the self-control of obesity. *J. Cons. Clin. Psychol.* 45:503, 1977.

5. Colletti, G., and Kopel, S. The relative efficacy of participant modeling participant observer and self-monitoring procedures as maintenance strategies following positive behaviorally based treatment strategies. Doctoral dissertation, Rutgers University, 1977.

6. Hall, S.M., Bass, A., and Monroe, J. Follow-up strategies in obesity treatment. Paper presented, Eleventh Annual Convention of the Association for the Advancement of Behavior Therapy, 1977.

7. Hall, S.M., and Hall, R.G. Outcome and methodological considerations in the behavioral treatment of obesity. *Behav. Ther.* 5:352-364, 1974.

8. Hall, S.M., Hall, R.G., Borden, B.L., and Hanson, R.W. Improvement of posttreatment performance via monitoring and limited contact in obese subjects. *Behav. Res. and Ther.* 13:167-172, 1975.

9. Hall, S.M., Hall, R.G., DeBoer, G., and O'Kulitch, P. External reinforcement and self-management in the treatment of obesity. *Behav. Res. and Ther.* 15:89-95, 1977.

10. Hanson, R.W., Borden, B.L., Hall, S.M., and Hall, R.G. Programmed versus nonprogrammed instruction and high and low therapist contact in self-management training. *Behav. Ther.* 7:366-373, 1976.

11. Harris, M.B. Self-directed program for weight control: A pilot study. *J. Abnorm. Psychol.* 74:263-270, 1969.

12. Janis, I.L., and Hoffman, D. Facilitating effects on daily contact between partners who make a decision to cut down on smoking. *J. Pers. Soc. Psychol.* 17:25-35, 1970.

13. Jeffrey, D.B. A comparison of the effect of external control and self-control in the modification and maintenance of weight. *J. Abnorm. Psychol.* 83:404-410, 1974.

14. Kingsley, R.C., and Wilson, G.T. Behavior therapy for obesity: A comparative investigation of long-term efficacy. *J. Cons. and Clin. Psychol.* 45:288-298, 1977.

15. Kopel, S. Effects of self-control, booster sessions, and cognitive factors in maintenance of smoking reduction. Doctoral dissertation, University of Oregon, 1974.

16. Kopel, S., and Arkowitz, H. The role of attribution and self-perception in behavior change: Implications for behavior therapy. *Genetic Psychol. Monographs* 92:175-212, 1975.

17. Levitz, L.S., and Stunkard, A.J. A therapeutic coalition for obesity: Behavior modification and self-help. *Am. J. Psychiatry* 131:423-427, 1974.

18. Lichtenstein, E., and Rodrigues, M.P. Long-term effects of rapid smoking treatment for dependent cigarette smokers. *Addict. Behav.* 2:109-112, 1977.

19. Lichtenstein, E., and Danaher, B.G. Modification of smoking behavior: A critical analysis of theory, research and practice, in M. Hersen, R.M. Eiseler, and P.M. Miller (eds.), *Progress in Behavior Modification.* New York: Academic press, 1973.

20. Ludwig, A.M., Wikler, A., and Stark, L.H. The first drink: Psychological aspects of craving. *Arch. Gen. Psychiatry* 30:539-547, 1974.

21. Mahoney, M.J., and Mahoney, K. Treatment of obesity: A clinical exploration, in B.J. Williams, S. Martin, and J.P. Foreyt (eds.), *Obesity: Behavioral Approach to Dietary Management.* New York: Brunner-Mazel, 1976.

22. Marlatt, G.A. Craving for alcohol, loss of control, and relapse: A cognitive behavioral analysis. Alcoholism and Drug Abuse Institute Technical REport No. 77-05, 1977.

23. McReynolds, W.T., Lutz, R.N., Paulsen, B.K., and Kohrs, M.B. Weight loss resulting from two behavior modification procedures with nutritionists as therapists. *Behav. Ther.* 7:283-291, 1976.

24. Stojiljkovi'c, S. Conditioned aversion treatment of alcoholics. *Quart. J. of Studies in Alcohol.* 30:900-904, 1969.

25. Stuart, R.B. Behavioral control of overeating. *Behav. Res. and Ther.* 5:357-365, 1967.
26. Stunkard, A.L. Behavioral treatment of obesity: Failure to maintain weight loss, in R.B. Stuart (ed.), *Behavioral Self-Management: Strategies, Techniques and Outcome.* New York: Brunner/Mazel, 1977, pp. 317-350.
27. Voegtlin, W.L., Lerﬁere, F., Broz, W.R., and O'Hallaren, P. Conditioned reflex therapy of chronic alcoholism. *Quart. J. of Studies on Alcohol.* 2:505-511, 1942.
28. Vogler, R.E., Lunde, S.E., Johnson, G.R., and Martin, P.L. Electrical aversion conditioning with chronic alcoholism. *J. Consult. Clin. Psychol.* 34:302-307, 1970.
29. Weiss, A.R. A behavioral approach to the treatment of adolescent obesity. *Behav. Ther.* 8:720-726, 1977.
30. Wikler, A. Conditioning of successive adaptive responses to the initial effects of drugs. *Conditional Reflex* 8:193-209, 1973.
31. Wollersheim, J.P. Effectiveness of group therapy based on learning principles in the treatment of overweight women. *J. Abnorm. Psychol.* 76:462-474, 1970.

Cost Accountability

In an era of increased accountability and increasing pressure to spend health–care dollars in the most efficient, effective way, it becomes necessary to look at the technology for determining cost effectiveness. Yates explores this seldom talked about and less often understood area in some detail. He points out the gloomy statistics that medical care is escalating in cost at almost an exponential rate, 2300% since 1940, and that it consumes approximately 8% of the gross national product. Clearly, this cannot continue. Behavioral medicine offers one way to institute preventive measures that may reduce health–care costs a great deal. However, this supposition that cost care will go down must be supported with detailed analysis. He describes the three types of analysis— cost–utility analysis, cost–benefit analysis, and cost–effectiveness analysis—and explores both the differences between these statistical approaches and each of their applications. As a sample analysis, he uses various weight control programs to demonstrate that on a cost–per–pound basis for immediate treatment results, perhaps no treatment at all is most beneficial to the population as a whole, and that behavioral treatment is extremely expensive. When data become available, similar analyses can be carried out for maintenance for continued behavioral change as a consequence of various intervention. Although on initial reading this area appears to be formidable, it is one that will be increasingly relevant to our work in the area of behavioral medicine, and one that will allow us to continue to develop new treatments and demonstrate their value as interventions beyond their novelty or research interest characteristics.

CHAPTER 8

The Theory and Practice of Cost-Utility, Cost-Effectiveness, and Cost-Benefit Analysis In Behavioral Medicine: Toward Delivering More Health Care for Less Money

Brian T. Yates

The use of behavioral and cognitive–behavioral techniques to mitigate what heretofore were considered exclusively medical problems is a major development in human services (21, 22, 23, 101, 102). Unfortunately, the rise of behavioral medicine coincides with a dramatic escalation in the cost of medical services. Health–care costs have risen 2300% since 1940 (57). Private and government expenditures for treatment and prevention of health problems in the United States consumed 8% of the gross national product in 1974 (7; total public and private direct and indirect expenses for mental health consume roughly 3% of the GNP, 15). In 1975 alone, health–care costs totaled $118.5 billion (1), compared to $20 billion for mental disorders (15). Health care cost an average of $638 per U.S. citizen in 1975 (31). About 1 out of every 14 dollars of the goods and services produced by our society at present is health care. Furthermore, the cost of health care is projected to increase to 10 to 12% of the U.S. GNP—1 out of every 9 or 10 dollars—by 1990 (17).

The cost of health care is extreme and increasing. If the acceptance of behavioral medicine is not to be eclipsed by the cost–cutting that probably will take place in the near future, it must be clearly demonstrated that applying behavioral techniques to preventing and mitigating health problems is "worth it" in terms of cost as well as outcome. We must also learn how to improve systematically the cost–outcome of delivering those services.

165

Intense concern about treatment efficacy and cost may provide fertile ground for the acceptance of new technologies like behavioral medicine because such techniques may well be more cost–beneficial than traditional medical procedures. However, there is also the danger that new technologies may be viewed as mere passing fads unless they demonstrate themselves to be more cost–beneficial than traditional technologies. To assess and, hopefully, demonstrate the superior cost–beneficiality of behavioral–medical technologies, it is essential for researchers and practitioners in behavioral medicine to evaluate and attempt to improve the cost as well as the effectiveness of treatment procedures.

THREE METHODS OF EVALUATING AND IMPROVING THE COST AND OUTCOME OF BEHAVIORAL–MEDICAL TREATMENTS

The most common methods of assessing, contrasting, and improving the cost and outcomes of delivery systems for human services are: a) cost–utility analysis, b) cost–benefit analysis, and c) cost–effectiveness analysis. All of these methods are part of an input–output approach to organizational management and decision–making termed *operations research* (2, 3, 5, 8, 13, 33, 90, 94, 100), which has been used extensively to improve the cost–outcome of delivering traditional health care (29). The five general steps in operations research as they are applied in social service systems are described in a model of cost–outcome evaluation after some preliminary definitions.

Cost-Utility Analysis

Cost–utility analysis contrasts estimates of the cost of different treatment options to estimates of the outcomes that would result from implementing those options (26, 79). Cost–utility analysis usually is conducted *before* an option is selected for implementation, requiring rough estimates of option costs and option outcomes. This type of analysis is useful for making decisions if funds or time for data collection are short, or if outcomes or costs cannot be measured by other methods. A cost–utility analysis of alternative obesity reduction strategies is presented later in this chapter.

Cost-Benefit Analysis

Cost–benefit analysis contrasts the monetary costs of a treatment program to the monetary value of treatment outcomes. The contrast often takes the form of a ratio of benefits over costs. If benefits exceed costs by a substantial margin (say, two to one), a treatment is termed "cost beneficial." Different treatment strategies can be compared in terms of their benefit/cost ratios. In cost–benefit analysis, the outcomes of behavioral–medical treatments might be measured as long–range increments in extrapolated lifetime earnings produced by treatment. Usually, cost–benefit analysis involves studies of ongoing programs to obtain information on direct outcomes and costs, as well as an estimation of indirect costs and outcomes. Elaborate formulas are used to transform psychological and physiological outcomes into monetary ones.

Cost–Effectiveness Analysis

Cost–effectiveness analysis contrasts treatment costs to *non*monetary meaures of treatment outcomes. In addition, cost–effectiveness analysis is based on studies of actual treatments, rather than on the guesstimates used in cost–utility analysis. Cost–effectiveness analysis seems particularly suited to evaluation of human services because such systems typically consume monetizable resources (such as therapist and client time, facilities, equipment, and materials), but produce changes in behavior, physiology, longevity, or satisfaction ratings that are difficult or inappropriate to translate into dollars and cents.

In most instances cost–effectiveness analysis compares the relative "worth" of different programs rather than assessing a single program. A single ratio of effectiveness over cost, or cost over effectiveness, does not give the sort of absolute index of treatment worth as does a benefit/cost ratio. A cost/effectiveness ratio such as "$5 per pound lost" does, however, indicate something more about treatment than effectiveness alone. Such cost–effectiveness indices also can be used to compare the combined cost and outcome of different treatment components. An analysis presented in this chapter describes how cost/effectiveness ratios could be used to decide how to blend the four components of a hypothetical cardiovascular risk reduction program so as to maximize risk reduction given information on the costs of using each treatment component, and the constraints imposed by budgets on each type of cost.

Cost–Effectiveness Analysis Vs. Cost–Benefit Analysis

Cost–effectiveness analysis is especially appropriate for evaluation situations in which information must be obtained in a relatively short period of time, or in which comparisons of cost–outcome statistics will be made between treatments that address similar behavioral–medical problems. For example, a cost–benefit analysis that measured outcome of obesity treatments as increments in lifetime earnings would involve extrapolation of questionable reliability from short–term follow–up data and obesity–longevity statistics. This analysis could be rendered invalid by unexpected recidivism and would be a better case as a cost–effectiveness analysis of the cost per pound lost, or the cost per pound loss maintained after follow–up (e.g., 53, 95, 96). There are many other circumstances in which cost–effectiveness analysis may be superior to cost–benefit analysis (43, 54, 59, 63, 64).

Generally, if comparisons are to be made between treatments for which outcomes all can be measured in the same nonmonetary units, cost–effectiveness analysis is appropriate. For alternative treatments of obesity, cost–effectiveness comparisons could be made between cost/pound–lost ratios. However, if one has several alternatives to consider—for example, deciding whether to fund smoking reduction or exercise facilitation—a common outcome measure must be found. This common measure will have to be more global than either measure used by the individual programs.

In deciding whether to fund a smoking or exercise program, measures of a) reduction in cardiovascular risk or b) increments in lifetime earnings due to increments in longevity could be used as common outcome measures, depending on treatment goals. The former measure would allow the cost–effectiveness analysis appearing later in this chapter. The latter measure mandates cost–benefit analysis. Some decisions call for cost–outcome comparisons that can be conducted only by transforming different effectiveness indices (e.g., cardiovascular risk reduction versus reduction of heroin addiction) into the lowest common metric—monetary benefits. In this type of decision–making situation, cost–benefit analysis is appropriate.

Cost Accounting

Cost accounting, the fourth type of cost–oriented evaluation method, is mentioned here because it is used widely and provides an additional perspective on the advantages of cost–utility, cost–effectiveness, and cost–benefit analyses. Cost accounting is often misrepresented as "cost–benefit" or "cost–effectiveness" analysis. It involves only the itemization of treatment costs (often as the mean cost per client; cf. 97), usually for the purpose of forecasting budgetary trends or for evaluation when no outcome measures are available.

In cost accounting, treatments are compared solely in terms of their cost, e.g., treatment A costs $1000 per client per month whereas treatment B costs $800 per client per month. Cost accounting is conducted as part of cost–effectiveness and cost–benefit analysis, as shown in later examples. Alone, however, it is simply not enough. The major argument against cost accounting as a separate evaluation method is that it ignores the possibility that different treatments may produce different outcomes. Thus, use of cost accounting as the only analytic procedure in an evaluation of behavioral–medical treatments is as serious an error in decision–making as ignoring the possibility that treatments may differ in their cost and only assessing the efficacy of alternative treatments.

There are many differences between cost–utility, cost–effectiveness, and cost–benefit analyses, yet there are similarities as well. Each technique shares basic procedures and deals with issues of measurement, administrative decision-making, and implementation, as noted in the following model of cost–outcome analysis in general.

A MODEL FOR COST–OUTCOME ANALYSIS

This model is a synthesis of cost–outcome evaluation procedures proposed by psychologists, educators, economists, and evaluation researchers (11, 12, 18, 19, 20, 45, 51, 64, 78, 79, 82, 92, 99). It has been tested through application in residential treatments for behaviorally disturbed children (91, 99) and in obesity treatments (95, 96). It currently is being introduced in several other psychological service systems (97). The model has two major types of parameters: a) parameters for designing cost–outcome analyses and b) parameters for implementing cost-outcome analyses. Major design parameters are listed and briefly described in Table 1; major implementation parameters are noted in Table 2.

Most models include a number of basic assumptions for this model. They are: 1) all human service systems consume a mixture of resources and produce a mixture of outcomes due to the operation of certain treatment processes; 2) some of these resources, processes, and outcomes can be measured reliably and validly; and 3) outcome must be maximized in the context of certain cost constraints (the *primal* problem) or costs must be minimized while adhering to particular outcome criteria (the *dual* problem).

Parameters in the Design of Cost–Outcome Analyses

Levels of Specificity

The level of specificity at which cost and outcome data are collected may depend on the diversity of the system being analyzed as well as the purpose of data collection (39, 41, 58). If the purpose of analysis is to improve the cost–to–outcome ratio via an operations research technique of model manipulation such as linear programming (90, 94), cost and outcome data should be collected at both a specific and detailed *micro* level for the program as a whole. The justification for microlevel cost–outcome data collection is that once costs and their relation to program outcomes are known for each component, a decision can be made as to which treatment components should be changed to increase outcome or decrease cost. For example, a microlevel cost–effectiveness analysis of a residential program for problem children might collect data on the

Table 1. Parameters in the Design of Cost–Outcome Analyses

1. *Levels of Specificity:* Macro (for interprogram evaluation or intraprogram assessment of outcome changes produced by treatment innovations). Micro (to provide detailed cost-effectiveness data for use in linear programming or other procedures for deciding how to improve treatment). Same for cost and outcome data.

2. *Interest–Group Perspectives:* Different definitions and preferences for measures of cost and outcome that are expressed by different interest groups involved in the analysis. Different perspectives on cost and/or outcome might be adopted by therapists, administrators, funding agencies, clients and their associates, advocacy organizations, taxpayers, researchers. Exemplary cost perspectives: Operations, client, social, present-value, fixed–variable. Exemplary effectiveness perspectives: Business–as–usual, goal, change, normative, marginal.

3. *Variables:* May be operationalizations of perspectives. Common major cost variables as "ingredients," e.g., personnel, facilities, equipment, and materials. Many minor cost variables. Exemplary outcome variables: Nonmonetary, monetary, composite indices. Outcome variables may differ greatly between treatments, depending on client population and interest groups involved. For cost–benefit analysis, outcome variables must be monetizable.

4. *Objective/Subjective Orientation:* A continuum crossing all other parameters, applicable to cost and outcome measurement. Objective orientation is most common in research; treatment and funding decisions inevitably include subjective as well as objective data. Examples of subjective data that are and should be integral to cost–outcome analyses are case anecdotes, client fears, the "hassle" in client implementation of treatment procedures, and the benefits of undergoing treatment as they are perceived by the client and concerned others.

5. *Certainty/Uncertainty:* Regardless of objectivity/subjectivity, data collected on costs and psychological and medical processes and outcomes naturally are associated with some uncertainty. When such data are used in operations research as a basis for crucial decisions, the uncertainty of the data should be taken into account by conducting sensitivity analysis of the cost–outcome findings. Sensitivity analysis involves reworking of the analysis with "worst case" and "best case" data expressing lower and upper bounds of treatment costs and outcomes. The results of sensitivity analysis illustrate the degree of "noise" in the cost–outcome indices.

---

cost of reducing, by one standard deviation, the difference between the frequencies at which a problem child and a normal child emit each of several important interpersonal behaviors (99).

To evaluate the success of changes in the treatment that were made on the basis of micro cost–outcome assessment, a more global macrolevel assessment is conducted to contrast overall long–term outcomes to total treatment costs (see Table 2). Yates et al. (99) performed this sort of analysis by comparing the total funds consumed by a residential treatment program to the number of rehabilitated children who did not relapse during the year following treatment.

Interest-Group Perspectives

The way in which cost and outcome data are to be collected is a function of the interest groups involved in the analysis as well as the level of specificity (36, 42, 76). Each of the following interest groups may have different and, in some cases, conflicting views on what and how cost and outcome data should be collected: a) therapists; b) treatment administrators (48); c) funding agencies (55); d) clients who receive treatment; e) relatives and close associates of clients (38, 103); f) advocacy organizations that represent past, present, or potential clients (6, 81); g) taxpayers; and h) researchers (56). Barriers to the cost–outcome analysis are sometimes erected by pressures from conflicting interest groups. Some of these "political problems" can be mitigated by measuring costs and outcomes from the perspectives of several groups and then forming composite cost, outcome, and cost–outcome indices that are the weighted averages of measures advocated by different interest groups (20, 34, 49, 68, 80).

Costing Perspectives.   Some perspectives are adopted so commonly that it is useful to assign them particular names. In measurement of service costs, the operations, client, social, present–value, and fixed/variable perspectives are commonly considered. From the *operations* perspective, cost is measured simply as the cost shown in accounting records. Operations cost values include monetary expenditures, employee benefits, and depreciation of facilities and equipment. *Clients* and the friends and relatives of clients may be more concerned with their own expenses for treatment, including time devoted to treatment activities, forgone earnings, and the subjective cost or "hassle" of treatment (15, 56, 95). The *social* costing perspective takes the opportunity value position that resources donated to treatment (such as volunteers' time) actually cost society something because those resources are not available for alternative uses and should be measured along with operations costs to provide more comprehensive cost assessment.

The *present–value* perspective on costs is likely to be adopted when treatments may have long- as well as short-run costs. This perspective often is used in conjunction with others to quantify the cost of treatment as it is distributed over time. Basically, the present–value perspective modifies the total cost of a treatment by devaluing delayed costs according to a discount rate:

$$\text{Present Value Cost} = \sum_{t=1}^{N} [\$_{(t)}/(1 + d)^t] \tag{1}$$

where $\$_{(t)}$ is treatment cost during time period t, N is the total number of time periods required for treatment, and d is the discount rate (79). The discount rate that should be used in present–value costing is often debated, but usually is between .05 and .10 per year (10, 52). The higher the discount rate, the less effect delayed costs have on overall estimates of treatment costs. Use of the present-value perspective favors treatments that maintain the same cost over time or, better yet, spend more in the later than in earlier periods. For example, a program that requires $100,000 during the first year but only $50,000 for the remaining four years is more costly from the present-value perspective than is a program requiring $50,000 for the first four years but $100,000 in the fifth year ($245,932 versus $233,665—a difference of $12,267). Outcomes also can be present-valued. Of course, the present-value perspective favors service systems that produce the major outcomes quickly (97).

A final perspective relevant to cost measurement is the *fixed/variable* cost distinction. Fixed costs are overhead costs that must be paid regardless of the number of clients treated. Variable costs (food in inpatient programs, for example) are incurred in direct proportion to the number of clients treated. Programs with primarily variable costs are more flexible; they can adapt more rapidly to changes in funding and client load. On the other hand, if a high percentage of treatment costs are fixed, an economies-of-scale problem may occur in which only large client enrollments will allow the treatment to be cost-effective.

Effectiveness Perspectives.   Several perspectives unique to outcome measurement can be differentiated. The *business-as-usual* perspective considers outcome satisfactory unless proven otherwise by a dramatic event. The *goal* perspective assesses outcome relative to a priori goals, such as evaluating obesity treatment in terms of the proportional reduction in obesity (74, 96). The *change* perspective simply asks that some (positive) change occur. From the *normative* perspective, therapeutic outcome is measured relative to the normative state (an inappropriate measure for programs aimed at cardiovascular risk reduction, due to the normalcy of cardiovascular morbidity and mortality; cf. 60, 99). *Marginal* perspectives compare the outcome of treatment to the outcome of alternatives such as traditional regimens or no treatment. The marginal perspective is often adopted to measure treatment costs as well. Use of the marginal perspective on effectiveness in cost-oriented assessments is sometimes called "cost-efficiency analysis" (61).

Variables

The variables used in measurement of cost and outcome are determined largely by the level of specificity and perspective selected in analysis design, but again there are a number of different cost and outcome variables.

Cost Variables.   The variables used in measuring resources consumed by treatment can be best selected by noting what goes into treatment. This *ingredients* approach (25, 45, 87) typically yields three major cost variables: a) personnel, b) facilities, and c) equipment and materials (see 75). Each major cost variable may contain many minor variables, the exact nature of which is determined by the specificity and perspective parameters adopted. For example, from the operation perspective, the cost variable of personnel is composed of salaries paid to different types of personnel. From the social perspective, personnel subvariables might itemize personnel costs by educational background and experience. The value of the social subvariables for personnel might be the product of the number of hours the staff member (volunteer or paid) spent in any treatment-related activity, times the going hourly payrate for staff of that background and educational level (e.g. 99). Viewed from the client perspective, personnel time would amount to the time spent by the client in treatment-related activities.

If microlevel analysis is being conducted and cost data are available only at a macrolevel, the macro cost data have to be broken down until they are at the same microlevel as are effectiveness data. The micro cost variables should be developed so that they can be combined with outcome variables when calculating cost-outcome indices (e.g., 99).

Outcome Variables.   Although the same basic cost variables are used in most types of cost-outcome analysis, the outcome variables selected depend on the type of analysis being performed, the levels of specificity used, the perspectives chosen, and the purposes of the treatment program. If a cost-utility or cost-effectiveness analysis is to be conducted within a single treatment program, outcome variables can be specific to the treatment (e.g., reduction in number of cigarettes smoked for smoking reduction programs). Cost-utility and cost-effectiveness analyses that include alternative treatments for the same health problem also can use highly specific outcome variables. However, if the cost-utility or cost-effectiveness analysis is to compare diverse treatments, a more general outcome variable that is shared by both should be used.

If a cost-benefit analysis is being designed, outcome variables that can be transformed into monetary values should be selected. For example, in cost-benefit analysis of alternative heroin treatments, the outcome variable of opiate-free days might be used if the analysts had derived a procedure for assessing the monetary savings to society of each opiate-free day (65, 66). Other monetizable outcome variables are reduced absenteeism or accident rates observed for an industrial program that helped employees deal with alcoholism and family problems (40).

Objective/Subjective Orientation

In order to depict all cost–outcome analyses, the present model must recognize that outcomes and costs can be and are assessed on a continuum of objectivity–subjectivity. Some evaluators may advocate dispensing with subjective assessments; yet to do so is to wish away human nature and the nature of the political processes that control the funding of human services (34, 50). "Objective" assessments of costs and outcomes can ignore important variables such as morbidity (instead of mortality). Furthermore, subjective costs and outcomes experienced by the client may well determine which recommended treatment procedures (e.g., medication, exercise) are actually adhered to by the client (95).

Techniques can be borrowed from social and personality psychology to measure subjective assessments of treatment costs and outcomes (96). In this way, subjective costs and subjective outcomes can be considered explicitly in decisions. Weinstein and Stason (82), for example, consider the subjective outcome of *quality* of life sufficiently important to include it in their equation for quantifying treatment outcome in medicine:

$$\Delta E = \Delta Y_{Morbidity} - \Delta Y_{Side-Effects} \qquad (2)$$

where ΔE is change in outcome in quality–adjusted life-years produced by treatment, ΔY is positive change in duration of life, $\Delta Y_{Morbidity}$ is positive change in the quality of life years due to reduction of morbidity risks, and $\Delta Y_{Side-Effects}$ is negative change in the quality of life–years due to increases in morbidity or other negative side effects of treatment. Although there is room for error in such qualitative measurements (28), they seem terribly important to measure in analysis of programs in behavioral medicine.

Certainty/Uncertainty

Data collected for cost–outcome analysis always will have some uncertainty associated with them. For cost–oriented analyses, the degree of uncertainty in cost and outcome data is considered explicitly in *sensitivity analysis*. Basically, sensitivity analysis is a reworking of the cost–outcome analysis based on the worst–case and best–case scenarios of cost and outcome. In the operations research technique of linear programming, sensitivity analysis is conducted in a sophisticated manner to discover which cost constraints could be slackened so as to produce the cheapest increase in oveall system productivity (37). Thus, explicitly recognizing the inherent certainty/uncertainty of cost and outcome data not only allows more rational decision–making, but also provides a method of determining how to obtain maximal increases in treatment outcome from minimal increases in treatment costs.

The model presented above can serve as a conceptual device for conducting cost–outcome analysis. The following cost–utility, cost–effectiveness, and cost–benefit analyses provide concrete demonstrations of how the model can be applied in behavioral medicine.

Parameters in the Implementation of Cost–Outcome Analyses

Steps for Implementation

Levels of specificity, perspectives on measurement, and variables for cost and outcome measurement are important in designing cost–outcome analyses. The steps outlined in Table 2 indicate how implementation of a complete cost–outcome analysis might proceed in the context of the operations research approach to systematically improving (instead of summarily "evaluating") treatment.

Table 2. Parameters for Implementing Complete Cost–Outcome Analyses: Steps

a. Assess macro cost–outcome.

b. Determine contribution of each treatment component to treatment outcome.

c. Assess micro (process) cost–outcome of each treatment component for each resource type consumed.

d. Estimate maximum amount of each resource type available.

e. Use data from steps 2, 3, and 4 to decide, via linear programming or other procedure, how to best improve the macro cost–outcome of treatment by changing execution levels of treatment components.

f. Implement treatment innovations on a small scale.

g. Assess macro cost–outcome again and determine if it has been improved by decision-making procedure.

h. If macro cost–outcome is not improved after implementation of solution, return to Step *b* and revise the model of the service system. If macro cost–outcome is improved, increase scope of innovation implementation with periodic assessment of macro cost–outcome.

The same basic steps are followed for cost–utility, cost–effectiveness, and cost–benefit analyses. The primary difference is that steps b, c, and d involve data collection in actual treatments for cost–effectiveness or cost–benefit analysis; in cost–utility analysis these steps involve collection of etimates from experts. Implementation begins in all three types of analysis with assesment of the overall cost/outcome ratio of the treatment system, step a. Analysis proceeds through steps b, c, and d to compose a model (usually mathematical) of the service system. Next, the model is manipulated mathematically to find ways to increase outcome while holding costs constant, or ways to decrease cost while holding outcome constant (e). The analysis then tries out the way that appears best (f). If the innovation is successful in the pilot version, step g, it is implemented on a broader scale (i). If not, the model is reconstructed (h). Accountability is built into the analysis itself; if cost–outcome analysis no longer produces outcomes that are worth the cost of analysis, analysis is terminated.

EXEMPLARY COST–OUTCOME ANALYSES

A Cost–Utility Analysis of Obesity Reduction Treatments

The problem focused on by this analysis is optimization of the cost–utility of alternative obesity reduction methods. Assessment was conducted at the macrolevel because the data lacked specificity. Manipulation of a macro cost–utility model was used to decide which treatments should be used within a set of cost or effectiveness constraints.

Model–Building Method and Results

Obtaining Cost and Outcome Estimates.   Participants at a behavioral–medical conference were asked to supply the following objective and subjective outcome and cost estimates for obesity reduction techniques with which they were familiar: a) "long–term success rate per 100 clients (achievement of substantial to complete loss of excess weight)"; b) "monetary cost of full implementation of technique per client"; c) "rating of subjective *benefits to client* of successful technique application" (a rating of "1" indicates "no benefit," a rating of "10" indicates "extreme benefit" on a 10–point scale); and d) "rating of subjective *costs to client* of successful technique application (a rating of "1" indicates "no subjective cost," a rating of "10" indicates "extreme cost" on a 10–point scale)."

In each of their four responses, participants were asked to provide their 1) "best guess," 2) *"upper bound* of estimate," and 3) *"lower bound* of estimate." Participants were informed that their data would be used in a presentation, but were not told the exact way in which it would be manipulated. Participants were later assured that their techniques would not be connected in any publication with the data they provided; hence, the particular treatments assessed cannot be described. Objective and subjective cost and outcome data were provided by 11 of the 17 participants.

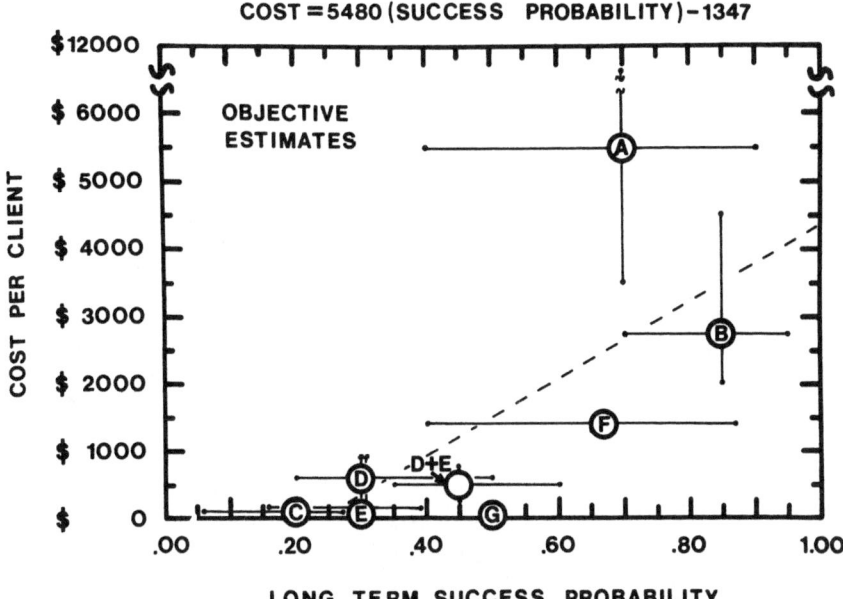

Fig. 1. Cost–utility analysis: Objective cost per client and success rates for obesity treatments, as estimated by experts (circles denote best–guess estimates, axes are formed by upper– and lower–bound estimates).

Responses.   All responses to the cost–utility questionnaire are listed in Table 3. Responses to upper– and lower–bound queries are parenthesized and weight reduction techniques are denoted by capital letters. Probability estimates of long–term success were the result of dividing each participant's response to question a by 100.

Calculating Cost–Utility Indices.   For each obesity reduction technique, the average cost per successful client was estimated by dividing the monetary cost estimate (b) in Table 3 by the long–term success probability estimate (a). The resulting Objective Cost–Utility Indices are listed in column (e) of Table 3. The indices formed by using upper– and lower–bound cost and success estimates are listed within parentheses. Figure 1 provides a graphic presentation of the way in which lower– and upper–bound estimates of cost and success combine to form objective cost–utility indices. Graphing the range of the cost and success estimates for each obesity reduction technique produces cost–utility areas for each technique. Figure 1 shows considerable overlap in objective cost–utility space for techniques that cost under $1000/client.

Table 3. Results of the Cost–Utility Questionnaire

Obesity Reduction Technique	Questionnaire Responses					Derived Indices	
	(a) Long–Term Success Probability Estimate. best guess (lower bound–upper bound)	(b) Monetary Cost best guess (lower bound–upper bound)	(c) Subjective Utility to Client Rating. (1 = no benefit 10 = extreme benefit)	(d) Subjective Costs to Client Rating. (1 = no cost, 10 = extreme cost)	(e) Objective Cost–Utility Index. Estimated Cost per Successful Client. (b/a)	(f) Subjective Utility–Cost Estimate (c/d)	(g) Composite Cost–Utility Index. (e/f)
A1	.65 (.50–.79)	$6000 (none)	8 (3–8)	5 (3–8)	$9231 ($7595–$12,000)	1.6 (0.8–3.0)	$5769 ($2532–$15,000)
A2	.75 (.40–.90)	$5000 ($3500–$12,000)	9 (4–10)	none	$6667 ($3889–$30,000)	—	—
Mean of A's	.70 (.40–.90)	$5500 ($3500–$12,000)	8.5 (4–10)	5 (3–8)	$7857 ($3889–$30,000)	1.7 (0.5–3.3)	$4622 ($1178–$60,000)
B1	.90 (.70–.95)	$2000 (none)	8 (6–10)	6 (4–8)	$2222 ($2105–$2857)	1.3 (0.8–2.5)	$1709 ($842–$3571)
B2	.80 (.70–.90)	$3500 ($3000–$4500)	8 (7–9)	3 (2–4)	$4375 ($3333–$6429)	2.7 (1.8–4.5)	$1620 ($741–$3572)
C	.20 (.05–.30)	$10 ($5–$15)	8 (5–10)	8 (5–10)	$50 ($17–$300)	1.0 (0.5–2.0)	$50 ($9–600)
D	.30 (.20–.50)	$600 ($400–$800)	7 (6–8)	5 (4–6)	$2000 ($800–$4000)	1.4 (1.0–2.0)	$1429 ($400–$4000)
E	.30 (.15–.40)	$500 ($400–$800)	8 (6–10)	5 (none)	$1667 ($1000–$5333)	1.6 (1.2–2.0)	$1042 ($500–$4444)
D + E	.45 (.35–.60)	$500 ($300–$700)	5 (4–8)	1 (1–2)	$1111 ($500–$2000)	5.0 (2.0–8.0)	$222 ($63–$1000)
F	.67 (.40–.87)	$1400 (none)	8 (6–10)	3 (1–5)	$2090 ($1609–$3500)	2.7 (1.2–10.0)	$774 ($161–$2917)
G	.56 (none)	$50 (20–$100)	none	none	$89 ($36–$179)	—	—

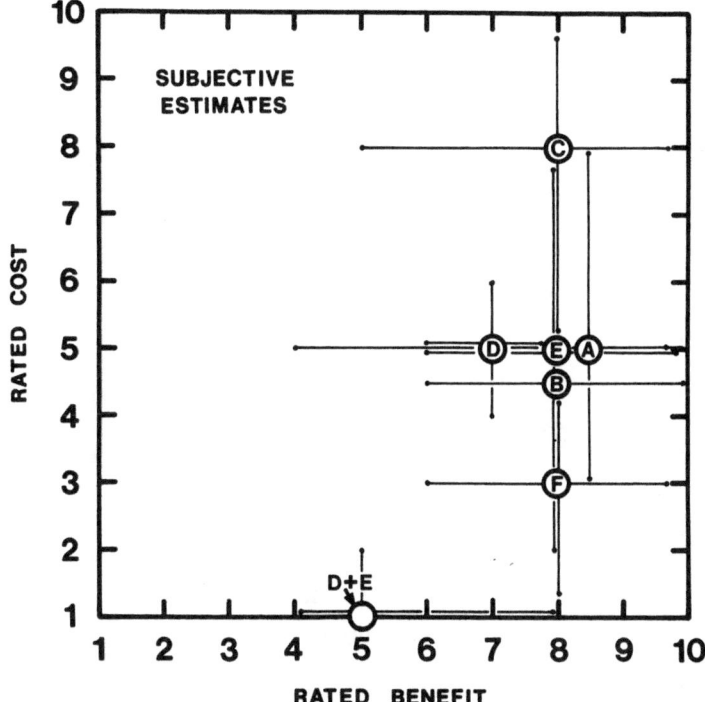

Fig. 2. Cost–utility analysis: Subjective cost and subjective benefit for obesity treatments, as estimated by experts (circles denote best–guess estimates, axes are formed by upper- and lower-bound estimates).

Subjective Cost–Utility Estimates (column f in Table 3) were the quotients of the subjective utility rating (c) over the subjective cost rating (d). Upper and lower bounds were calculated in the same way as for Objective Cost–Utility Indices. These indices were greater than one if rated utility exceeded rated cost and were less than one if rated cost exceeded rated utility. The subjective cost–utility areas are shown in Figure 2. The extreme overlap of the subjective cost–utility areas may be a natural product of the high uncertainty in estimates of subjective costs and outcome. Alternatively, the researchers who provided the subjective (to the client) cost and success estimates may have been unfamiliar with the subjective costs and outcomes experienced by the clients.

The Composite Cost–Utility Index (g in Table 3) was formed by dividing the Objective Cost–Utility Index by the Subjective Cost–Utility Index for each treatment strategy. This procedure decreased the value of the Objective Index if subjective utility exceeded subjective cost; otherwise the Objective Index

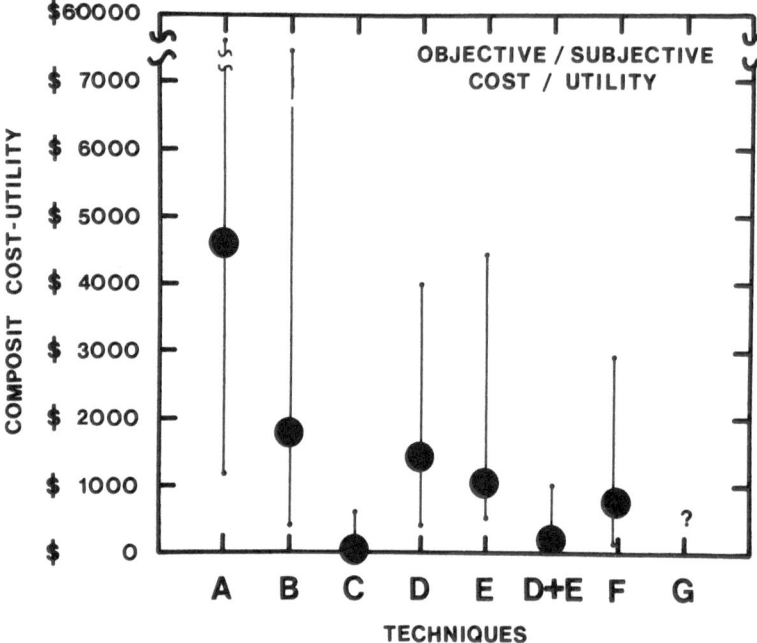

Fig. 3. Cost–utility analysis: Composite objective/subjective cost–utility indices (circles denote best–guess values, axes are for upper– and lower–bound values).

increased. Figure 3 presents the Composite Indices resulting from the best–guess, lower–bound, and upper–bound estimates for each obesity reduction technique.

Relationship Between Cost and Outcome Estimates.   Before a description of how cost–utility indices are used in decision–making can be given, the relationship between the cost and outcome estimates obtained should be examined. It was found that the "best guess" values of objective cost and objective outcome were significantly and strongly related, $r = 0.67, p = <.05$, as were the subjective cost and outcome estimates, $r = .67, p <.05$. The striking similarity of these correlations might be interpreted as indicating a relationship between subjective and objective estimates. However, this interpretation is not supportd by correlations between objective and subjective outcome estimates, $r = .25$, (n.s.), or between objective and subjective cost estimates, $r = -.15$ (n.s.). Apparently, the objective and subjective estimates are somewhat independent for cost and for outcome.

Model Manipulation: Decision–Making with Cost–Utility Information

Treatment Cost Given Outcome Constraints.   Given the moderate linearity of best–guess cost and outcome estimates in both objective and subjective cases (as indicated by their .67 correlations), we can interpolate the costs of different success rates. On the basis of the objective estimates, the intercept of the cost–success function for obesity reduction techniques is −$1347 with a slope of $548 per 10% increment in success rate (see Figure 1). If this function is correct, a 50% success rate requires an average of $1393 per client, and a 90% success rate would cost $3585/client. The interception of the line function with the technique cost–utility areas in Figure 1 indicates that techniques D, F, G, or hybrid technique D+E could be used to achieve the 50% success rate. This type of information might be useful in the design and implementation of weight control programs.

Treatment Outcome Given Cost Constraints.   The objective linear function also can be used to decide whether a program should be implemented by comparing the minimal acceptable success rate to the success rate predicted by the linear function for a cost figure. For example, if a business wished to spend no more than $500 per overweight employee for obesity reduction, it could expect a 34% success rate based on the cost–utility data. Techniques E, G, or D+E could be used to obtain this outcome, according to Figure 1. If a 34% success rate was at or above the success criterion adopted by the business, treatment would be recommended; if not, it would not be "worth it" to initiate the weight reduction program. Similar decision–making procedures could be used to help individual clients decide which obesity program to use (97).

Discussion

According to the linear equation, a success rate of approximately 24% can be produced without *any* monetary expenditures. This result may seem ludicrous at first glance, but it may actually represent the success rate achievable by self–initiation and self–run obesity reduction programs (27).

Subjective costs and outcomes and composite indices generally can be used in decision–making in the same way that objective costs and outcomes were used in the above example. The subjective and composite indices generated in this analysis have such high uncertainty (as indicated by the wide ranges between upper– and lower–bound estimates in Figures 2 and 3), however, that decisions based on them probably would be too uncertain to be of value.

Table 4. Sensitivity Analysis of Objective Cost–Utility Estimates for Obesity Reduction Techniques

	Predictions of Cost, Given a Criterion of 50% Success	Predictions of Success Rate, Given a Criterion of $500 Spent per Client
"Best Guess" (using best–guess cost and utility estimates)	$1393	34%
"Worst Case" (using upper–bound cost and lower–bound utility estimates)	$3437	1%
"Best Case" (using lower–bound cost and upper–bound utility estimates)	$ 445	51%

Caveats.   There are, of course, a number of qualifications to be attached to any cost–oriented analysis, and the present one is no exception. First, the output of analysis is only as valid as the data used in the analysis. Because cost–utility analyses are based on estimates rather than actual observations of ongoing treatments, the data put into the analysis may be less valid than data used in cost–effectiveness and cost–benefit analyses. Second, implicit in the above analysis was the somewhat simplistic assumption that the techniques assessed are equally applicable to all obese clients. In fact, some of the techniques were surgical and are designed only for the grossly overweight. A more complete analysis would obtain cost and success estimates for more treatments and would specify separate cost–success functions for different obese subpopulations. Even the most experimentally rigorous cost–outcome analysis may have low external validity if it does not include many different treatment techniques, because some of the techniques may greatly affect the cost–outcome equation.

Sensitivity Analysis.   Given the magnitude of monetary investment called for in the above decision analyses, it is important to conduct a sensitivity analysis of the cost–utility equation on which decisions will be based. A relatively simple sensitivity analysis was performed by first calculating linear equations for the worst– and best–case scenarios of cost–utility relationships for the obesity treatments. The worst–case equation was computed on the basis of the upper–bound cost estimates and lower–bound success estimates in Table 3; the best–case equation was based on lower–bound cost and upper–bound success estimates. Contrasting for the same success rate, the treatment costs derived from the worst–case, best–case, and best–guess equations show that a 50% success rate might cost as little as $445 or as much as $3437 per client. Success rates calculated from the three equations and a fixed cost also are highly variable (see Table 4).

The results of this sensitivity analysis suggest that the cost and success rates inferred from these particular cost and outcome estimates are too uncertain to be of practical use. The results are only suggestive. Solicitation of more carefully defined data from a larger pool of experts may yield more reliable cost–utility functions (98). The large differences between best– and worst–case cost and success rates suggest that actual data from ongoing treatments, as would be obtained in cost–effectiveness and cost–benefit analyses, could provide a firmer basis for treatment decisions.

A Hypothetical Cost–Effectiveness Analysis of a Multi–Component Cardiovascular Risk Reduction Program

The previous cost–utility example illustrated not only cost–utility analysis but also the consideration of subjective as well as objective indices of cost and outcome. Objective/subjective parameters can be employed explicitly in cost–effectiveness or cost–benefit analysis as well. The following example illustrates the use of two additional parameters of the cost–outcome analysis model that can be included in any type of analysis—marginal perspectives on cost and outcome, and micro– and macrolevels. The cost–effectiveness analysis shows how micro– and macrolevel assessment of cost–effectiveness can be used in linear–programming sensitivity analyses to optimize effectiveness within certain cost constraints and to minimize cost given specific effectiveness criteria. Although the following example uses largely hypothetical data, it illustrates basic procedures for cost–effectiveness analysis.

Model–Building Method and Results

The hypothetical program had four components, each designed to reduce a particular behavior or physiological state that is strongly related to cardiovascular risk (16): a) serum cholesterol, b) systolic blood pressure, c) relative weight [100 × (actual weight/median weight for sex and height)], and d) cigarette smoking. The program used behavioral techniques delivered by media and mail advertising, as well as direct therapist–client contact with adjunct bibliotherapy to modify the four risk factors listed above. The hypothetical study involved an

Table 5. Micro– and Macro– Level Effectiveness Data for the Four Components of a Hypothetical Cardiovascular Risk Reduction Program

Treatment Group		Serum Cholesterol (mg/100 ml)	Systolic Blood Pressure (mm Hg)	Relative Weight (see text for units)	Cigarettes Smoked
			Program Components		
Experimental	Pre	250	150	128.6	20
	Post	230	140	120.7	13
	Δ	20	10	7.9	7
Control	Pre	250	152	127.9	20
	Post	249	151	125.7	22
	Δ	1	1	2.2	-2
Marginal Effectiveness		19	9	5.7	9

Note: In this hypothetical study, the average age of participants is 45 years.

experimental group of 100 high–risk males between 40 and 49 years of age and employed a control group of 100 males matched to members of the experimental group in age and levels of risk factors. Physiological and behavioral measures were obtained for each participant in both experimental and control groups on the four program components before and after bibliotherapy.

Macrolevel Cost–Effectiveness. Information obtained in a follow–up indicated that the experimental group would experience 15 cardiovascular morbidity or mortality events per 1000 participants in the six years following treatment. The control group was expected to experience 28 such events per 1000 over six subsequent years. This marginal decrement of 13 morbidity/mortality events per 1000 cost a total of $76,900 in program funds; $5915 per expected event avoided or 1.7 events avoided per $10,000 spent, on the average.

Microlevel Effectiveness. Effectiveness is measured for each participant and for each risk–reduction component first in terms of units specific to that component (i.e., serum cholesterol in mg/100 ml, systolic blood pressure in mm Hg, relative weight, and cigarette smoking as mean number of cigarettes per day for the most recent week). The resulting average effectiveness values for groups are shown in Table 5 along with effectiveness values for the treatment versus the control groups.

Micro– and Macrolevel Cost. The ingredients approach and operations perspective are used in this cost asessment. The major resource ingredients are

Table 6. Micro- and Macro- Level Cost Data for the Four Components of a Hypothetical Cardiovascular Risk Reduction Program

	Program Components				
	Serum Cholesterol	Systolic Blood Pressure	Weight	Cigarette Smoking	Totals
Costs of Ingredients					
Advertising					
Specific	$ 300	$ 600	$ 600	$ 1,500	$ 3,000
Share of Overall	$ 200	$ 200	$ 200	$ 200	$ 800
Bibliotherapy	$ 200	$ 300	$ 500	$ 800	$ 1,800
Therapists	$ 3,600	$ 7,200	$10,800	$14,400	$36,000
Measurement	$ 1,100	$ 600	$ 100	$ 1,500	$ 3,000
Program Administration	$ 8,000	$ 8,000	$ 8,000	$ 8,000	$32,000
	Summary Component Costs				
Fixed	$ 8,200	$ 8,200	$ 8,200	$ 8,200	$32,800
Variable	$ 5,200	$ 8,700	$12,000	$18,200	$44,100
Total	$13,400	$16,900	$20,200	$26,400	$76,900
% of Total	18%	22%	26%	34%	100%

listed at the top of Table 6, with itemizations for each component listed. Some advertising and all administrative costs are not attributable to any particular component. These fixed costs were divided equally over the components. Bibliotherapy, therapist, and measurement costs vary between components. These fixed and variable costs are listed and summed in the lowest columns in Table 6. The *marginal micro cost* of each component is the variable cost of that component (the increment over fixed treatment costs spent for component execution). Table 6 indicates that therapists are the most expensive resource, accounting for 47% of the total, macrolevel treatment cost of $76,900. Inspection of Table 6 shows that the smoking reduction component is the most expensive component.

Adjusting Cost and Effectiveness Indices.   The next step in cost–effectiveness analysis is to form cost–effectiveness ratios for each component and for each type of resource consumed. Typically, cost data are available only for entire components of a program, and must be transformed into per–client per–com-

Table 7. Microlevel Cost-Effectiveness Indices (Cost Per Unit Factor Reduction) for Linear Programming in a Hypothetical Cardiovascular Risk Reduction Program

Resource Types	Components				Cost Constraints
	Serum Cholesterol	Systolic Blood Pressure	Weight	Smoking	
Advertising (Specific)	$15.79 (per 1 mg/ 100 ml)	$66.67 (per 1 mm Hg)	$105.26 (per 1% decrease)	$166.67 (per ciga- rette)	⩽ $3,000
Bibliotherapy	$10.53 (per 1 mg/ 100 ml)	$33.33 (per 1 mm Hg)	$87.72 (per 1% decrease)	$88.89 (per ciga- rette)	⩽ $1,800
Therapists	$189.47 (per 1 mg/ 100 ml)	$800.00 (per 1 mm Hg)	$1,894.74 (per 1% decrease)	$1,600.00 (per ciga- rette)	⩽ $36,000
Measurement	$57.89 (per 1 mg/ 100 ml)	$66.67 (per 1 mm Hg)	$17.54 (per 1% decrease)	$166.67 (per ciga- rette)	⩽ $3,300
Maintenance of Ideal Risk Factor Labels					
I_{chol}	1	0	0	0	⩽ 30
I_{bld}	0	1	0	0	⩽ 30
I_{wt}	0	0	1	0	⩽ 28.6
I_{smk}	0	0	0	1	⩽ 21.0
Y Unit Reduction in Risk Factor Level	−.007	−.009	−.027	−.043	

ponent costs. In some programs it may be necessary to itemize the cost of treating specific clients (cf. 99). For the purpose of illustrating cost–effectiveness analysis and linear programming, however, analysis is performed for the group as a whole (effectiveness and cost will be maintained at a per–group instead of per–client level).

Micro Cost–Effectiveness Indices for Linear Programming. Microlevel cost-effectiveness indices are calculated separately for each treatment component and for each type of resource consumed by components (Table 7). These ratios are calculated by dividing the variable cost values (given in Table 6) for components and resource types (i.e., advertising—specific only, bibliotherapy, therapists, and measurement) by the marginal effectiveness values listed for each component

(Table 5). The units of these cost–effectiveness indices are the same in the numerator, but component-specific in the denominator (e.g., dollars per 1 mg/100 ml decrease in serum cholesterol). (Only variable costs were used in these calculations because it was assumed that the fixed, overhead costs of nonspecific advertising and program administration would have to be borne in approximately the same amount regardless of the exact nature of components used.)

Risk–Reduction Constants for Different Components.   The final step in the microlevel cost–effectiveness analysis is to specify the contribution of different components to the program of cardiovascular risk reduction. In the present example, the reduction in cardiovascular risk that could be expected as a result of one unit movement, e.g., 1 mg/100 ml decrease in serum cholesterol, is computed and is shown in the Table 7, row "ΔY." (Change in Y was used instead of a change in R in the following equation, 3a, because Y is linearly related to the risk factors—a necessary assumption of linear programming—and R is not.)

The decrement in risk is calculated from a set of equations adapted from Cornfield and Mitchell (16) for persons between 40 and 49 years of age. The first equation expresses the number of persons per 1000 who are predicted to experience morbidity or mortality due to cardiovascular dysfunction in the six years following measurement. The second equation, which must be solved for Y in order to solve the first equation, weights risk as a function of the client's current level on each major risk factor.

$$R = \text{Clients}/1000 = \frac{100}{(1 + e^{(-Y)})} \tag{3a}$$

where e is the exponential constant (2.71828),

$$Y = 13.7 + .007 \ x_{chol} + .009 \ x_{bld} + .027 \ x_{wt} + .434 \ x_{smk} + .120 \ x_{age} \tag{3b}$$

and x_{chol} is mg/100 ml of cholesterol, x_{bld} is blood pressure in mm of Hg, x_{wt} is relative weight, i.e. [(100 × (actual weight/median weight in population of same sex and height)], x_{smk} is amount of smoking (0 = never smoked, 1 = less than 1 pack/day, 2 = 1 pack/day, 3 = more than 1 pack/day), and x_{age} is the client's age in years.

Equations 3a and 3b express risk at fixed risk–factor levels. Change in risk is calculated as the difference between the "clients/1000" values produced by using the pretreatment levels and a 1–unit decrease in risk–factor level for a given factor. For example, risk is 30 cardiovascular events/1000 persons with the same characteristics/6 years at 250 mg/100 ml of serum cholesterol (Table 5), the i unit decrease value is 249 mg/100 ml of serum cholesterol, and Y changes from −.860 to −.867 when serum cholesterol drops from 250 to 249 mg/100 ml. In a nonhypothetical study one would have to demonstrate the applicability of the

**Table 8. Cost of Avoiding One Cardiovascular
Mortality/Morbidity Event/1000 Persons/6 Years for Different
Resources and Different Treatment Components
(Hypothetical Data)**

Resource Types	Components			
	Serum Cholesterol	Systolic Blood Pressure	Weight	Smoking
Advertising (Specific)	$ 42.80	$ 198.70	$ 150.75	$ 43.30
Bibliotherapy	28.50	99.30	125.65	23.10
Therapists	513.60	2384.10	2713.55	415.70
Measurement	156.90	198.70	25.15	43.30

Note: These ratios were calculated by dividing the cost data provided in Table 8 by the ΔR values for specific components.

equations to predicting risk reduction before cost–effectiveness analysis could be performed.*

The data provided in Table 7 allow estimation of the amount of each resource type that was expended in each component for risk reduction. For example, $42.80 of component–specific Advertising, $28.50 of Bibliotherapy, $513.60 of Therapists, and $156.90 of Measurement could be used to produce a risk reduction of 1 event/1000/6 years via a 2.71 mg/100 ml reduction of serum cholesterol. These cost–effectiveness ratios (see Table 8) provide an intuitively appealing array of data that may be used in decision–making. However, when one is faced with cost constraints, the ratios would be difficult to use in deciding how to maximize macrolevel outcome—i.e., risk reduction—by dictating specific changes in risk–factor levels. Linear programming does this job reasonably well; it indicates how much each component should be implemented to reduce risk to the lowest possible level, given budget limitations on use of each resource.

---

* In Cornfield and Mitchell's equation, the coefficient of smoking is .434, and x_{smk} could be only 0 (never smoked), 1 (less than 1 pack/day), 2 (1 pack/day), or 3 (more than one pack per day). The present ΔY coefficient of .043 for smoking is an attempt to express risk as a function of exact number of cigarettes smoked, and was derived and calculated ΔY as ... + .434[s − (1/20 of 21)] ... or ... + .434(1.9) + ... to express ΔY as a function of a 1–cigarette-per–day reduction in smoking.

Model Manipulation: Deciding How to Improve Effectiveness or Reduce Costs

The model-manipulation technique of linear programming involves solution of a model of a service system that can be quantitatively expressed in terms of equations (4a) and (4b):

$$\text{Maximize Z, where } Z = \sum_{j=1}^{n} (c_{(j)}x_{(j)}) \qquad (4a)$$

where Z is treatment outcome, j is one of n treatment components, $c_{(j)}$ expresses the contribution to treatment outcome of a unit of execution of component j (c is ΔY in the present example), and $x_{(j)}$ is the number of units of component execution to be solved for. Equation 4a must be solved for x_j within the resource expenditure constraints:

$$\sum_{j=1}^{n} (a_{(i. j)}x_{(j)}) \leq b_{(c)} \qquad (4b)$$

$b_{(c)}$ is the maximum of resource type i that can be expended during execution of all treatment components combined, $a_{(i+ j)}$ is the amount of resource type i that is required to produce a unit of execution of component j ($a_{(i. j)}$ is the cost figures in Table 7 for the present example), and $x_{(j)}$ again is the units of component execution to be solved for (see *8* for a good, simple discussion of linear programming that does not assume a background in algebra).

Table 9 provides the linear programming equations for the present cost-effectiveness analysis. Because it would be undesirable to further exacerbate risk factors, the constraints $x_{(j)} \geq 0$ on component execution were added. Since component execution that moved risk-factor levels below ideal levels also was not desirable, an additional set of resource constraints that limited risk-factor reduction to ideal levels was used. Resources I_{chol}, I_{bld}, I_{wt}, and I_{smk} were entered into the linear programming matrix, as shown in Tables 8 and 9, with constraints of ≤ 30 (to 220 mg/ 100 ml), ≤ 30 (to 120 mm Hg), ≤ 28.6 (to 100.0 relative weight), and ≤ 21 (to 0 cigarettes per day), respectively.

The linear equations first are solved to maximize treatment effectiveness given cost constraints by using a packaged computer program commonly available in business and economics courses (9). Treatment effectiveness is quantified as $-Y$ because increases in $-Y$ produce decreases in risk (Y itself is usually negative, so $-Y$ usually becomes positive when calculated—see Equation 3a). The cost constraints used in linear programming were the amounts of money spent in the different categories during the hypothetical treatment.

The computer solution indicates that an optimal risk reduction of $\Delta Y = -.825$ (15.6/ 1000/ 6) could be produced by executing a decrease in 17.8 mg/ 100 ml in serum cholesterol, *no* decrease in blood pressure, a 5.1% decrease in relative weight, and a 13.1 cigarette/ day decrease in smoking. This is an increase of less than $1/1000/6$ over the present treatment outcome with a total expenditure of $42,122 in variable costs—$1978 less than in the current budget. In this solution, costs would be less than constraints only for the therapist resource type, indicating that the cost of the program could be decreased to $42,122 in variable costs without decreasing its present effectiveness. If the relationship between current funding levels and the present structure of each component is known, production of the suggested changes in physiology and behavior can be prescribed in an exact manner.

Solution of the dual (cost reduction) problem indicates that budget cuts would produce the largest reduction of therapeutic outcome if they were made in bibliotherapy ($\Delta Y = +.00017$ per dollar reduction), with advertising being the next most critical resource ($\Delta Y = +.00011$ per dollar reduction). If we change the equations so that all cost constraints were raised 25%, linear programming indicates that risk reduction could be changed to $\Delta Y = -1.032$, down $2/1000/6$ from 15 to $13/1000/6$, with a total of $52,653 in variable costs. The next question is whether the $10,531 increase needed to save an additional two events should be spent. This moves the analysis into the realm of cost–benefit analysis and complex politics.

Discussion

The subsequent step in this improvement–oriented cost–effectiveness analysis would be to implement some of the above suggestions on a preliminary basis. After testing, the model can be revised or implemented on a broader scale (see Table 2). This would be a true operations research of a behavioral–medical treatment program. Some potential problems would be noted, however.

Table 9. Linear Programming Equations for Maximizing Reduction of Cardiovascular Risk Given Cost Constraints (From Table 8 and Equations 4a and 4b)

$$\text{Maximize} -Y = .007x_1 + .009x_2 + .027x_3 + .043x_4$$

Given the constraints:

$$15.79x_1 + 66.67x_2 + 105.26x_3 + 166.67x_4 \leqslant 3,000$$

$$10.53x_1 + 33.33x_2 + 87.72x_3 + 88.89x_4 \leqslant 1,800$$

$$189.47x_1 + 800.00x_2 + 1,894.74x_3 + 1,600.00x_4 \leqslant 36,000$$

$$57.89x_1 + 66.67x_2 + 17.54x_3 + 166.67x_4 \leqslant 3,300$$

and

$$30 \geqslant x_1 \geqslant 0, \ 30 \geqslant x_2 \geqslant 0, \ 28.6 \geqslant x_3 \geqslant 0, \ 21 \geqslant x_4 \geqslant 0.$$

See Table 8 and text for details.

Unfortunately, the metric in which the smoking component was measured by Cornfield and Mitchell only has four levels. The attempted adjustment of this metric described in the footnote may be accurate; it would be preferable to use risk equations that were built on a continuous scale. Also, linear programming assumes linearity of relationships between outcome (as indicated by Y) and process measures (units of change in risk factors). If the relationships deviate greatly from linearity, nonlinear programming techniques would be needed (see 37).

The present analysis also assumes that the cost of unit decreases in different risk factors is a linear function that can be extrapolated from the results of using the technologies applied to the experimental group. This may not be the case. For example, a different and more costly technology might be required to produce the 13.1 cigarette reduction called for in the programming solution (27). In addition, an actual treatment program might not include a weight reduction component because the relationship between weight loss and cardiovascular risk mitigation is questionable (35,85). Finally, the above calculations deal with treatment groups as if they were one individual. In an actual cost–effectiveness analysis of such a program, the equations would take into account individual differences in risk–factor levels. This could necessitate separate linear programming for each client, but it would provide an opportunity for inclusion of data on client–specific subjective costs and outcomes.

A Cost–Benefit Analysis of Alternative Heroin Addiction Treatments

The linear programming procedure used in the cost–effectiveness analysis can be used in cost–utility and cost–benefit analyses as long as the data in the analyses meet the assumptions of linear programming. The mathematical cost–outcome model used in the cost–effectiveness analysis was complex, as were the solution procedures. A simpler model that lumps all resource types into a single global cost is used more frequently (perhaps because of the psychological costs incurred by cost–outcome analysts when going through complex equations). As shown in the following cost–benefit analysis, the simpler model can be solved more or less intuitively once benefit/cost ratios are calculated. However, this reduction in precision can result in reduced power and lower chances of success for the cost–outcome improvements suggested by analysis.

Model–Building Methods and Results

The general problem examined in a cost–benefit analysis conducted by Rufener, Rachal and Cruze (66, 67) is similar to that examined in the above cost–effectiveness analysis, i.e., how does one maximize treatment outcome

Table 10. The Economic Costs of Drug Abuse
Fiscal Year 1975
($ Millions)

Cost Item	Assumed Number of Addicts*		
	Low	Middle	High
Direct Costs	$4,265	$4,932	$5,599
Medical Treatment	494	494	494
Law Enforcement	1,342	1,342	1,342
Judicial System Use	296	296	296
Corrections	294	294	294
Nondrug Crime	667	1,334	2,001
Drug Traffic Control	93	93	93
Drug Abuse Prevention	995	995	995
Housing Stock Loss	84	84	84
Indirect Costs	$4,167	$5,406	$6,644
Unemployability	1,239	2,478	3,716
Emergency Room Treatment	0.4	0.4	0.4
Impatient Hospitalization	20	20	20
Mental Hospitalization	8	8	8
Drug-related Deaths	12.5	12.5	12.5
Absenteeism	1,594	1,594	1,594
Incarceration	1,205	1,205	1,205
Treatment Costs	88	88	88
TOTAL COSTS	$8,432	$10,338	$12,243

From Brent L. Rufener, Alvin M. Cruze, and J. Valley Rachal, *Management Effectiveness Measures for NIDA Drug Abuse Treatment Programs, Volume II: Costs to Society of Drug Abuse,* Table 1, p. 13. See reference 67.
*The assumed numbers of heroin addicts were 250,000, 500,000, and 750,000.

given cost restraints? The cost–effectiveness analysis examined how treatment components of varying costs might be mixed to maximize effectiveness, i.e., maximize cardiovascular risk reduction. The cost–benefit analysis below determines which of several alternative heroin treatment programs to use. The alternative treatments on which cost–benefit data were derived are: a) methadone maintenance, b) therapeutic community, c) outpatient drug–free treatment, d) outpatient detoxification, and e) inpatient detoxification (cf. 66). Benefit was estimated from a societal perspective by 1) itemizing costs incurred by society as a result of heroin use, 2) estimating the reduction in costs that would be produced by rehabilitating a heroin abuser, and 3) adjusting benefits for the relative effectiveness of the different programs (this last step was executed after preliminary benefit/cost ratios were calculated). Cost was measured exclusively from the operations perspective for each treatment. This difference in the perspective that was used to estimate monetary benefit and costs may have mildly inflated the benefit/cost ratios.

Marginal Benefits. To determine what benefits (cost savings) might be produced for society as a result of ceasing heroin use, Rufener et al. first itemized the present costs to society of heroin abuse, as shown on the leftmost column of Table 10. Because the number of heroin addicts in the United States is uncertain, three separate addict figures were used to estimate cost savings. The three resulting costs of heroin use for U.S. society in the estimation year (1975) are listed in Table 10. Total costs of heroin abuse were $8.4, $10.3, or $12.2 billion in 1975, depending on estimates of heroin user population size. Assuming that the costs listed in Table 10 would not be incurred by rehabilitated users, the next task was to estimate the average benefits (cost savings) per treated heroin user.

A yearly relapse rate of 12% was used in cost savings estimation on the basis of Fuji's research (30). This rate is higher than most estimates but serves the analysts' purpose of estimating benefits conservatively while estimating treatment costs liberally (66). Given this rate, marginal benefits were estimated as present–valued costs to society for nonrelapsed clients over those clients' lifetimes, minus the present–valued sum of a) the costs that would have occurred if the client had not been treated, and b) the costs occurring due to relapse to heroin use over those clients' lifetimes:

$$\sum_{t=1}^{m} \frac{C_{(t)}(1 - r)^t}{(1 + d)^t} - \sum_{t=1}^{n} \frac{S_{(t)}(1 - r)^t}{(1 + d)^t} \tag{5}$$

where $C_{(t)}$ is the cost to society produced by continued or relapsed heroin use, $S_{(t)}$ is the cost to society produced by rehabilitated heroin users, m is the expected number of years remaining in a continued or relapsed users' life following treatment, n is the number of years remaining in the life of a rehabilitated heroin user, t is a particular year in the addict's life, r is the relapse rate per year, and d is the discount rate used in present–valuing of costs.

It would have been desirable to calculate benefits separately for each treatment using the relapse rate observed for that treatment, but such data were not available. The value "S" is included in Equation 5 because rehabilitated users may still impose some costs due to judicial system use, law enforcement, and hospitalization costs either as a result of their prior addiction or simply as a result of normal life. Details on the exact method by which each cost savings was calculated are available from Rufener et al. (66, 67).

Total present–valued cost savings per treated heroin abuser are shown in Table 11 for discount rates of .06, .08, and .10 used over expected lifetimes, based on Equation 5. The estimated benefits of heroin user rehabilitation are substantial, with estimates ranging from about $45,000 to $68,000 per client lifetime.

Table 11. Total Lifetime Benefits Per Rehabilitated Heroin Abuser

		$d = 0.06$	$d = 0.06$	$d = 0.06$
Estimated	low	$68,071	$62,987	$58,675
Heroin User	middle	56,531	52,224	48,595
Population Size	high	52,686	48,639	45,250

From Rufener et al.

Treatment Costs. The operation costs of alternative heroin treatments were calculated by adjusting the monetary expenditures per client in treatment for the relapse rate (clients who leave treatment decrease treatment costs) and then present–valuing treatment cost if treatment lasted more than one year. The leftmost column of figures in Table 12 is the average cost per client per year for the different treatments. Next to this column is the average duration of the different treatments. The rightmost column of Table 12 lists the total cost of each treatment, adjusted for relapse rate and present–valued by the same three discount rates used in marginal benefit estimation. Relapse adjustment and present–valuing were conducted by Rufener et al., as:

$$\sum_{t=1}^{q} \frac{(1 - r_{(t)})^t}{(1 + d)^t} T_{(t)} \qquad (6)$$

where q is the number of years required for treatment, $r_{(t)}$ is the cost of treatment in year t. It would have been much more desirable to calculate costs with the specific relapse rate generated by a particular treatment, but such data were not available.

Benefit/Cost Ratios. Division of the present–valued marginal benefit estimates for different sizes of heroin user population (Table 11) by the relapse–adjusted present–valued costs for different treatments (Table 12) yields the benefit/cost ratios listed in Table 13. Outpatient drug–free treatment clearly has the best and largest benefit/cost ratio, followed by outpatient and inpatient detoxification and methadone maintenance. A simple sensitivity analysis was conducted on these ratios; benefit/cost was calculated for the first year after treatment completion (Table 14) instead of for client lifetimes. The resulting benefit/cost ratios generally are lower than those calculated for client lifetimes, but still are substantial and retain the same basic ordering with outpatient drug–free treatment again being the most cost–beneficial.

Adjustment For Relative Effectiveness. Finally, Rufener et al. adjusted their client–lifetime benefit/cost ratios for the relative effectiveness of different

Table 12. Cost Per Client Per Year of Alternative Heroin Rehabilitation Treatments, Adjusted for Relapse Rate and Present-Valued

Treatment	Simple Cost Per Client Per Year	Years Required for Treatment	Relapse-Adjusted and Present-Valued Treatment Costs, Different Discount Rates		
			$d = .06$	$d = .08$	$d = .10$
Methadone Maintenance	$6,000	Remainder of Client's Life	$12,942	$11,874	$10,997
Therapeutic Community	6,000	4 years	28,105	27,451	26,836
Outpatient Drug Free	1,200	2 years	2,196	2,178	2,160
Outpatient Detoxification	2,200	4 years	6,801	6,643	6,494
Inpatient Detoxification	30,000	1/3 year	11,030*	11,030*	11,030*

Note: A relapse rate of 12% was used in calculating the costs listed in the three rightmost columns (see Equation 6 and text).

From Rufener et al.

*These values do not differ as a function of discount rate because treatment lasted only 1/3 year, thus removing the necessity to preent-value the cost.

treatments. To measure treatment effectiveness, the average number of opiate–free, nonopiate–free, and legitimate support/employment days per client were summed for each treatment (as shown in the second leftmost column of figures in Table 15). The average number of trouble–free days, 542.4/client, was then divided into the number of trouble–free days separately for each treatment to produce an "adjustment factor" (shown in Table 15). Benefit/cost ratios for a 10% discount rate and the "middle" assumption of heroin user population (from Table 13) were multiplied by the appropriate adjustment factor. This procedure produced benefit/cost ratios weighted for the relative efficacy of different treatments (see the rightmost column of Table 15). Again, outpatient drug–free treatment is more cost–beneficial than the other treatments by a wide margin, followed by outpatient detoxification. Inpatient detoxification, methadone maintenance, and therapeutic community come in as distant thirds.

Table 13. Benefit/Cost Ratios* of Drug Treatment Programs
for Multiyear Period

Treatment	Discount Rate	Assumed No. of Abusers		
		Low	Middle	High
Methadone	.06	5.26	4.37	4.07
Maintenance	.08	5.30	4.40	4.10
	.10	5.34	4.42	4.11
Therapeutic	.06	2.42	2.01	1.87
Community	.08	2.29	1.90	1.77
	.10	2.19	1.81	1.68
Outpatient	.06	31.00	25.74	23.99
Drug Free	.08	28.92	23.98	22.33
	.10	27.16	22.50	20.94
Outpatient	.06	10.01	8.31	7.75
Detoxification	.08	9.48	7.86	7.32
	.10	9.04	7.48	6.97
Inpatient	.06	6.17	5.12	4.78
Detoxification	.08	5.71	4.73	4.41
	.10	5.32	4.40	4.10

*Benefit-cost ratios are calculated by dividing present value of benefits by present value of costs.
From Rufener et al.

Discussion

Because costs were not itemized separately for different program components in the present cost–benefit analysis, and because budget constraints are not being considered, the decision–making situation is simpler than it was in the preceding cost–effectiveness analysis. The macro–type of data used in the cost–benefit analysis also leads to a simple treatment choice instead of a more complex decision about how to improve treatment. To maximize the ratio of benefits to costs, one chooses the highest benefit/cost ratio—in this case, outpatient drug–free treatment. In reality, however, considerations such as neighborhood pressure for inpatient rather than outpatient treatments may dictate alternative choices by additionally weighting ratios for different treatments.

The cost–benefit analysis described above illustrates not only some of the general procedures of cost–benefit analysis, but also some of its faults. As the authors of the analysis note, the adjustment factor probably is an imperfect way of measuring the benefits produced by alternative treatments. In addition, relapse rates for each treatment might have been used instead of a single overall relapse rate, unless treatments had been shown not to have different relapse rates. The relapse rate used in the present analysis, in fact, seems unusually low.

Table 14. Sensitivity Analysis: Benefit-Cost Ratios of Drug Treatment Programs, Benefits and Costs for Different Abuser Population Assumptions

	Assumed No. of Abusers		
Treatment	Low	Middle	High
Methadone Maintenance	5.40	4.46	4.15
Therapeutic Community	1.31	1.08	1.00
Outpatient Drug Free	9.91	8.19	7.61
Outpatient Detoxification	5.40	4.46	4.15
Inpatient Detoxification	1.08	0.89	0.83

From Rufener et al.

Table 15. Adjusting Benefit/Cost Ratios for Relative Efficacy of Alternative Treatments

Treatment	Nonadjusted* Benefit/Cost Ratio	Average†** Trouble-Free Days Per Client	Adjustment Factor	Final Benefit/ Cost Ratio
Methadone Maintenance	4.42	539	.99	4.39
Therapeutic Community	1.81	667	1.23	2.23
Outpatient Drug Free	22.50	309	.57	12.82
Outpatient Detoxification	7.48	517	.95	7.14
Inpatient Detoxification	4.40	680	1.25	5.53

*10% discount rate, middle assumed heroin user population size.

†Trouble-free days were the sum of opiate-free, nonopiate-free, legitimate support, and legitimate employment days.

**Average number of troulb free days is 542.4.

From Rufener et al.

Furthermore, apparently there was not random assignment to different treatments. Finally, cost savings estimates are based on many projections—e.g., addict versus rehabilitated addict lifetime—that may not be accurate. These problems are typical of many cost–benefit analyses currently in the literature—ones that were conducted in response to funding agency mandates or other imperatives that seldom allow the time or money necessary for a thorough and experimentally sound cost–benefit analysis. Of course, cost–benefit analysis does not have to be like this. It can be conducted at the same high level of sophistication as cost–effectiveness analysis and can be used in conjunction with linear programming to systematically improve the outcome and reduce the cost of treatment programs.

PROBLEMS AND PROMISE IN COST–OUTCOME ANALYSES AND BEHAVIORAL MEDICINE

Politics and Cost–Outcome Analyses

The principal focus of this paper has been on the instrumental aspects of three kinds of cost–outcome analysis, rather than on its political, expressive aspects (58). These latter elements deserve discussion however, as they seem to be an inevitable part of any cost–outcome analyses (32, 70, 83, 84).

One view on the politics of cost–outcome analyses is that politics should be minimized because it can impede an analysis (69). One method for minimizing the political nature of an analysis is to combine some of the perspectives whose conflicts are responsible for the political situation, as in a composite effectiveness or cost index. Another way in which the politics of cost–outcome analysis can be mitigated is to emphasize that the purpose of the analysis is to *improve* treatment delivery. Such emphasis on the *formative* aspects of the analysis may engender fewer political impediments than emphasis on the purely evaluative or *summative* aspects of the analysis (62, 71, 89). Analyses that are primarily summative may produce changes in personnel or resource allocation that have little to do with the improvement of cost outcome (14, 24, 44, 77, 88).

Political aspects of cost–outcome analysis also can be reduced by designing the analysis to be primarily "in-house," i.e., conducted by treatment personnel as a routine activity. If cost–outcome analysis is conducted once a year by "outsiders," the analysts can be easily misperceived as ignorant intruders who deserve to have their data falsified and innovations sabotaged (4, 86). The in-house analysis team could mitigate political problems and could produce sophisticated analyses by occasionally calling in a cost–outcome consultant (72). If data collected from the in-house analysis were to be provided to outside agencies, validity of the data could be assessed by surreptitious checks.

Whereas the political aspects of cost–outcome analysis may be viewed as something to be minimized, concern also has been voiced that the findings of cost–outcome analyses do not have sufficient impact in the realm of political action. For example, cost–effectiveness analysis and other forms of evaluation research may be and have been funded not for program facilitation, but for the implicit purpose of delaying indefinitely the implementation of social service programs (47, 77). Concern also has been expressed about the power that may eventually be assimilated by cost–effectiveness analysts and other evaluation agents (46). Perhaps the latter concern will become important once there is less reason for the former concern. Our primary focus at present should be the discussion and use of cost–outcome analyses in behavioral medicine, for the purpose of reducing monetary and psychological costs and improving the efficacy of delivering present behavioral–medical technologies and developing new ones that are more cost–effective.

A Plan for Integrating Cost–Outcome Analysis Into Behavioral Medicine

To increase the scientific and political impact of the behavioral–medical movement, it seems imperative that we collect and analyze data on the costs of our treatments with the same concern for reliability and validity that we have shown for the effectiveness of our treatments. Translation of these data into benefits that are valued in the same units as cost, as in cost–benefit analysis, should increase further the political impact of behavioral medicine by providing the means for decision–making that may favor behavioral as opposed to traditional medical technologies. Decision–making also may be aided by the use of collected estimates of probable costs and outcomes of alternative strategies for mitigating behavioral–medical problems, as in cost–utility analysis.

A major question remaining is how to implement in general behavioral medicine the techniques of cost–outcome analysis that were described in this chapter. My answer is threefold: a) training, b) routine (perhaps required) cost as well as outcome data collection and reporting, and c) establishment of a cost–outcome network in behavioral medicine or in the larger area of behavioral psychology.

Training

A number of evaluation research training programs exist at present, but these are primarily designed to produce profesional evaluators. Perhaps it would serve the present purpose better to include a cost–outcome analysis course in required behavioral–medical curricula. Those who have completed their formal education could receive continuing education courses or workshops in cost–outcome analysis (e.g., 93).

Routine Data Collection

Given the scientific orientation of behavioral medicine, most researchers and many practitioners already collect data on treatment outcomes. Collection of data on treatment costs usually is easier than collection of data on outcomes. Treatments may differ significantly in costs, despite not infrequent nonsignificant differences in outcome (73). Ideally, editors would welcome these data in addition to the outcome data reported in most journals.

Forming a Cost–Outcome Data Network

Training in cost–outcome analysis could provide the skills necessary for cost–outcome data collection and analysis; requirements to report cost as well as outcome data in publications would facilitate application of these skills. However, only a centralized compilation of cost and outcome analyses can provide the information bank needed to influence potential funders and decision–makers in medicine and in political spheres. We could either form interfaces with other evaluation research networks or establish our own. Some coordination of cost–outcome analysis is necessary to meet our dual accountability of treatment cost and treatment outcome for the people who fund our work and for the people whose health depends on our efforts.

ACKNOWLEDGMENTS

I wish to acknowledge the assistance of Dr. Curtis Wilbur and Marjorie Dauphin in formulating some of the exemplary analyses. Dr. Albert Stunkard served as an inspiration for many of the concepts included in this paper, although he should not be blamed for any. Dr. Jim Ferguson served as an understanding and insightful editor. Daniel Najjar was a most patient typist and mind–reader.

REFERENCES

1. Abelson, P.H. Cost–effective health care. *Science* 192:1, 1976.
2. Ackoff, R.L. The development of operations research as a science. *Operations Research* 4:265f, 1956.

3. Ackoff, R.L. Systems, organizations, and interdisciplinary research, in D.P. Eckman (ed.), *Systems: Research and Design.* New York: John Wiley & Sons, 1961, pp. 26–42.
4. Ackoff, R.L., and Rivett, P. *A Manager's Guide to Operations Research.* New York: John Wiley and Sons, 1963.
5. Ackoff, R.L., and Sasieni, N.W. *Fundamentals of Operations Research.* New York: Wiley, 1968.
6. Adams, S., and Orgel, M. *Through the Mental Health Maze.* Washington, D.C.: Health Research Group, 1975.
7. American Psychological Association task force on health research. Contributions of psychology to health research: Patterns, problems, and potentials. Unpublished manuscript, Washington, D.C., A.P.A., 1975.
8. Anderson, D.R., Sweeney, D.J., and Williams, T.A. *An Introduction to Management Science: Quantitative Approaches to Decision Making.* St. Paul, Minn.: West Publishing, 1976.
9. Bartfeld, C.I., Burns, K.L., Ivison, S.H., May, J.O., Logan, J., Rowe, J.D., Selman, V., and Shahin, G. *Computer procedures for American University business programs,* vol. 1. Manuscript, The American University, Washington, D.C., 1977.
10. Baumol, W.J. On the social rate of discount. *American Economic Review* 58:788–802, 1968.
11. Burwell, B.A., Reiber, S.E., and Newman, F.L. *The client oriented cost/outcome system of the Fayette County Mental Health/Mental Retardation Clinic, Inc.* Paper presented at the meeting of the Association of Mental Health Administrators, Washington, D.C., September 1975.
12. Carter, D.E., and Newman, F.L. *A Client Oriented System of Mental Health Service Delivery and Program Management: A Workbook and Guide.* Philadelphia: Eastern Pennsylvania Psychiatric Institute, 1974.
13. Chin, R. The utility of systems models and developmental models for practitioners, in W.G. Bennis, K.D. Benne, and R. Chin (eds.), *The Planning of Change.* New York: Holt, Rinehart & Winston, 1969, pp. 297–312.
14. Cicarelli, W. The impact of Head Start: Executive summary, in *The Impact of Head Start: An Evaluation of the Effects of Head Start on Children's Cognitive and Affective Development,* vol. 1. Bladensburg, Md.: Westinghouse Learning Corporation, 1969.
15. Conley, R.W., Conwell, M., and Arrill, M.P. An approach to measuring the cost of mental illness. *Am. J. Psychiatry,* 124:755–762, 1967.
16. Cornfield, J., and Mitchell, S. Selected risk factors in coronary disease. *The Archives of Environmental Health* 19:382–394, 1969.
17. Council on Wage and Price Stability (1976).
18. Doherty, N.J., and Hicks, B.C. The use of cost–effectiveness analysis in geriatric day care. *Gerontologist* 15:412–417, 1975.
19. Dressel, P.L. (ed.). *Handbook of Academic Evaluation.* San Francisco: Joseey–Bass, 1976.
20. Edwards, W., and Guttentag, M. Experiments and evaluations: A reexamination, in C.A. Bennett and A.A. Lumsdaine (eds.), *Experiments and Evaluations: Some Critical Issues in Assessing Social Programs.* New York: Academic Press, 1975.
21. Epstein, L.H., ad Cincirpini, P.M. Behavioral medicine III: Health care delivery. *Association for the Advancement of Behavior Therapy Newsletter* 4(5):7–9, 1977.
22. Epstein, L.H., and Martin, J.F. Behavioral medicine. *Association for the Advancement of Behavior Therapy Newsletter* 4(3):5–6, 1977.
23. Epstein, L.H., and Parker, L.H. Behavioral medicine II: Treatment. *Association for the Advancement of Behavior Therapy Newsletter* 4(4):9–10, 1977.
24. Evans, J.W. Head Start: Comments on the criticisms. *Britannica Review of American*

Education 1:253–260, 1969. Chicago: Encyclopedia Britannica, 1969.
25. Fanshel, D., and Shinn, E.B. *Dollars and Sense in the Foster Care of Children: A Look at Cost Factors.* New York: Child Welfare League of America, 1972.
26. Fisher, G.H. The role of cost–utility analysis in program budgeting, in D. Novick (ed.), *Program Budgeting.* Washington, D.C.: U.S. Government Printing Office, 1964.
27. Flaxman, J. Quitting smoking, in W.E. Craighead, A.E. Kazdin, and M.J. Mahoney (eds.), *Behavior Modification: Principles, Issues, and Applications.* Boston: Houghton Mifflin, 1976.
28. Francis, W.J. Notes from HEW: What social indicators don't indicate. *Evaluation* 1(2):79–83, 1973.
29. Fries, B.E. Bibliography of operation research in health care systems. *Operations Research* 24(5):801–814, 1976.
30. Fuji, E.T. Public investment in the rehabilitation of heroin addicts. *Social Science Quarterly* 55:49–50, 1974.
31. Gibson, R.M., and Mueller, M.S. *Research and Statistics Note 27.* December 1976.
32. Glennan, T.K. Jr. Institutional and political factors in social experimentation, in H.W. Riecken and R.F. Boruck (eds.), *Social Experimentation as a Method for Planning and Evaluating Social Intervention.* New York: Academic Press, 1974.
33. Goldman, T.A. (ed). *Cost–Effectiveness Analysis.* New York: Praeger, 1967.
34. Guttentag, M. Subjectivity and its use in evaluation research. *Evaluation* 1(2):60–65, 1973.
35. Halperin, M., Gordon, T., Kjelsberg, M., Neaton, J., and Sherwin, R. Statistical design considerations in the NHLI Multiple Risk Factor Intervention Trial (MRFIT). *J. Chron. Dis.* 30:261–275, 1977.
36. Hilbert, S. Who benefits from the program? Criteria selection, in P.O. Davidson, F.W. Clark, and L.A. Hamerlynck (eds.), *Evaluation of Behavioral Programs: In Community, Residential, and School Settings.* Champaign, Ill.: Research Press, 1974.
37. Hillier, F.S., and Lieberman, G.J. *Operations Research,* 2nd ed. San Francisco: Holden–Day, 1974.
38. Kahn, A. *Theory and Practice of Social Planning.* New York: Russell Sage Foundation, 1969.
39. Katz, D., and Kahn, R.L. *The Social Psychology of Organizations.* New York: John Wiley & Sons, 1966.
40. Kennecott Copper Corporation. Insight. Unpublished report, Utah Copper Division, Salt Lake City, 1975.
41. Krapfl, J.E. Accountability through cost–benefit analysis, in D. Harshbarger, and R.F. Maley (eds.), *Behavior Analysis and Systems Analysis: An Integrative Approach to Mental Health Programs.* Kalamazoo, Mich.: Behaviordelia, 1974.
42. Krause, M.S. Construct validity for the evaluation of therapy outcomes. *J. Abnorm. Psychol.* 74:524–530, 1969.
43. Leveson, I. Cost–benefit analysis and program target population: Narcotics addiction treatment. *Am. J. Econ. Soc.* 32:129–142, 1973.
44. Levin, H.M. Cost effectiveness evaluation of instructional technology: The problems, in S. Tickton (ed.), *To Improve Learning—An Evaluation of Instructional Technology,* vol. 2. New York: R.R. Bowker, 1971.
45. Levin, H.M. Cost–effectiveness analysis in evaluation research, in M. Guttentag and E. Struening (eds.), *The Handbook of Evaluation Research,* vol. 2. Beverly Hills, Cal.: Sage Publications, 1975.
46. Levine, D. The dangers of social action, in D. Harshberger and R.F. Maley (eds.), *Behavior Analysis and Systems Analysis.* Kalamazoo, Mich.: Behaviordelia, 1974.

47. Levy, L. The use of evaluative research in creating accountability, in D. Harshberger and R.F. Maley (eds.), *Behavior Analysis and Systems Analysis.* Kalamazoo, Mich.: Behaviordelia, 1974.

48. McIntyre, M. Theoretical overview: The role of the front-line worker in program evaluation, in R. Coursey (ed.), *Evaluations in Mental Health.* New York: Wiley, 1976.

49. McIntyre, M., Attkisson, C., and Keller, T. Components of program evaluation capability in community mental health centers, in W. Hargreaves, C. Attkisson, M. McIntyre, and L. Siegel (eds.), *Resource Materials for Community Mental Health Program Evaluation* (Pt. 1). San Francisco: NIMH, 1974.

50. McNerney, W.J. The quandary of quality assessment. *N. Eng. J. Med.* 295:1505-1511, 1976.

51. Macy, B.A., and Mirvis, P.H. A methodology for assessment of quality of work life and organizational effectiveness in behavioral-economic terms. *Administrative Science Quarterly* 21:212-226, 1976.

52. Marglin, S.A. The social rate of discount and the optimal rate of investment. *Quart. J. Econ.* 77:95-112, 1963.

53. Marston, A.R., Marston, M.R., and Ross, J. A correspondence course behavioral program for weight reduction. *Obesity/Bariatric Medicine* 6:140-147, 1977.

54. May, P.R.A. Cost-efficiency of mental health delivery systems. *Am. J. Public Health* 60:2060-2067, 1970.

55. Mazade, N., Surles, R., and Atkin, J. Fiscal resource development for state mental health agencies. *Admin. Mental Health* 2:180-185, 1976.

56. Midlarsky, M., and Midlarsky, E. Analysis of research efficiency: Costs and information gain. *Psychol. Rep.* 37:607-617, 1975.

57. Mueller, M.S., and Gibson, R.M. National Health Expenditures, fiscal year 1975. *Social Security Bulletin*, 1976, *39*, 3ff.

58. Neufeldt, A.H. Considerations in the implementation of program evaluation, in P.O. Davidson, F.W. Clark, and L.A. Hamerlynck (eds.), *Evaluation of Behavioral Programs: In Community, Residential and School Settings.* Champaign, Ill.: Research Press, 1974.

59. Noble, J.H. Jr. The limits of cost-benefit analysis as a guide to priority-setting in rehabilitation. *Evaluation Quart.* 1:347-380, 1977.

60. Patterson, G.R. Interventions for boys with conduct problems: Multiple settings, treatments, and criteria. *J. Consult. Clin. Psychol.* 42:471-481, 1974.

61. Pennypacker, H.S., Koenig, C.H., and Seaver, W.H. Cost efficiency and effectiveness in the early detection and improvement of learning abilities, in P.O. Davidson, F.W. Clark, and L.A. Hamerlynck (eds.), *Evaluation of Behavioral Programs: In Community, Residential, and School Settings.* Champaign, Ill.: Research Press, 1974.

62. Reinke, W.A. Methods and measurements in evaluation, in W.A. Reinke (ed.), *Health Planning: Qualitative Aspects and Quantitative Techniques.* Baltimore: Waverly Press, 1972.

63. Rivlin, A.M. *Systematic Thinking for Social Action.* Washington, D.C.: The Brookings Institution, 1971.

64. Romans, J.T. The economic evaluation of mental health programs. *Internat. J. Mental Health* 2:38-50, 1973.

65. Rufener, B.L., Cruze, A.M., and Rachal, J.V. *Management Effectiveness Measures for NIDA Drug Abuse Treatment Programs: Costs to Society of Drug Abuse.* Research Triangle Park, N.C.: Research Triangle Institute, 1977.

66. Rufener, B.L., Rachal, J.V., and Cruze, A.M. *Management Effectiveness Measures for NIDA Drug Abuse Treatment Programs* (Vol. 1): *Cost Benefit Analysis.* (NIDA Technical Paper), U.S. DHEW Public Health Service, GPO Stock No. 017-024-00577-1,

1977.
67. Rufener, B.L., Rachal, J.V., and Cruze, A.M. *Management Effectiveness Measures for NIDA Drug Abuse Treatment Programs* (Vol. 2): *Costs to Society of Drug Abuse.* (NIDA Technical Paper), U.S. DHEW, Public Health Service, GPO Stock No. 017-024-00578-9, 1977.
68. Rust, M.A. *Endorsement of accountability components in community mental health centers.* Doctoral dissertation, University of Michigan, 1976.
69. Salancik, G.R., and Lamont, V.C. Conflicts in societal research: A study of one RANN project suggests that benefiting society may cost univerities. *J. Higher Education* 46:161-176, 1975.
70. Sarri, R.C., and Selo, E. Evaluation process and outcome in juvenile corrections: Musings on a grim tale, in P.O. Davidson, F.W. Clark, and L.A. Hamerlynck (eds.), *Evaluation of Behavioral Programs.* Champaign, Ill.: Research Press, 1974.
71. Scriven, M. The methodology of evaluation, in C.H. Weiss (ed.), *Evaluating Action Programs: Readings in Social Action and Education.* Boston: Allyn & Bacon, 1972.
72. Sechrest, L. The psychologist as program evaluator, in P.J. Woods (ed.), *Career Opportunities for Psychologists: Expanding and Emerging Areas.* Washington, D.C.: American Psychological Association, 1976.
73. Siegert, F., and Yates, B.T. The cost-effectiveness of individual and group behavior therapy for parents of problem children. *Evaluation & the Health Professions,* 1980, in press.
74. Smith, D. Goal attainment scaling as an adjunct to counseling. *J. Couns. Psychol.* 23:22-27, 1976.
75. Sorensen, J.E., and Phipps, D.W. *Cost-Finding and Rate-Setting for Community Mental Health Centers.* National Institute of Mental Health, DHEW Publication No. (ADM) 76-291, U.S. GPO, Washington, D.C., 1975.
76. Strupp, H.H., and Hadley, S.W. A tripartite model of mental health and therapeutic outcomes. *Am. Psychol.* 32:187-196, 1977.
77. Suchman, E.A. Action for what: A critique of evaluative research, in C.H. Weiss (ed.), *Evaluating Action Programs: Readings in Social Action and Education.* Boston: Allyn & Bacon, 1972.
78. Temkin, S. Making sense of benefit-cost analysis and cost-effectiveness analysis. *Improving Human Performance* 3:39-48, 1974.
79. Thomas, J.A. *The Productive School: A Systems Analysis Approach to Educational Administration.* New York: Wiley, 1971.
80. Tripodi, T. *Uses and Abuses of Social Research in Social Work.* New York: Columbia University Press, 1974.
81. Trotter, S. Nader group releases first consumer guide to psychotherapists. *APA Monitor* 6(12):11-13, 1975.
82. Weinstein, M.C., and Stason, W.B. Foundations of cost-effectiveness analysis for health and medical practices. *N. Engl. J. Med.,* 296(13):716-721, 1977.
83. Weiss, C.H. *Evaluation Research: Methods of Assessing Program Effectiveness.* Englewood Cliffs, N.J.: Prentice-Hall, 1972.
84. Weiss, C.H. *Evaluating Action Programs: Reading in Social Action and Education.* Boston: Allyn & Bacon, 1973.
85. Wilbur, C. Personal communication, NIH, November 1, 1977.
86. Williams, W., and Evans, J.W. The politics of evaluation: The case of Head Start, in P.H. Rossi and W. Williams (eds.), *Evaluating Social Programs: Theory, Practice, and Politics.* New York: Seminar Press, 1972.
87. Wolins, M. *A Manual for Cost Analysis in Institutions for Children.* New York: Child

Welfare League of America, 1962.
88. Worchel, S., Lind, E.A., and Kaufman, K.H. Evaluations of group products as a function of expectations of group longevity, outcome of competition, and publicity of evaluations. *J. Personality Soc. Psychol.* 31:1089–1097, 1975.
89. Wortman, P.M. Evaluation research: A psychological perspective. *Am. Psychol.* 30:562–575, 1975.
90. Yates, B.T. *The use of operations research to improve psychological treatments: Prescriptions from a historical perspective.* Paper presented at the meeting of the Western Psychological Association, Los Angeles, April 1976.
91. Yates, B.T. A cost–effectiveness analysis of a residential treatment program for behaviorally disturbed children, in P. Mitter (ed.), *Research and Practice in Mental Retardation,* vol. 1. Baltimore: University Park Press, 1977.
92. Yates, B.T. Cost–effectiveness analysis: Using it for our own good. *State Psychological Association Affairs Newsletter* 8:6, 1977.
93. Yates, B.T. *How to conduct cost–effectiveness and cost–benefit analysis of social service programs.* Two–day workshop presented at the 101st annual meeting of the American Association on Mental Deficiency, New Orleans, May 1977.
94. Yates, B.T. How to improve, rather than evaluate, cost–effectiveness. *Counseling Psychologist, 8,* 72–75, 1979.
95. Yates, B.T. Three ways to improve the cost–effectiveness of behavioral programs for obesity reduction. *International Journal of Obesity, 2,* 249–266, 1978.
96. Yates, B.T. Three basic strategies for improving the cost–effectiveness of social services. In G. Lansberg et al. (Eds.), *Evaluation in practice.* Washington, D.C.: U.S. Government Printing Office, 1979.
97. Yates, B.T. *Improving effectiveness and reducing costs in mental health.* Springfield, Ill.: Charles C. Thomas, 1980.
98. Yates, B.T., Hurley, L., and Hugonnet, M. *Using operations research to improve the cost–effectiveness of behavioral-medical therapy: Self Management.* Paper presented at the meeting of the Association for Advancement of Behavior Therapy, San Francisco, December 1979.
99. Yates, B.T., Haven, W.G., and Thoresen, C.E. Cost–effectiveness at Learning House: How much change for how much money?, in J.S. Stumphauser (ed.), *Progress in Behavior Therapy with Delinquents.* Springfield, Ill.: Charles C. Thomas, 1979.
100. Zifferblatt, S.M. Analysis and design of counselor–training systems: An operant and operations research perspective. *The Counseling Psychologist* 3:12–31, 1972.
101. Zifferblatt, S.M. Increasing patient compliance therapy through the applied analysis of behavior. *Prevent. Med.* 4:173–182, 1975.
102. Zifferblatt, S.M., and Wilbur, C.S. Maintaining a healthy heart: Guidelines for a feasible goal. *Prevent. Med.,* in press.
103. Zussman, J. Mental health service quality control: An idea whose time has come. *Comprehensive Psychiatry, 13,* 497–506, 1972.

Addictions
and Their Treatment

Addictions to harmful substances are more common in our society now than ever before. More than nine–million people are considered to be "alcoholics" and it is estimated that six percent of high school seniors consume alcohol–containing beverages daily. Eight percent of all deaths in this country are alcohol related (1). An increase in heroin addiction seems to be occurring following its leveling off during the mid–seventies (2). Despite massive media campaigns, designed to educate the public to the dangers of smoking, the absolute number of smokers (over 55 million) remains constant, as younger smokers replace the older ones who quit. Most alarming, the percentage of high school females who smoke is almost equal to that of their male peers (1). Behavioral medicine research has already provided some useful techniques to reduce the use of harmful substances; like controlled drinking, which is an alternative to abstinence for some alcoholics, and rapid–puffing which may help some smokers quit their smoking habit. In this section, we review the behavioral approaches to alcohol, narcotic, and tobacco addiction.

The section begins with Sobell and Sobell's discussion of nonproblem drinking. Of the many controversies raised by behavioral techniques, none has generated as much heated discussion as the controversy over whether or not alcoholics can learn to control their drinking. Pioneer studies by Lovibond and Caddy (3) and Sobell and Sobell (4) showed that chronic alcoholics could learn to control their drinking and maintain "nonproblem drinking rates." These studies were in opposition to the basic philosophy of many abstinence–oriented programs. Sobell and Sobell review the issues and controversies of nonproblem drinking and report the results of studies that have appeared since their original one. Despite the evidence that some alcoholics can develop nonproblem drinking, the mainstay of treatment is abstinence. Smith discusses many of the abstinence–oriented approaches and the techniques used to achieve abstinence. Several clinic trials with long–term outcome indicate that abstinence–oriented techniques, combined with other techniques, can be very useful in treating alcoholics.

Several studies not discussed in either of these chapters have demonstrated the usefulness of extending an alcohol–treatment program into the community, and reinforcing non–drinking behaviors in this environment. Hunt and Azrin (5) developed a program where "time–out" from vocational, family and social reinforcers occurred when a patient would drink. They developed a very comprehensive program to provide these reinforcers: Patients were given vocational and job–seeking skills; marital and family counseling was provided if desired; and clients were taught to avoid drinking friends and to establish non–drinking social relationships. Release from the hospital was contingent upon finding a job, and the participants developed their own community social club. The treated group showed significantly less drinking, less time away from home, less institutionalization, and significantly more employment than control subjects at six months post–treatment.

In another study, goods and resources from a community agency were provided to clients, contingent upon their sobriety (6). The ten chronic public–drunkenness offenders in the program had significantly fewer arrests and greater hours of employment than ten control subjects during the two months that the program was in effect. These two studies provide models for how alcohol–treatment programs can become more effective.

Callner and Ross discuss many of the theories of the etiology of addiction. They point out, in behavioral terms, the complexity of addictive behaviors; drug–taking and drug–seeking. The environmental interactions of these affected individuals involve classical and operant conditioning, positive and negative reinforcement, multiple discriminative stimuli, modeling, peer pressure, punishment and threatened punishment, etc. The authors use the animal literature to point out that reinforcement, schedules, drug dosage, inter–injection intervals, and medication strength, all play a vital role in determining a narcotic habit.

Many types of treatment have been used in an attempt to free people of a narcotic addiction. These have included counter–conditioning using chemical, electrical, and covert aversion therapies; and desensitization paradigms, designed to extinguish the craving for narcotics with and without chemical adjuncts such as methadone, and contingency contracting. To date, the best programs appear to be combinations of all these techniques. Maintenance of a drug–free state appears to depend on developing skills in the patient that will enable him to integrate into a "drug–free" culture and resume life as a "drug–free" individual.

Although behaviorally oriented treatment programs combined with community interventions, full integration into a drug–free culture, and appropriate psychopharmacological interventions offer the best and most efficient treatment approach to narcotic addiction to date, these treatments are far from ideal. To date, outcome studies have not been overwhelmingly positive. The authors make recommendations for future research that will hopefully change the poor state of the art. Most research has not been with "street" addicts, the efficacy of generalizing techniques, such as covert sensitization, which require the complete and enthusiastic cooperation of the patient, is questioned. Better methods for data collection are suggested, arguing for greater experimental control, and long–term follow–up studies with *in vivo* assessment of efficacy. The authors suggest continuing-therapy-outcome research along current lines, with more emphasis on biochemical approaches, and more attention to behaviors that covary with drug taking such as drug seeking behaviors.

Behavioral research on smoking cessation has focused largely on the effectiveness of particular techniques or the effectiveness of combinations of techniques. With the exception of rapid puffing, the results are uniformly discouraging. Most smokers quit with most techniques and start smoking again within six months. Even rapid puffing seems less effective when used outside of a research setting. An overview of the research on smoking cessation and controlled smoking is presented by Pechacek and McAlister, along with some practical suggestions for health care professionals, who wish to help their clients change their smoking habits. There is a clear need for new approaches to the problem of preventing smoking behavior from developing, and maintaining non–smoking for those who have quit. Pechacek and McAlister present recent work in the areas of prevention, community–wide programs, and mediated programs which may be effective and cost–effective interventions.

Particularly exciting is the work done in high schools to dissuade adolescents from beginning smoking. A behavioral analysis of the initiation of smoking behaviors in adolescents (primarily because of modeling the behaviors of peers and adults, and social reinforcement), and techniques designed to reduce these effects, appear promising in decreasing the incidence of high–school–age smokers.

Nash and Farquhar (Chapter 14) describe the study of three communities which focused on a community–wide health–education program designed to change smoking behavior. Some of the most significant changes in that study occurred in smokers' given face–to–face intensive instruction on quitting. Zlutnick and Corley's chapter, describing the treatment for chronic pain and strategies for withdrawing patients addicted to analgesic medication, is also relevant to the topic of smoking cessation.

REFERENCES

1. Drug use, patterns, consequences and the federal response: A policy review. Office of Drug Abuse Policy, Executive Office of the President, March, 1978.
2. Frank, B., Schneider, J., Johnson, B., and Lipton, D.S. Seeking truth in heroin indicators: The case of New York City. *Drug and Alcohol Dependence*, 3:345–358, 1978.
3. Hunt, G.M. and Azrin, N.H. A community reinforcement approach to alcoholism. *Behav. Res. T.*, 11:91–104, 1973.
4. Lovibond, S.H. and Caddy, G. Discriminated aversive control in the moderation of alcoholics' drinking behavior. *Behav. Ther.*, 1:437–444, 1970.
5. Miller, P.M. A behavioral intervention program for chronic public drunkenness offenders. *Arch. Gen. Psychiat.*, 32:915–918, 1975.
6. Sobell, L.C. and Sobell, M.B. A self–feedback technique to monitor drinking behavior in alcoholics. *Behav. Res. T.*, 11:237–238, 1973.

Chapter 9

Nonproblem Drinking As a Goal in the Treatment Of Problem Drinkers

Mark B. Sobell
Linda C. Sobell

Knowledge about the nature of alcohol problems has grown tremendously in recent years (26). Understandably, the research findings that comprise this new body of knowledge have often conflicted with traditionally accepted concepts of alcoholism. Facts are replacing conjecture, and the process is painful for those who for several years have based their notions of clinical treatment on popular, but nevertheless empirically unsupported, suppositions.

In this brief chapter, we examine in some detail one area of recent clinical research that has had substantial impact on the clinical treatment of persons with drinking problems. This topic—the extent to which alcohol problems are reversible—has pragmatic implications which have forced a reconsideration of appropriate ways to treat persons with drinking problems. This chapter also: 1) summarizes several reasons why a more flexible approach to the development of treatment goals as opposed to a blanket prescription of lifelong abstinence is now necessary; 2) examines the present state of the art with regard to making treatment goal decisions; and 3) reviews selected clinical issues regarding how to effect such goals.

THE EVIDENTIAL BASE

Presently, there are almost 100 studies documenting that some persons have recovered from drinking problems without having to be totally abstinent. While the vast majority of these studies have been cited and reviewed in other papers

(12, 17, 23, 25, 26, 31, 34), some reports have only recently appeared in print (e.g., 18). Interestingly, until recently the majority of these studies were follow–up reports of alcoholics who had been treated in traditional programs oriented toward a singular treatment objective of total abstinence. Moreover, many of the subjects in these studies were reported to have been previously addicted to alcohol [*gamma* alcoholics, in the taxonomy devised by Jellinek (9)]. Additionally, several dozen studies have also demonstrated beyond doubt that even severely chronic alcoholics are capable of drinking in a highly controlled manner within a laboratory setting, if provided with appropriate incentives (reviewed in 14, 17, 23, 26, 38).

Although these findings had been accumulating in the literature for at least two decades, it took the publication of two major behavioral treatment studies to direct serious attention to the possibility that nonabstinent treatment goals might be advantageous in the treatment of some individuals with alcohol problems. In the first study, conducted in 1970 in Australia by Lovibond and Caddy (13), outpatient alcoholics and problem drinkers were treated through behavioral counseling and blood alcohol level discrimination training. The goal of the treatment program was to engender skills in these individuals, so that they could drink alcohol in a limited fashion, defined by the authors as seldom, if ever, exceeding a blood alcohol level of .07% (mg/100 ml blood). The authors reported that for many of the subjects, this goal was attained.

The second influential and controversial study was first reported in 1972 by Sobell and Sobell (36). In that study, chronic alcoholics in a state hospital participated in an individualized multicomponent behavioral treatment program which involved experimental intoxication, videotape replay of drunken behavior, intensive behavioral analysis of the circumstances controlling the subjects' drinking (antecedent and consequent stimuli), and training in alternative nondrinking behaviors by which the subjects could effectively deal with situations where previously they had drunk to excess. In addition, while some subjects were trained to be abstinent, others were trained to drink in a limited, or controlled, manner. A major strength of this study was that appropriate control groups were used for each experimental treatment.

Highly detailed follow–up of subjects in the Sobell and Sobell study found that subjects treated with the experimental controlled drinking goal functioned significantly better than their control subjects and engaged in a substantial amount of limited nonproblem drinking (33, 34, 35, 37). Those same subjects, surprisingly, also spent more time abstinent than all other subjects during the two–year follow–up interval.

One can but speculate as to why these particular studies were to promote a greater acceptance of nonabstinence goals. Perhaps the studies' impact related to the fact that both incorporated an *explicit* treatment objective of nonproblem drinking; but they were not the first studies to have explored such a goal. For example, in 1954, Shea (29) reported the successful use of such a goal in conjunction with the psychoanalytic treatment of an alcoholic. Furthermore, during the 1960's, Mukasa and his colleagues (21, 22) in Japan reported the successful use of cyanamide to achieve limited drinking in several hundred alcoholics. The literature also shows that studies that have reported successful nonabstinent outcomes for alcoholics have not been totally ignored, as evidenced by the caustic and bountiful criticisms (7) directed at Davies' now classic report of traditionally, abstinence–oriented, treated alcoholics who were engaging in normal drinking several years following treatment (6).

It also seems likely that an increasing interest by behavioral researchers in the treatment of alcohol problems may have lent substantial support to the consideration of alternative goals to abstinence. However, the most important reason why alternatives to abstinence have received attention probably relates to the rapid growth of empirical research in alcohol studies, research which gained its impetus from the pioneering work of Mendelson and his colleagues (15) in studies of experimental intoxication. These early studies made clear that much knowledge could be gained from studying intoxicated alcoholics under controlled conditions. Thus, attention to nonabstinent goals might well be considered as an inevitable consequence of the direct scientific study of alcoholics.

CAN ALCOHOLICS EVER DRINK SAFELY?

Frequently, it is asked in retrospect whether individuals who are able to achieve successful nonabstinent outcomes were actually alcoholics in the first place. In this regard, some have even gone so far as to suggest that anyone capable of learning to drink without encountering further problems must, *ipso facto,* never have been a "true" alcoholic (1, 11, 39). This objection raises a problem which complicates any interpretation of whether some "alcoholics" can or should learn to drink in a nonproblem manner, namely, the chronic lack of consensus about an appropriate definition of alcoholism.

Historically, the search for a scientifically acceptable definition of alcoholism has been complex and elusive. As a result, this topic will not be addressed in detail here. For our purposes, two examples will suffice. The definition favored by Jellinek (9), a leader in the formulation of traditional notions of alcoholism, was that alcoholism referred to any "use of alcoholic beverage that causes any damage to the individual or society or both" (p. 35). The adverse consequences could be physical, social, or psychological in nature. In contrast, the American Medical Society on Alcoholism (AMSA) has recently proposed that the designation "alcoholism" be reserved for those conditions "characterized by tolerance and physical dependency or pathologic organ changes, or both—all direct or indirect consequences of the alcohol ingested" (28, p. 764). The AMSA definition is obviously much less inclusive than the commonly and professionally accepted definition used by Jellinek. According to the AMSA formulation, many individuals who suffer adverse consequences related to their use of alcohol but do not manifest "physical dependency or pathologic organ changes" cannot be considered to be "alcoholic." These individuals, whom national surveys suggest are more numerous than "alcoholics" (3), are left uncategorized. In this chapter, they will be referred to as "problem drinkers," consistent with the AMSA definition of alcoholism.

Returning now to our original question, are some alcoholics, as defined above, capable of drinking without incurring further liabilities? Research evidence suggests unequivocally that this is not only possible but actually occurs for many more individuals than has been generally recognized. Several studies (4, 8, 24, 27) have reported that individuals who achieve successful nonabstinent outcomes are unlikely to maintain contact with clinicians or treatment programs strongly oriented toward abstinence. Whether an explicit treatment objective of limited consumption of alcohol for such an individual is ever a justified goal (i.e., "should" it, rather than "can" it be done), however, is a separate issue which will be considered shortly.

Considering problem drinkers, the evidence is similarly clear—alcohol problems are not necessarily progressive (5, 26). In fact, one of the major contentions of this chapter is that problem drinkers constitute the population most likely to benefit from nonabstinent treatment goals. It should also be noted that while the highest reported incidence of drinking problems (mostly those problems *not* involving physical dependence) in the United States occurs for males in their twenties, few people under the age of 30 participate in Alcoholics Anonymous (10).

Of course, several additional criticisms of reports that some alcoholics and problem drinkers can function well and still drink in moderation have appeared in the literatue, as have a number of arguments in favor of nonabstinent treatment objectives. These arguments, which actually have more to do with ideologies than facts, have been summarized elsewhere (e.g., 12, 25, 26, 31, 34).

WHO SHOULD DRINK?

We now turn our attention to the important issue of for whom a nonproblem drinking outcome might be appropriate as a treatment objective. First, however, let us briefly consider the general topic of treatment goals. Rather than impose an artificial dichotomy upon treatment goals, we prefer and encourage others to use one general treatment goal for all cases—a reduction in drinking to a nonproblem level. For this paper, drinking problems will be defined as any adverse consequences deriving from an individual's use of alcohol, including physical, psychological, and social consequences. For many, an absence of alcohol problems might only be achieved through total abstinence (e.g., for persons who suffer from cirrhosis). For others, however, it might be accomplished within a context of drinking which does not result in adverse consequences. While this definition does not avoid the difficult problem of delineating for whom nonproblem drinking might be feasible, it clearly acknowledges that specific treatment objectives should be flexible and subject to modification, should the client experience adverse circumstances.

The evidence presently available regarding which types of individuals can achieve nonproblem drinking is, unfortunately, largely either correlational or anecdotal. Furthermore, most of these results have derived from follow-up studies of traditional (abstinence-oriented) treatment programs. Until recently, random assignment of persons to treatment goals was difficult, if not impossible, to justify; consequently, only one study has been reported in which subjects were randomly, rather than selectively, assigned to goals (27). However, although lacking experimental test, the correlative findings reported in the literature to date (reviewed in 31) suggest some subject characteristics which may be predictive of individuals who can attain successful nonabstinent outcomes. Keeping in mind that correlational evidence must be interpreted cautiously, the literature suggests that individuals who have less serious drinking problems at entry into treatment are more likely to acquire a posttreatment pattern of nonproblem drinking. In particular, this relationship is suggested by characteristics of less pretreatment alcohol intake, less prior symptomatology, especially physical dependence, and a shorter self-reported history of drinking problems. It remains to be determined, of course, whether these characteristics also describe the same individuals who are most likely to succeed at abstinence. Only controlled research can answer these questions.

Little research has been reported which is useful in identifying isolated treatment factors conducive to nonproblem drinking outcomes. There is some scant evidence suggesting that treatment oriented toward nonabstinent outcomes is related to successful nonabstinent outcomes (27, 33, 34, 35, 36, 37). However, such studies are too limited in scope to allow firm conclusions to be drawn. There is also some evidence indicating that individuals who attain nonproblem drinking outcomes following treatment in abstinence-oriented programs tend to spend relatively less time in treatment than individuals who do not attain such outcomes. The significance of this finding is presently unknown.

These same correlational data also provide valuable insights into the nature of nonproblem drinking outcomes. For example, it has often been the case that individuals experience some drinking problems shortly following treatment, and then overcome those problems. Also, as with abstinence, successful drinking outcomes are frequently, but not necessarily, associated with improvement in other areas of life, e.g., interpersonal functioning. Finally, it has been suggested by some that the onset of nonproblem drinking is often preceded by a significant positive change in an individual's life circumstances. Although the present evidence does not support such a relationship, these studies have rarely gathered data relevant to this question.

At this point, it should be emphasized that the term nonproblem drinking—drinking which does not engender adverse consequences—must be distinguished from an outcome of attenuated drinking, which can be used to describe those cases where persons with severe drinking problems manage to modify their drinking so as to minimize potential adverse consequences. Attenuated drinking might well be considered a feasible goal in recalcitrant cases of chronic alcoholism, but it is far removed from a treatment objective of nonproblem drinking.

As noted earlier, persons with drinking problems of lesser severity and who have never suffered alcohol withdrawal symptoms might be excellent candidates for nonproblem drinking. In addition to the data suggesting that such individuals may be more able to acquire the necessary skills to achieve nonproblem drinking, it is also the case that very few services presently exist for treatment of the problem drinker as compared to the "chronic alcoholic." Moreover, it is possible that traditional treatment programs, with their strong emphasis on abstinence, may have inadvertently prevented many persons, such as problem drinkers, from seeking treatment. Despite the proclamations to the contrary, the diagnostic label "alcoholic" has frequently been indiscriminately applied, and it is still distasteful to many people. It seems unlikely that its negative connotation will change in the near future. On the other hand, it is probable that more persons would admit having a drinking problem if the outcome of this type of problem were not depicted as emasculating with a requirement for a permanent life style of abstinence. Preferably, one could offer an alternative orientation, where recovery is viewed as possible for some or many, and where it is recognized that one can minimize future handicaps by early, and less intense, interventions.

Elsewhere, Miller and Caddy (19), and we ourselves (36), have addressed several other possible criteria which might be used to determine whether nonproblem drinking is a feasible goal for a given case; the reader is advised to consult those references prior to enacting any nonabstinence–oriented treatment strategy. Basically, certain factors, such as evidence of serious health problems which would be exacerbated by alcohol consumption, or strong external demands for abstinence, can be readily seen as apparent contraindications to a treatment goal of nonproblem drinking. Similarly, it seems unreasonable to attempt to convince a 20–year–old who has had some, but few serious, alcohol problems and who lives within an environment and social setting supportive of moderate drinking, that he is probably a fledgling alcoholic and should immediately abandon alcoholic beverages for the rest of his life. Furthermore, it should be kept in mind that treatment goal decisions, like treatment progress, should be frequently assessed, and modifications in either the goals or the methods introduced if the evidence indicates a lack or reversal of progress.

ACHIEVING AND MAINTAINING NONPROBLEM DRINKING

Assuming that a nonproblem drinking objective is selected as a treatment goal in a given case, how then does one go about achieving that goal with a client? Many of the questions addressed in this short chapter cannot be answered sufficiently, and nowhere is this limitation more pronounced than concerning the topic of treatment methods. We can only mention some of the more prominent issues and approaches to treatment and caution the reader that the task is difficult, perhaps more arduous than the pursuit of total abstinence. We implore practitioners to study the existing literature intensively before attempting to treat patients with these techniques.

Although a few cases have been reported where a nonbehavioral approach to treatment has been used to seek a nonabstinent goal, the major advances in achieving and maintaining nonproblem drinking have derived almost totally from behavioral research. While not discounting the possible contributions of biological factors, the majority of these approaches has considered that environmental factors and learning play key roles in the development of drinking patterns which result in adverse consequences. Even Jellinek, in his classic formulation of the disease concept of alcoholism (9), stated that a learning process "is a prerequisite to bring about the conditions which are necessary for the development of addiction in the pharmacological sense" (p. 77).

In most modern formulations (e.g., 17, 34), the acquisition of particular drinking behaviors is considered to be a discriminated operant response; that is, a behavior which only occurs in the presence of certain antecedent stimuli (including internal physiological factors, cognitions, and environmental factors) and which is acquired and maintained because of its consequences. These consequences are typically conceptualized as consisting of short-term rewards, followed by delayed but adverse consequences, such as feelings of remorse, physical ailments, alcohol withdrawal symptoms, etc. In this way the immediate consequences are hypothesized to exert control over the drinking response. Combined with the phenomenon of tolerance, where an individual needs to drink a greater and greater amount of alcohol simply to achieve an equivalent degree of effect, this provides an appealing explanation of the development of a pattern of excessive drinking. Parenthetically, this explanation has yet to be soundly supported by empirical evidence.

Behavioral treatments have often incorporated a set of techniques with particular methods tailored to the characteristics of each case. From a research perspective, a broad–spectrum approach does not allow precise examination of the contribution of specific components to the overall treatment outcome. For clinical purposes, however, the broad–spectrum approach seems prudent in terms of maximizing potential treatment effects. This is particularly true if the selected methods derive from a careful evaluation of an individual's treatment needs. In many respects, the specific treatment components are often well-known behavior therapy techniques. For example, a client may need assertive training in combination with systematic desensitization to provide him with alternative skills for dealing with situations which have typically led to excessive drinking. Another method which is more cognitively based includes training clients in problem–solving skills (35, 36). This is a four–step procedure: problem identification, delineation of behavioral alternatives to problem drinking, evaluation of those alternatives and their probable outcomes (including immediate and delayed consequences), and training in any skills which may be necessary to enact those alternatives.

Other methods have been developed to deal specifically with drinking behavior. For example, self–monitoring of drinking behaviors using written records can be an easily implemented and highly valuable component of treatment (30). Self–monitoring involves the client directly and immediately in the analysis of his drinking or potential drinking, facilitates discussion of instances when drinking has occurred, and allows early therapeutic intervention if a pattern of increasing or problem drinking becomes evident. The maintenance of drinking records is especially useful when nonabstinent goals are pursued, since problem drinking has possible serious, immediate consequences. Self–monitoring can also be used in conjunction with behavioral contracting, as demonstrated by Miller (16).

The efficacy of self–monitoring can be enhanced by using a portable breath tester, for example the Mobat (32), to provide the patient with feedback about his blood alcohol level (BAL). Clients can be trained to estimate their BAL fairly accurately using this device for discrimination training (2). Although there is some controversy regarding whether a person can base such estimates on internal cues, e.g., facial warmth, numbing, etc., or must rely on external factors, e.g., knowledge of what amount of ethanol has been consumed over what period of time, this is irrelevant to the value of the technique since its utility is dependent on the fact that persons do learn to estimate their BALs correctly. Finally, although early studies investigated the utility of electric shock avoidance conditioning to shape appropriate drinking behaviors (20), it has since become clear that these methods are unnecessary, and less aversive methods are equally or more effective.

Before concluding our discussion, some related issues deserve further elaboration. First, the attitude of the therapist as communicated to the client may be an important factor in achieving nonabstinent goals. The therapist in these cases occupies a precarious position. He not only must remain alert to the possibility that treatment objectives might need to be changed if they become clearly unrealistic, but he also must be able to concurrently reinforce the client's approximations to success. This requires considerable skill and experience. We have found that rewarding the client's sharing of drinking experiences—e.g., reporting of instances of problem or nonproblem drinking, even if those experiences resulted in adverse consequences—is very useful. The obvious correlate of this process is to explore at length with the client the consequences of his drinking. It is seldom necessary for the therapist to appear judgmental even if problem drinking occurs, for the facts when fully explored usually speak for themselves.

Second, there are many subtleties to the treatment of alcohol problems, especially if the treatment goal is nonproblem drinking. For example, clients often encounter unanticipated and countertherapeutic resistance from friends, relatives, and others in the community (e.g., physicians, judges) with regard to their nonproblem drinking. It is the therapist's responsibility to become thoroughly familiar with these subtle problems before attempting to treat a client. Similarly, it is relatively easy to confuse the treatment goal of nonproblem drinking with treatment methods, or to perceive that goal as a panacea. It is neither. Treatment is a process directed toward attaining specified objectives. Goals tell us how to evaluate progress with respect to those objectives, and sometimes it is appropriate for goals to be revised. A decision to change goals, however, should not result from superficial considerations, but rather from a careful examination of all the clinical data available to the therapist. Although we have emphasized a need for caution in pursuing nonabstinent treatment objectives, there are also occasions when the goal of abstinence may be inappropriate. Careful consideration of individual case circumstances should be prerequisite to all treatment goal decisions.

REFERENCES

1. Block, M. Comment on "Normal drinking in recovered alcohol addicts," in D.L. Davies, Normal drinking in recovered alcohol addicts. (Comment by various correspondents). *Q. J. Stud. Alc.* 24:109–121, 321–332, 1963.
2. Caddy, G.R. Blood alcohol concentration discrimination training: Development and current status, in G.A. Marlatt and P.E. Nathan (eds.), *Behavioral Approaches to Alcoholism.* New Brunswick: Rutgers Center for Alcohol Studies, 1978, NIAAA–RUCAS Treatment Series No. 2, pp. 114–129.
3. Cahalan, D., and Room, R. *Problem Drinking Among American Men.* Monograph No. 7. New Brunswick: Rutgers Center of Alcohol Studies, 1974.
4. Chaney, E.F., O'Leary, M.R., and Marlatt, G.A. Skill training with alcoholics. (Doctoral dissertation, University of Washington, 1977). *Dissertation Abstracts Intl.,* 1977, 37.
5. Clark, W.B., and Cahalan, D. *Changes in problem drinking over a four-year span.* Paper

.

28. Seixas, F.A., Blume, S., Cloud, L.A., Lieber, C.S., and Simpson, R.K. Definition of alcoholism. Letter in *Ann. Int. Med.* 85:764, 1976.

29. Shea, J.E. Psychoanalytic therapy and alcoholism. *Q. J. Stud. Alc.* 15:595–605, 1954.

30. Sobell, L.C., and Sobell, M.B. A self-feedback technique to monitor drinking behavior in alcoholics. *Behav. Res. and Ther.* 11:237–238, 1973.

31. Sobell, M.B. Alternatives to abstinence: Evidence, issues and some proposals, in P.E. Nathan, G.A. Marlatt, and T. Loberg (eds.), *Alcoholism: New Directions in Behavioral Research and Treatment.* New York: Plenum Press, 1978, pp. 177–209.

32. Sobell, M.B., and Sobell, L.C. A brief technical report on the Mobat: An inexpensive portable test for determining blood alcohol concentration. *J. Appl. Behav. Anal.* 8:117–120, 1975.

33. Sobell, M.B., and Sobell, L.C. Alcoholics treated by individualized behavior therapy: One year treatment outcome. *Behav. Res. and Ther.* 11:599–618, 1973.

34. Sobell, M.B., and Sobell, L.C. *Behavioral Treatment of Alcohol Problems: Individualized Therapy and Controlled Drinking.* New York: Plenum Press, 1978.

35. Sobell, M.B., and Sobell, L.C. Individualized behavior therapy for alcoholics. *Behav. Ther.* 4:49–72, 1973.

36. Sobell, M.B., and Sobell, L.C. Individualized behavior therapy for alcoholics: Rationale, procedures, preliminary results and appendix. *California Mental Health Research Monograph, No. 13,* Sacramento, 1972.

37. Sobell, M.B., and Sobell, L.C. Second year treatment outcome of alcoholics treated by individualized behavior therapy: Results. *Behav. Res. and Ther.* 14:195–215, 1976.

38. Sobell, M.B., and Sobell, L.C. The need for realism, relevance and operational assumptions in the study of substance dependence, in H.D. Cappell and A.E. LeBlanc (eds.), *Biological and Behavioral Approaches to Drug Dependence.* Toronto: Addiction Research Foundation. 1975, pp. 138–167.

39. Weisman, M. Letter in *News and Views.* Alcoholism Council of Greater Los Angeles, January 1975, p. 4.

Chapter 10

Abstinence–Oriented Alcoholism Treatment Approaches

James W. Smith

Alcoholism has troubled mankind since earliest recorded times, when Hippocrates and other early Greek and Roman physicians wrote extensively about its association with brain dysfunction (23). As each new field of medicine and behavioral science developed, workers in each discipline have dutifully (if not eagerly) attempted to explain alcoholism in terms of their own science and have formulated treatment programs, some elaborate, others starkly simple, based on their particular viewpoints. The fact that now, centuries later, members of the helping professions are still arguing heatedly among themselves about its etiology—e.g., is it an inherited, constitutional biochemical defect or a bad habit?—the proper method of treatment; and, perhaps even more surprisingly, the goal of treatment—shall it be abstinence or controlled drinking?—is immensely frustrating and disappointing to those working in the field. This confusion points out the lack of reliable information about the basic nature of alcoholism, including its etiology, the natural history if untreated, and the long–term course when comparable alcoholic patients are treated with different therapeutic modalities.

Part of the problem undoubtedly stems from the fact that alcoholism is not a unitary disorder. Instead, it appears to be a collection of several different entities which all have alcohol consumption as one of several damaging symptoms. Jellinek (26) attempted to bring order into the field by dividing the alcoholisms into five types which he labeled with the Greek letters alpha through epsilon. Others, e.g. Schuckit (39), divide the field into primary alcoholics who seem to be normal in all respects except for their inability to control their alcohol intake, and secondary alcoholics who have a preexisting psychiatric disorder, usually sociopathy in males and depression in females, in which excessive alcohol intake is secondary to their psychopathology. In secondary alcoholics, the disease tends to mirror the course of the psychopathology rather than the course of primary alcoholism.

Abstinence–oriented programs assume that alcoholics must remain "dry" and target nondrinking as the primary goal. At Schick's Shadel we use a comprehensive clinical program that is focused on changing a variety of problems. We conceptualize alcohol problems as falling into one or a combination of the following categories, each of which has a standard treatment approach:

1. Deficiencies in information or required behavior.
2. Behavioral excesses.
3. Inappropriate environmental stimulus control.
4. Inappropriate self–generated stimulus control.
5. Inappropriate reinforcement contingencies.

Deficiencies of Information or Required Behaviors

The first category includes general lack of information, or misinformation, about alcoholism. Education with appropriate information about alcohol, its effects, and alcoholism is included in most alcoholism treatment programs, usually in didactic group meetings.

The alcoholic may be deficient in interpersonal skills, or basically unassertive. For example, he may be unable to turn down a drink gracefully. For these deficiencies, assertiveness training, behavioral rehearsal, role playing, etc. are often useful.

A third common area of deficit is the patient's inability to realistically evaluate his own performance and achievements, usually accompanied by a lack of self–esteem or poor self–image. Alcoholics often have difficulty viewing their positive attributes and accomplishments favorably. They tend to depreciate these attributes and project an "I'm no good" self–image while at the same time striving, sometimes excessively hard, to do a good job at work or elsewhere. Failing to achieve goals that they feel are realistic—e.g., taking only two drinks at a party—may reinforce their poor self–image. From these repeated failures, they receive the implicit message "I am weak." Training in self–monitoring of positive behaviors and achievements and rehearsal in tangible or cognitive self–reward can help change these behaviors. Sometimes alcohol has been used as a self–administered reward for many years. If he did a good job he would treat himself to "a few drinks." Treatment emphasizes substitution of an alternate more appropriate reward for alcohol.

Another behavioral deficit often seen in alcoholic patients is a lack of healthful ways to deal with tension. Alcohol or other drugs may be the sole recreational outlet for these patients. Encouraging the patient to sample a wider range of outlets may help provide behaviors that will take over the tension–reducing function of alcohol and enhance change. Making a social commitment, like phoning a friend *today* and setting up a specific appointment, e.g., Thursday at 2:00 P.M., for a game of golf rather than making a global statement of "I'm going to start playing golf" is a useful self–management tool to increase the likelihood that the intent is carried out to a specific action.

Behavioral Excesses

The most obvious excess of alcoholics involves the amount of alcohol consumed. The change method most often used in behavior therapy programs is covert or overt (chemical or electrical) aversion conditioning, which will be described in detail later.

Other problems may include excessive conditioned anxiety to objects or events or excessive self–observation. Conditioned anxiety in alcoholics may take the form of fear, or considerable discomfort, in social settings, which they often treat by self–medication with alcohol. Relaxation training and self–hypnosis may be useful for these patients. Assertiveness training or other types of social skill training has proved useful for relieving discomfort specifically related to social gatherings. Excessive self–observation may take the form of rumination about one's impact on others and anxiety about what others may be thinking or saying about him. Thought stopping and the development of incompatible responses have been useful for patients with these fears.

Inappropriate Environmental Stimulus Control

Poor environmental stimulus control tends to be a common finding in alcoholic patients. Alcoholics encounter many environmental stimuli such as times of day, days of the week, or interpersonal situations where the thought of a drink comes to mind immediately. Once areas associated with frequent thought of a drink have been identified, a variety of methods to control them can be implemented. Some strategies may be as simple as taking a different road home from work so as not to pass a familiar bar. In other cases, more complex incompatible responses must be designed. For instance, a nonpracticing nurse who was recently divorced and whose children were grown and out of the home, experienced strong urges to drink from 6:00 to 8:00 P.M., a time that was formerly "family time," but now was empty. She was encouraged to take a refresher course in nursing. She then obtained a job on the 3:00 to 11:00 P.M. shift at the hospital and eliminated the alcohol craving from 6:00 to 8:00 P.M.

Inappropriate Self-Generated Stimulus Control

Inappropriate self-generated stimulus control may take the form of inaccurate self-labeling of one's capabilities with consequent self-fulfilling prophecies, e.g., an alcoholic who views himself as weak and lacking will power or ability to withstand temptation will have this self-impression confirmed when he compares his lack of ability to limit his alcohol intake once he has begun drinking, to a nonalcoholic friend who has no trouble with control and no alcohol addiction. Appropriate change methods include information about the nature of addiction and reconditioning attitudes by rehearsing positive self-statements, etc.

Faulty labeling of internal stimuli is another form of inappropriate stimulus control. For example, when a person is hungry his blood sugar level is usually low. If he has an alcoholic drink at this point, it causes a slight rise in blood sugar level and temporarily eliminates the hunger. After many repetitions of this sequence, the alcoholic may begin to misinterpret normal craving for food caused by low blood sugar as a craving for alcohol. A similar sequence may occur when slight dehydration causes a normal sensation of thirst which becomes misinterpreted as "a cold beer would taste good." Patients can be educated about normal physiology and taught to drink fruit juice or eat food at a time when craving is experienced. Covert techniques like self-instruction and reattribution may also be helpful.

Inappropriate Reinforcement Contingencies

An alcoholic's environment may fail to support or positively reinforce appropriate behaviors. For example, the spouse of a newly abstinent alcoholic may not give positive reinforcement like compliments or positive comments for his maintenance of sobriety and appropriate new behaviors. Instead, the spouse may remind the alcoholic of all the bad things he did while drinking in the past. Family counseling, spouse education, and contracting between the couple members help resolve this problem. Continued or renewed drinking may be subtly reinforced by people in the patient's home environment. For example, a spouse who has through necessity taken over the reins of the family may feel threatened when the alcoholic sobers up and begins to reassume some of her new functions. She may sabotage his efforts to remain sober by telling him that it is all right to have one or two drinks now that he is sober, even though she knows that in the past this has always led to a binge; that he was much more fun when he was drinking; that he has a terrible personality when not drinking, etc. To change these behaviors, it is necessary to change the social environment by educating and counseling the spouse. In extreme cases, when the spouse is unwilling to change, it may be necessary to recommend divorce.

AVERSIVE TREATMENTS

For the specific problem of alcohol addiction, avesive conditioning techniques offer the most thoroughly researched treatment approach with the longest period of follow-up.

Perhaps the oldest approach to abstinence treatment is aversion conditioning. The Romans placed spiders or other repellent objects in the bottom of the wine cup to be discovered by the drinker after draining the vessel. In more modern times, Kantorovich (27) reported on the aversion conditioning treatment of alcoholism using electrical aversion in 1929. In the United States, Voegtlin (42) developed a chemical aversion technique in the mid-1930's. In 1950, Lemere and Voegtlin (29) reported on a series of 4096 fee-paying, voluntary patients treated over a 13-year period with emetine-induced nausea which was paired with the sight, smell, and taste of a variety of alcoholic beverages. His preferred beverages were emphasized but treatment also included other types of liquor in order to aid in generalization of the conditioned response. They emphasized the temporal relationship between the unconditioned stimulus (nausea) and the conditioned stimuli (sight, smell, and taste of alcoholic beverages). The patients received from four to six treatments over an average hospital stay of ten days. Booster treatments were given six months after the initial treatment or sooner if the desire to drink returned. In addition to aversion therapy, patients received "support and encouragement" from the staff and engaged in informal discussions with other patients. Discharge interviews stressed the patients' responsibility for maintaining abstinence. They were informed that their aversion to alcohol would eventually wear off, and they were given suggestions for dealing with drinking associates, boredom, fatigue, and other environmental hazards which might be associated with a return to drinking (40). A heavy emphasis was placed on maintaining lifelong abstinence from alcohol. Lemere and Voegtlin (29) reported that 60% of their patients remained abstinent for one year or longer, 51% remained abstinent two years or longer, 38% for five years or longer, and 23% for ten years or longer. Of those patients who were retreated after relapse (N = 878) 38% remained abstinent.

Beaubrum (5) reported on a series of West Indies alcoholics in which emetine aversion conditioning was used as an adjunct to an Alcoholics Anonymous (AA) treatment program. He reported that, of those patients available for follow-up, 39.1% treated with emetine alone and 38.1% of those treated with AA alone were abstinent two years later while 77.5% of those treated with emetine and AA were abstinent. A control group which received neither AA nor emetine was reported to have an abstinence rate of 33.3% at follow–up.

Emetine aversion therapy has been used in much the same fashion as described by Lemere and Voegtlin (29) at Schick's Shadel Hospital continuously since the treatment was devised in 1935 with the addition of "pentothal interviews" on alternate days instead of an aversion treatment (15). The pentothal interview is used to facilitate uninhibited discussion by the patient of personal problems that may have contributed to his drinking and may relieve feelings of tension. Suggestions can be given to the patient in this state to support the patient's resolve to remain sober and to remind the patient of the aversive consequences he has experienced in treatment and elsewhere when he has used alcohol (41).

Four hundred seventy–seven patients treated in 1976 were sent a follow–up questionnaire to which 284 patients responded. One hundred eighty–three of these (64.4%) indicated they had remained totally abstinent for 12 months after treatment, and another 81 (28.6%) were abstinent at the time of follow–up but had consumed alcohol on at least one occasion since treatment. Wiens et al. (47) reported a series of 261 first admissions for alcoholism (53 women and 208 men) treated at Raleigh Hills Hospital in Portland, Oregon in 1970. They used an emetine aversion therapy similar to that described by Lemere and Voegtlin (29). At one–year follow–up, 63% of their 261 patients had remained abstinent.

Emetine is the drug that has been used most frequently in chemical aversion therapy, however, some researchers have used apomorphine as the nausea-inducing drug. Voegtlin, Lemere, and Broz (43) argue that apomorphine is unsuitable for two reasons. First, the nauseant action of the drug is too short, about two or three minutes, and second, the "narcotic euphoric phase that immediately follows the nauseant phase" interferes with the development of successful aversion.

Along other lines, in 1934, Dent first reported on the beneficial aspects of apomorphine used in subemetic doses in the treatment of chronic alcoholism (13, 14). He believed it eliminated craving by physiologic action on the brain rather than the development of conditioned aversion. More recently, Schlatter and Samarthyji (38) used an approach similar to Dent's in a nonblind study which found that patients treated with oral apomorphine reported a decreased craving for alcohol, but resumed drinking at a rate little different from those treated without apomorphine.

Poor results from aversion conditioning programs may result from so–called backward conditioning, where alcohol is given after nausea develops. Franks (20, 21) considers "backward conditioning" a most difficult form of conditioning to develop and a form easily extinguished. Elkins (16) suggested that backward conditioning, since it pairs alcohol with decreasing nausea, could actually increase the reward value of the alcohol. Green and Garcia (22) report animal studies which support this concept. Finally, Rachman and Teasdale (34) report that well–conducted chemical aversion therapy is associated with one–year abstinence rates of approximately 60%, but they feel that the procedures are arduous and, because of this, the number of possible pairings of nausea with the sight, smell, and taste of alcoholic beverages in a reasonable period of time is limited.

Sanderson, Campbell, and Laverty (37) reported on a different type of pharmacological aversion treatment. They studied twelve hospitalized alcoholics who were told they would undergo an unpleasant experience designed to produce a beneficial change. An intravenous infusion of normal saline was started after placing the patient on a stretcher and connecting polygraph leads to him. After his physiological responses (GSR, muscle tension, heart rate, respiratory rate) had stabilized, the patient was given a bottle of his favorite alcoholic beverage, instructed to hold the bottle, look at it, smell and taste the contents, and then to return it to the experimenter. After several repetitions of these behaviors, 20 mg of succinylcholine, a muscle paralyzing agent used in surgical anesthesia, was added to the intravenous infusion out of sight of the patient. When a characteristic GSR pattern indicated that the drug was about to paralyze the patient, the patient was again presented the bottle of liquor and instructed to drink some of it. At about the time he put it to his lips he would become paralyzed, unable to move or breathe. When the apnea lasted over 60 to 90 seconds the patient was artificially ventilated. Patients describe this experience as terrifying. When offered the bottle again four refused to handle it and the others completed the task in a brisk, perfunctory manner. At follow–up the authors reported that six of the 12 were not drinking, three were drinking, and three could not be located for evaluation.

Farrar et al. (19) report a similar experiment with 12 male psychiatric hospital volunteers. At follow–up one year later only two were abstinent. In a series of 23 cases treated with succinylcholine aversion, Holzinger et al. (24) found at follow–up averaging 4.2 months after treatment (range 3 days to 7.5 months) only two patients were abstinent. Mandill et al. (30) randomly assigned 45 alcoholic inpatients to three experimental groups: apneic conditioning; apneic pseudoconditioning (paralysis without alcohol); and placebo treatment (alcohol alone). They concluded that apneic conditioning did not produce changes in drinking behavior which were sufficiently great or stable enough to recommend it as a treatment technique.

It should be noted that this treatment is potentially lethal. Persons with abnormal variants of cholinesterase, the enzyme which breaks down succinyl-choline, or low plasma cholinesterase levels from cirrhosis, malnutrition, severe anemia, etc., may have greatly prolonged paralysis and require artificially supported ventilation for long periods of time.

Faradic stimulation, or electrical aversion, was first reported by Kantorovich (27), who treated 20 alcoholics in 1929 by pairing faradic stimulation with alcoholic beverage presentation in 5 to 20 sessions. He reported that 14 (70%) were abstinent at follow–up, which ranged from 3 weeks to 20 months. In contrast he reported failure in a similar percentage (7 out of 10) alcoholics in a "control group" receiving hypnosis or medication.

Blake (6) treated 25 patients with faradic stimulation which was paired with sipping an alcoholic beverage and terminated when the patient spit it out. They received from 3 to 36 sessions over 4 to 8 days. A matched group received the same therapy and was also given relaxation training. At one–year follow–up, he reported that 23% of patients treated by faradic aversion conditioning alone were abstinent, while 46% of those receiving aversion conditioning plus relaxation training were abstinent. He also reported that 27% and 13% respectively were "improved." The abstinence rates suggest that relaxation training enhances the treatment success of faradic aversion therapy.

Elkins (17) pointed out a number of weaknesses in the design of Blake's studies (6, 7), including nonrandom assignment of patients to treatment groups, sequential treatments, absence of no–treatment and no–faradic–aversion control groups, etc. He concludes that although the efficacy of faradic conditioning and the interactive effect between relaxation and aversive conditioning has not been clearly demonstrated, the clinical results justify further experimentation.

McChance and McChance (31) reported no significant differences in outcome at 9 and 12 months' follow–up when 89 patients were randomly assigned to either faradic aversion therapy or insight–oriented group psychotherapy in addition to general ward treatment which included weekly patient–staff meetings, occupational therapy, AA meetings, and recreational activities. Register (36) was similarly unimpressed with the contribution of faradic aversion conditioning in a group of 60 patients treated at a VA Hospital. Vogler et al. (45, 46) showed statistically significant improvement in faradic aversion treated patients when compared with sham conditioned and ward control patients. However, the results were of little practical significance because the overall duration of abstinence was short: A mean of nine days to relapse for the control groups vs. 19.5 days for the aversion group.

Jackson and Smith (25) reported more promising results. They compared faradic aversion therapy to chemical (nausea) aversion therapy at Schick's Shadel Hospital. Patients were assigned to the faradic aversion group if they were judged by the medical staff to be physically or emotionally unable to tolerate the more strenuous nausea aversion. Detailed descriptions of the chemical (15, 41) and faradic (12) aversion methods are published elsewhere. The chemical aversion patients received five treatment sessions where the sight, smell, and taste of alcoholic beverages was paired with nausea produced by an injection of emetine. Following each treatment session, the patient was given an oral dose of emetine which, together with the emetine injection, maintained nausea for an additioal three hours: a total of up to 15 hours of conditioning during the patient's ten days in hospital treatment. The faradic aversion patient received an aversive level of electrical stimulation to the forearm paired with the sight, smell, and taste of alcohol, with a random onset, with at least ten treatment trials per therapy session. On some occasions (free choice trials) they could prevent the shock by reaching for an alternate drink like orange juice. The complete faradic aversion session lasted from 20 to 45 minutes, depending on the selection speed of the individual patient, and the total time of exposure to aversive conditioning was no more than four hours during the patient's ten–day course of treatment. Two reinforcement conditioning sessions were scheduled for all patients at intervals of 30 and 90 days after the initial ten–day treatment.

At two–year follow–up, approximately 60% of both groups responded to a follow–up questionnaire. Fifty–seven percent of the chemical aversion group remained abstinent with no further treatment, 20% were abstinent at follow–up but had received further treatment, and 23% were drinking. In the faradic aversion group the results were, respectively, 55%, 30%, and 15%.

These results are from a clinical treatment program in which other treatments were also used, although used equally in both groups. Patient assignment to groups was the result of clinical decisions rather than random assignment, and the subjects in the faradic group were older (average of nine years) and medically more infirm than those in the chemical aversion group. Despite these experimental deficiencies, the results are promising.

Rachman (33) and Rachman and Teasdale (34) compare faradic aversion and chemically induced nausea aversion and point out that the timing of the presentation of electrical stimulation can be controlled with great precision, which allows it to be paired with alcohol precisely or at any point in the chain of behaviors involved in drinking. By contrast, chemically induced nausea, once set in motion, runs its course. They point out that the intensity of the aversive faradic stimulus can be varied to suit the requirements of the individual patient, and the physical effects on the patient (and staff) are less rigorous and permit many more pairings of alcohol and the aversive stimulus than would be practical using nausea. Because of their flexibility, faradic procedures also are useful for discrimination training during which the aversive stimulus is terminated for choosing a nonalcoholic beverage (12). Electrical stimulation also has the advantage of needing fewer technically trained treatment personnel than emetic aversion procedures, which require close medical supervision.

After reviewing both the basic physiology of acquired aversion and the chemical literature, Elkins (17) concludes that successful aversion therapy aimed at the elimination of alcohol consumption can be more efficiently achieved through the use of nausea than aversive shock. Nausea can be produced without the use of oral or injected drugs. Lazarus (28) used a mixture of foul–smelling chemicals which patients inhaled after tasting the material to which they were made averse (in this case food), and reported good results with two subjects.

Mellor and White (32) reported success using nausea from "motion sickness," induced by a specially designed rotary chair. They induced nausea in 10 blindfolded alcoholic patients who were rotated at 17.5 revolutions per minute while positioned 20 degrees off the vertical axis. Two trials a day were carried out for six consecutive days. During each trial an alcoholic beverage was presented to taste and swallow a small amount. After each presentation the patient was rotated until nausea (but not vomiting) occurred. Eight of the ten experienced severe nausea. At follow–up six months later, two were totally abstinent since treatment and four had aversive reactions when they drank. Two of these later were abstinent at the time of follow–up. Two did not develop an aversion during the initial treatment. Despite a relatively low abstinence rate, the procedure avoids most of the hazards involved in the chemically induced nausea procedures and may be of some therapeutic use.

Aversive techniques have been developed based on imagery. Since nausea, rather than vomiting, is the aversive stimulus (35), these methods may be of use in some instances where physical disability precludes the use of chemical aversion therapy. In the technique described by Cautela (9, 10, 11), the therapist determines the patient's favorite alcoholic beverages and typical drinking settings and then instructs the patient in muscular relaxation techniques (49). The relaxed patient is directed to imagine himself in his usual drinking setting about to drink his favorite drink. This imagined scene is elaborated on by the therapist, who gives nausea inducing suggestions until the patient fantasizes becoming nauseated and vomiting. Cautela stresses that inducing real nausea during the verbal presentation is necessary and can be obtained with only a few conditioning trials.

Cautela's technique punishes the patient for the *intention* to take a drink and for all the links in the chain of behaviors leading to bringing a drink up to the lips. The patient is asked *not* to imagine the taste of liquor, on the assumption that the thought of its taste may be reinforcing (48). Ten scenes pairing the intention to drink with the actual feeling of nausea induced by the imagined scene and imagined vomiting are alternated with ten scenes of escape conditioning during which the patient terminates the imagined urge to drink with its attendant nausea, by imagining a decision to not drink which is immediately followed by the disappearance of nausea and a feeling of well–being. After receiving instructions and training, the patient is told to imagine the scene twice a day by himself. Cautela reports that it takes 6 to 12 months to achieve successful treatment results and therefore should be used with other supplemental therapeutic efforts.

A similar treatment approach termed "verbal aversion therapy" has been described by Anant (3). Like Cautela, Anant first relaxed his patients and then had them imagine nausea and vomiting associated with alcoholic beverages in five "stages." In the first stage the patient is directed to imagine drinking an alcoholic beverage which is followed by changes in taste, a stomach ache, nausea, and vomiting. In stage two, the patient uses again the stage–one scenes and additional aversive scenes of embarrassing situations such as vomiting on close friends, the bar, all over one's own clothing, etc. During the third stage, the patient imagines that the smell of alcohol rather than drinking causes nausea. In the fourth stage, all references to alcohol are omitted and the patient imagines he feels abdominal pain and nausea after a strong desire for a drink. The aversive symptoms are described as leaving when he controls his urge and does not drink. The fifth stage involves discrimination training in which the patient imagines he feels nausea whenever he feels a desire for alcoholic beverages, but immediately feels better when he decides to have a soft drink instead. Anant (3) reported that of 14 patients treated in groups and 11 treated individually with this technique, all of whom completed treatment, all were totally abstinent at follow–up 8 to 15 months later. In a subsequent report (4), he noted that only 3 of the 14 treated in groups remained abstinent. He recommends periodic booster treatment sessions to prevent extinction of the aversion.

Elkins (17) describes a procedure similar to Anant's during which he measured GSR, respiratory rate, and heart rate. He found characteristic GSR and respiratory rate changes when imagined nausea occurred. After about four sessions of four to six scenes, he found that 22 of 24 patients developed feelings of nausea with physiological evidence during imagery and suggestion, and that 15 of 22 developed "conditioned" nausea to the thought of alcohol with further training (18). A similar failure to condition in some subjects has been reported in a minority of alcoholics treated with chemical (nausea) aversion (44).

A follow–up telephone contact was carried out with the patient and a "significant other" in 13 patients with conditioned nausea and 6 without conditioned nausea. Those with conditioned nausea were abstinent much longer (mean 14.9 months' abstinence) than those without conditioned nausea (mean 3.71 months' abstinence), who did not differ from patients who dropped out before receiving six treatment sessions and those who did not develop any nausea (mean 3.86 months' abstinence).

ALCOHOLICS ANONYMOUS (AA)

Although an increasing number of professionals in the field of behavioral therapy have become active in alcoholism treatment in recent years, lay persons, through the fellowship of Alcohlics Anonymous (AA), are still treating the largest number of alcoholic individuals. For this reason, behavior therapists should understand how AA works. This organization is committed to total abstinence as opposed to controlled ("nonproblem") drinking as the treatment goal. AA has 12 "steps" and 12 "traditions" which members are expected to practice. In this program, frequent group attendance is urged, self–revelation, and social reinforcement is given for adhering to treatment goals. Each member

234   SMITH

has a sponsor who reinforces his progress through the 12 steps and helps remind him of his goals. Affiliate AA organizations of Alanon and Alateen (8) work with the family to assist them in coping with living with an alcoholic. The interested reader should consult other sources (1, 2) for a more detailed description of AA. In summary, alcoholics exhibit many types of behavioral problems. These can be categorized as behavioral deficits, behavioral excesses, inappropriate environmental stimulus control, inappropriate self-generated stimulus control, and inappropriate reinforcement contingencies. Behavioral therapy strategies exist to make therapeutic changes in each of these categories. Aversion therapies are often used in abstinence-oriented alcoholism treatment programs. Chemically induced nausea has been the most extensively used aversive stimulant, and it appears to have the highest documented success rate. Other forms of aversive treatments, such as electrical stimulation and covert imagery, have also been used, but with less success. Successful alcoholism treatment programs all employ a large number and type of therapeutic interventions that include work with families, environmental change, job training or rehabilitation, and fellowship. The social reinforcing aspects of a program can be of significance in treatment maintenance, as can be seen in programs like Alcoholics Anonymous.

REFERENCES

1. *Alcoholics Anonymous.* New York: Alcoholics Anonymous World Service Inc., 1976.
2. *Alcoholics Anonymous Comes of Age.* A Brief History of A.A. New York: Alcoholics Anonymous World Service Inc., 1970.
3. Anant, S.S. A note on the treatment of alcoholics by a verbal aversion technique. *Canadian Psychol.* 8a (1):19, 1967.
4. Anant, S.S. Treatment of Alcoholics and Drug Addicts by Verbal Aversion Techniques. *Intern. J. Addictions* 33:381, 1968.
5. Beaubrum, M.H. Treatment of alcoholism in Trinidad and Tobago. *Br. J. Psychiatry* 112:643, 1967.
6. Blake, B.G. The application of behavior therapy to the treatment of alcoholism. *Behav. Res. and Ther.* 3:75, 1965.
7. Blake, B.G. A follow-up of alcoholics treated by behavior therapy. *Behav. Res. and Ther.* 5:89, 1967.
8. Burt, D.W. A behaviorist looks at A.A. *Addictions* 22(3):57, 1975.
9. Cautela, J.R. Treatment of compulsive behavior by covert sensitization. *Psychol. Rep.* 16:33, 1966.
10. Cautela, J.R. Covert sensitization. *Psychol. Rep.* 20:459, 1967.
11. Cautela, J.R. The treatment of alcoholism by covert sensitization. *Psychother: Theory, Res. and Practice* 7(2):86, 1970.
12. Chapman, R.F., and Smith, J.W. Peripheral neuropathy and electrical aversion treatment of alcoholism. *Behav. Ther.* 3:469, 1972.
13. Dent, J.Y. Apomorphine in the treatment of anxiety states with special reference to alcoholism. *Br. J. Inebr.* 32:65, 1934.
14. Dent, J.Y. Apomorphine. *Med. Pr.* 212:141, 1944.

15. Dunn, R.B., Smith, J.W., Lemere, F., and Charalampous, K.D. A comprehensive intensive treatment program for alcoholism. *Southwestern Med.*, May 1971.

16. Elkins, R.L. *Aversion therapy for alcoholics: Chemical, electrical or imagery?* Paper presented at the meeting of the Southeastern Psychological Association, Miami Beach, April 1971.

17. Elkins, R.L. Aversion therapy for alcoholics: Chemical, electrical or verbal imagery? *International J. of the Addictions* 10(2):157, 1975.

18. Elkins, R.L., and Murdock, R.P. The contribution of successful conditioning to abstinence maintenance following covert sensitization (verbal aversion) treatment of alcoholism. *IRCS Medical Science: Psychology and Psychiatry; Social and Occupational Med.* 5:167, 1977.

19. Farrar, C.H., Powell, B.J., and Martin, L.K. Punishment of alcohol consumption by apneic paralysis. *Behav. Res. and Ther.* 6:13, 1968.

20. Franks, C.M. Behavior therapy, the principles of conditioning and the treatment of the alcoholic. *Quart. J. Stud. Alc.* 24:511, 1963.

21. Franks, C.M. Conditioning and conditioned aversion therapies in the treatment of the alcoholic. *Intern. J. Addictions* 1:61, 1966.

22. Green, K.F., and Garcia, J. Recuperation from illness: flavor enhancement for rats. *Science* 173:749, 1971.

23. Hankoff, L.D. Ancient descriptions of organic brain syndrome: The "Kordiakos" of the Talmud, *Am. J. Psychiatry* 129:233, 1972.

24. Holzinger, R., Mortimer, R., and Van Dusen, W. Aversion conditioning treatment for alcoholism. *Am. J. Psychiatry* 124:246, 1967.

25. Jackson, T.R., and Smith, J.W. A comparison of two aversion treatment methods for alcoholism. *J. Stud. Alc.* 39:187, January 1978.

26. Jellinek, E.M. *The Disease Concept of Alcoholism.* New Haven: Hillhouse, 1960, p. 36.

27. Kantorovich, N.V. An attempt at curing alcoholism by associated reflexes. *Novaye v Refleksoloqii Fiziologii Neronoy Sistemy* 3:436, 1929.

28. Lazarus, A.A. Aversion therapy and sensory modalities: Clinical impressions. *Percept. Motor Skills* 27:178, 1968.

29. Lemere, F., and Voegtlin, W.L. An evaluation of the aversion treatment of alcoholism. *Quart. J. Stud. Alc.* 11:199, 1950.

30. Mandill, M.F., Campbell, D., Laverty, S.G., Sanderson, R.E., and Vandewater, S.L. Aversion treatment of alcoholics by succinylcholine–induced apneic paralysis—an analysis of early change in drinking behavior. *Quart. J. Stud. Alc.* 27:483, 1966.

31. McChance, D., and McChance, P.F. Alcoholism in Northeast Scotland: Its treatment and outcome. *Br. J. Psychiatry* 115:189, 1969.

32. Mellor, C.S., and White, H.P. Taste aversion to alcoholic beverages by motion sickness. *Am. J. Psychiatry* 135(1):125, January 1978.

33. Rachman, S. Aversion therapy: Chemical or electrical? *Behav. Res. and Ther.* 2:289, 1965.

34. Rachman, S., and Teasdale, J. Aversion therapy: An appraisal, in C.M. Franks (ed), *Behavior Therapy: An Appraisal and Status.* New York: McGraw–Hill, 1969, p. 279.

35. Raymond, M.J. The treatment of addiction by aversive conditioning with apomorphine. *Behav. Res. and Ther.* 1:287, 1964.

36. Register, D.C. *Change in Autonomic Responsivity and Drinking Behavior of Alcoholics as a Function of Aversion Therapy.* Doctoral dissertation, University of Nebraska; University Microfilms, No. 71-19, 514, 1971.

37. Sanderson, R.E., Campbell, D., and Laverty, S.G. An investigation of a new aversive conditioning treatment for alcoholism. *Quart. J. Stud. Alc.* 24:261, 1963.

38. Schlatter, E.K.E., and Samarthji, L. Treatment of alcoholism with Dent's oral apomor-

phine method. *Quart. J. Stud. Alc.* 33:430, 1972.
39. Schuckit, M.A. Treatment of alcoholism in office and outpatient settings, in J.E. Mendelson and M.K. Mello (eds.), *Diagnosis and Treatment of Alcoholism,* in press.
40. Shadel, C.A. Aversion treatment of alcohol addiction. *Quart. J. Stud. Alc.* 5:216, 1940.
41. Smith, J.W., Lemere, F., and Dunn, R.B. Pentothal interviews in the treatment of alcoholism. *Psychosomatics* 12(5):330, 1971.
42. Voegtlin, W.L. The treatment of alcoholism by establishing a conditioned reflex. *Amer. J. Med. Sciences* 99:802, June 1940.
43. Voegtlin, W.L., Lemere, F., and Broz, W.R. Conditioned reflex therapy of alcohol addiction. III. An evaluation of present results in the light of previous experiences with the method. *Quart. J. Stud. Alc.* 1(3):501, 1940.
44. Voegtlin, W.L. Conditioned reflex therapy of chronic alcoholism. Ten years' experience with the method. *Rocky Mountain Med. J.* 44:807, 1947.
45. Vogler, R.E., Lunde, S.E., Johnson, G.R., and Martin, P.L. Electrical aversion conditioning with chronic alcoholics. *J. Consult. Clin. Psychol.* 34:302, 1970.
46. Vogler, R.E., Lunde, S.E., and Martin, P.L. Electrical aversion conditioning with chronic alcoholics: Follow-up and suggestions for research. *J. Consult. Clin. Psychol.* 36:450, 1971.
47. Wiens, A.N., Montague, J.R., Manough, T.S., and English, T.J. Pharmacological aversive counterconditioning to alcohol in a private hospital: One year follow-up. *J. Stud. Alc.* 37:1320, 1976.
48. Wisocki, P.A. The empirical evidence of covert sensitization in the treatment of alcoholism: An evaluation. Paper presented at the AABT Convention, Miami, 1970.
49. Wolpe, J. *Psychotherapy by Reciprocal Inhibition.* Stanford, Cal.: Stanford University Press, 1958.

Copyright 1980, Spectrum Publications, Inc.
The Comprehensive Handbook of Behavioral Medicine, Volume 3

CHAPTER 11

Behavioral Treatment Approaches to Drug Abuse

Dale A. Callner
Steven M. Ross

In addition to a large body of literature devoted to the sociological and pharmacological aspects of drug abuse, there have been many investigations of treatment for drug abusers. The most recent trend in the drug treatment literature has emerged from therapy approaches based on both classical and operant learning principles. This review is designed to describe and appraise behavioral treatments of drug abuse, identify common problems associated with operation and measurement of these treatments, and propose recommendations for the refinement of future treatment.

For this review of behavioral strategies to treat drug abuse, we will limit our discussion to studies involving the human use of legal and illegal drugs taken chronically and in excess amounts without a medical prescription. Common classes of abused drugs include opiates (primarily heroin), barbiturates, amphetamines, cocaine, psychedelics, and toxic inhalants. Treatment approaches to other commonly used drugs, such as marijuana, alcohol, nicotine, and caffeine, will not be considered in this review. While treatment approaches to caffeine and marijuana abuse are rare, the reader is referred to Bernstein (5) and Marston and McFall (69) for reviews of the behavioral approaches to nicotine abuse, and to Franks (35, 36) and MacCulloch, et al. (66) for reviews of the behavioral approaches to alcohol abuse. Before we review the treatment research, it is necessary to briefly present the major behavioral theories proposed to explain chronic drug abuse.

BEHAVIORAL THEORIES OF DRUG ABUSE

It is beyond the scope of this chapter to comprehensively review the many nonbehavioral theories and methods that have been introduced to explain and treat drug abuse [see Isball (44), and Siegler and Osmond (87) for reviews of theories and treatment approaches to drug abuse]. Historically, treatments of drug abuse developed from the philosophy that "enforced abstinence," prolonged periods either in prisons or sanitaria, would allow the drug user to free himself from his addiction (10). Later treatment approaches developed from psychodynamic concepts such as the "addictive personality," oral dependency, and disrupted psychosexual development (34, 39, 41, 80, 101, 106). Social psychological concepts such as social alienation, existential hopelessness, and the need for group acceptance (21, 22, 110) led to residential halfway house programs employing a "therapeutic community" as their major treatment approach (33, 47, 48, 59, 71, 99). Finally, biochemical theories of drug abuse, which suggest that the structure and action of the drug on the human nervous system are responsible for drug abuse, have initiated several chemical treatment and maintenance procedures, such as methadone (27, 28, 29) and narcotic antagonist drugs (19, 32).

With the exception of the recent investigation into the biochemical basis of drug abuse, nonbehavioral treatment approaches to drug abuse do not appear to be overwhelmingly promising. On the contrary, drug abusers are usually seen as poor candidates for traditional psychotherapy, and treatment attempts have seldom reported long–term success rates (12, 37, 40, 72).

Theories associated with both classical and operant conditioning represent the most recent attempts to explain and alter drug abuse. In general, conditioning theories suggest that chronic drug use is comprised of many behaviors that are acquired and maintained by a variety of learned internal and environmental stimuli. Although many behavioral theorists suggest that both classical and operant conditioning occur in the acquisition and maintenance of excessive drug use, the following sections summarize the major principles of each form of conditioning as they have been applied to explain drug abuse.

Classical Conditioning Components of Drug Abuse

Stating that both classical and operant processes play a role in the acquisition and maintenance of excessive drug use, Wikler (102, 103) suggests that classical conditioning is primarily responsible for both long–term drug use and posttreatment relapse. He maintains that the drug user initially uses drugs to relieve tension, which is associated with various emotional states such as guilt, anxiety, anger, and depression. Because drug use is repeatedly reinforced by tension reduction, drug use is maintained while physical dependence quickly develops. In his theory, initial drug use (prior to physical dependence) is explained by the operant principle of negative reinforcement, i.e., drugs are originally used to reduce aversive emotional states. After physical dependence has developed, subsequent drug use primarily alleviates the aversive symptoms associated with the drug withdrawal syndrome. With the development of physical dependency, many environmental stimuli in the drug user's life become classically conditioned to the aversive aspects of the withdrawal syndrome. That is, drug use is maintained by repeated temporal contiguity between physical withdrawal symptoms (unconditioned stimulus) such as peers, familiar neighborhoods, and music (101, 102). When the drug–induced withdrawal reactions are repeatedly experienced in specific environmental surroundings, the surroundings themselves eventually begin to elicit withdrawal symptoms. It has been suggested that recurrence of withdrawal symptoms, even after detoxification, occurs as a result of internally elicited reactions to the conditioned environmental elements of the addict's life that have never been fully extinguished (65). The effects of this classically conditioned withdrawal syndrome can only be relieved by drug ingestion, which leads to continued drug use or relapse following detoxification. Wikler used the term *conditioned abstinence* to refer to this recurrence of withdrawal symptoms resulting from classically conditioned environmental stimuli (111).

Wikler has suggested that extinction of both the conditioned abstinence syndrome as well as operantly reinforced drug–using behavior must occur. For example, in the case of opiate dependence, narcotic antagonist drugs could be used to block the usual effects produced by heroin, or other opiates, both in the treatment setting as well as the addict's natural environment. Because the persistence of the conditioned abstinence syndrome may depend on occasional reinforcement by actual withdrawal symptoms, opiate–seeking behavior is extinguished because injections of opiates are blocked by the narcotic antagonists (104, 105). Although the use of narcotic antagonists to test Wikler's theories of drug abuse and treatment is still in the preliminary stage, this approach suggests a promising area for future research. As recommended by Krasnegor and Boudin (57), future research directed toward a more comprehensive understanding of the conditioned abstinence syndrome will add considerably to our knowledge of chronic drug use, the relapse phenomenon, and possible treatment approaches.

Operant Conditioning Components of Drug Abuse

Explanations of drug abuse emphasizing operant principles have concentrated on several types of reinforcement contingency in the acquisition and maintenance of drug use (11, 23, 26, 45, 102, 103, 104, 105). In general, these reinforcement contingencies can be summarized as follows: a) positive reinforcement associated with the social aspects of drug use, e.g., acceptance by drug–using peer groups, music and language associated with drug use, excitement of hedonistic street life and manipulatory behavior, and acting out toward the "establishment"; b) positive reinforcement associated with the pharmacological properties of the drug, e.g., euphoria, anxiety reduction, "rushes," relaxation; c) negative reinforcement associated with aversive aspects of the environment, e.g., relieving boredom, reduction of aversive aspects of family life and living conditions; d) negative reinforcement related to nondrug–induced aversive physical states, e.g., relief from chronic or acute pain due to injury or illness; and e) negative reinforcement related to drug–induced aversive physical states, e.g., relief from physical discomfort of withdrawal symptoms.

Kraft (51, 52, 53, 54, 55, 56) has elaborated on the operant principle of negative reinforcement by suggesting that "social anxiety" is the major factor associated with repeated drug use. That is, the drug user can eliminate the anxiety he feels in social situations and deal more appropriately with it by taking drugs. Kraft maintained that reduction of social anxiety will also result in a reduction or elimination of drug use. Treatment procedures are aimed at relieving the drug user's anxiety by desensitizing him to the presence of progressively larger numbers of people.

BEHAVIOR THERAPIES FOR DRUG ABUSE

From these notions of classical and operant learning theory have come several treatment approaches to drug abuse. These can be grouped into three general categories: counterconditioning, contingent reinforcement, and combined behavioral techniques.

Counterconditioning

The majority of behavioral treatment approaches to drug abuse have been based on the principle of counterconditioning. In general, counterconditioning involves a variety of techniques designed to pair either incompatible or aversive consequences with specific problem–related stimuli (3). In the behavior therapy literature, noxious chemical, electrical, and covert stimuli have been used in the presence of problem–related stimuli for aversive counterconditioning, and relaxation has been most commonly used as an incompatible response paired with anxiety–provoking stimuli, as in systematic desensitization.

Chemical Aversion Therapy

Chemical aversion therapy involves administering chemical compounds to the patient which eventually produce noxious effects such as nausea, vomiting, or temporary paralysis. Once the time for the noxious effects of the chemical to take effect is determined, the patient is instructed to engage in various aspects of his problem behavior, thereby pairing problem–related stimuli with the onset of the aversive experience. Attempts to reduce drug abuse by chemical aversion techniques closely resemble earlier work done with alcoholic patients (98, 100). Raymond (81) and Liberman (63) paired apomorphine with self–administrations of drugs to produce a conditioned nausea and vomiting response in drug abusers. In a large group study, Thomson and Rathod (96) used scoline to produce a temporary paralysis which was timed to coincide with self–administration of heroin. Although all of these studies sought to reduce subsequent drug use, it was hoped that the unpleasant responses produced by the chemicals would generalize to other related aspects of the drug user's life, such as thought of drug use or watching another person use drugs.

More recently, Kurland, McCabe, and Hanlon (58) gave paroled heroin users escalating 500 mg doses of the opiate antagonist naloxone (to 2000 mg per day) when they gave more than two "dirty" urines or missed two clinic appointments for treatment, and discontinued naloxone administration after four consecutive "clean" urines. When compared to a nonchemotherapy group after six months, 37% of the drug–free group required reinstitutionalization whereas only 8% of the naloxone group were reinstitutionalized, and 38% of the naloxone group ($N = 108$) remained totally abstinent for six months compared to only 12% of the control group ($N = 371$).

Electrical Aversion Therapy

The use of electric shock as the noxious stimulus paired with drug use has the advantage of greater stimulus control, versatility, and safety when compared with chemically induced noxious stimulation. Like chemical aversion, electrical aversion techniques attempt to link a noxious stimulus with the behavioral and subjective components associated with drug taking, e.g., subjective drug urges, preparing the paraphernalia, actual sensations produced by the drugs. Electric shock can be administered directly after the onset of the behavior to which aversion is to be conditioned. Furthermore, portable shock units permit *in vivo* counterconditioning, which enables the procedure to deal with important environmental stimuli that may be difficult to reproduce in a hospital or clinic setting.

Electrical aversion techniques are similar to the procedures used in earlier studies with alcoholic patients (7, 43, 66, 70). Wolpe (109) was apparently the first to use electric shock in an attempt to reduce drug use, when he trained a single patient to use a portable shock unit to help him deal with the various environmental and internal stimuli that naturally occur in conjunction with drug use. Although electric shock is used in association with other behavioral techniques, Lesser (60), O'Brien and Raynes (73), and Spevack, Pihl, and Rowan (89) have also used it as the principal means of therapeutic intervention in drug abuse. In an interesting combination of covert and verbalized drug experiences paired with mild electric shocks, Copeman (24) demonstrated that electrical aversion therapy can be effectively applied to counterconditioning drug–related experiences reported or imagined by addicts. Two other studies (8, 75) have employed electrical aversion as a secondary behavioral intervention. Although not yet tested in a controlled manner, an "electric needle" designed by Blachly (6) delivers a shock from an electrically charged syringe to one or more patients when the plunger is pressed.

Covert Sensitization

Covert sensitization, also referred to as verbal aversion of aversive imagery therapy, uses imagined scenes as aversive events. The behavior to which aversion is to be conditioned is presented in the form of an imagined scene. This technique for establishing an aversive response to a particular stimulus by imaginally induced noxious scenes has been used in the treatment of many clinical problems such as smoking, obesity, and alcoholism (15, 16, 17, 18).

In the treatment of drug abuse, Anant (2) and Steinfeld (90, 91, 92) have used covert sensitization to produce a conditioned avoidance response to many of the behaviors involved with drug seeking and use. In these studies, the patients were asked to imagine a series of scenes in which they first feel like taking a drug, then travel to the place where they usually obtain it, prepare to inject it, inject it, feel sick, vomit, and then finally, gradually feel better as they move progressively farther away from the place where they took the drug. More recently, Snowden (88) used a wider variety of aversive imagined stimuli, nausea, depression, skin abscesses, etc., to countercondition addicts in a methadone maintenance clinic. Many of these studies also used relaxation training techniques to enhance the patient's ability to vividly imagine the scenes presented. Covert sensitization has also been used in conjunction with several other behavior therapy techniques by O'Brien et al. (75) and Wisocki (107).

Covert sensitization requires no apparatus or drugs, and the patient can be trained to use it in naturalisitc settings. Although the validity of a patient's self–reported covert images can never really be known and should always be seriously questioned, covert sensitization appears to be a particularly applicable counterconditioning technique in training self–control for a variety of drug–related behaviors.

Systematic Desensitization

Systematic desensitization pairs an incompatible response, usually relaxation, with stimuli that normally elicit anxiety and might otherwise lead to drug use. The patient is first relaxed by verbal training in muscle relaxation, by drugs, or by hypnosis. Imagined situations that elicit anxiety are then ranked according to the amount of anxiety they elicit. Relaxation is then paired with the various anxiety-eliciting images on the hierarchy by asking the patient to imagine each situation while maintaining a high degree of relaxation.

Systematic desensitization has been used to treat a wide variety of clinical problems (3, 77, 108, 111). It has been studied most extensively as a treatment for drug abuse by Kraft (51, 52, 53, 54, 55), who suggested that social anxiety is a major factor associated with drug abuse and that a treatment which relieved the patient's anxiety in social situations would also eliminate his drug use. His treatment procedures first desensitized the patient to being around progressively larger groups of people and gradually reduced the patient's dependency on the therapist by having him spend progressively greater periods of time away from the therapist. In this treatment, the patient actually lives through each step in the hierarchy rather than imagining it.

Spevack et al. (89) report a case study in which several desensitization hierarchies were used to reduce the fears associated with an unpleasant LSD experience. Separate hierarchies were constructed to desensitize the patient to several activities thought to produce aversive LSD "flashback" experience, e.g., rock music produced uncomfortable feelings similar to those experienced while the patient was in the drug state.

Contingent Reinforcement

The second general category of behavioral drug treatments uses techniques designed to reinforce specified social behaviors. Contingent reinforcement programs have been used for individual outpatients and in large-scale inpatient treatment programs. When used individually, contingency contracting involves an agreement between the patient and the therapist which specifies behaviors to be reduced or increased in frequency, and reinforcing or aversive consequences. In an inpatient or residential setting, tokens which can be traded for privileges or reinforcing objects are often used for reinforcement.

Contingency Contracting

Contractual agreements to specify appropriate and inappropriate behaviors and consequences have been used with several populations, such as students (42), delinquents (94), and married couples (50). Several investigators (8, 9, 82, 86) have used contingency contracting to treat specific drug–related behaviors by contingent application of reinforcing and aversive consequences. Although decreasing drug abuse was part of each of these studies, other behaviors—such as reducing hospital dress violations, increasing spontaneous group–therapy verbalizations, decreasing subjective feelings of frustration, and increasing physical activity—were included in the contingency contracts. Recreational privileges and money were often used as reinforcers. Beatty (4) compared the effects of written contracts with behavioral contingencies to written contracts without contingencies on managerial behaviors, e.g., attending meetings, keeping daily logs, or male heroin addicts. The reinforcers in the program were apparently less powerful than those inherent in drug taking, and the two treatment interventions had little effect on the dependent measures.

Token Economy Programs

Glicksman, Ottomanelli, and Cutler (38), O'Brien, Raynes, and Patch (74), and Ottomanelli (76) have used token economies in the treatment of drug abusers in hospital settings. Glicksman et al. (38) allowed drug abuse patients to earn their hospital discharge by accumulating points based on program performance. O'Brien et al. (74) developed a system employing the Premack Principle (79) in which narcotic–abusing patients engaged in desired activities—e.g., acquiring passes, being allowed visitors, TV and radio privilege—contingent upon increasing the occurrence of various low frequency behaviors, e.g., punctuality, adherence to program rules, cleanliness, etc. Ottomanelli (76) gave heroin users points for the quality of their participation in group and educational therapy and allowed them to earn hospital releases by accumulating points. Unfortunately, follow–up data at 9– and 12–month intervals indicated that 75% of the subjects discharged from treatment had been reinstitutionalized, had not reported to their aftercare officers, or had absconded.

Many studies do not specify abstinence as a goal and instead emphasize the other problem behaviors commonly found in residential drug programs. In an attempt to individualize large programs, the use of a token economy to help manage the general program rules may be supplemented by individually tailored contingency contracts which deal with the specific problems of each patient.

Combined Behavioral Treatments

Perhaps the greatest recent effort has been devoted to applying a combination of behavioral methods to the treatment of drug abuse—for example, a combination of relaxation training, electrical aversion, contingency contracting, and covert sensitization (75). Wisocki (107) used a combination of covert reinforcement to teach the patient to reinforce himself for imagined drug refusals, covert sensitization, and thought stopping, to interfere with persistent thoughts of heroin use. The immediate value of this combined treatment approach is that it can be readily taught and practiced outside the immediate treatment setting.

Callner and Ross (13, 14) addressed the problem of identifying and training the specific assertion and communication skills needed by addicts to reintegrate into "drug-free" society. Specific assertion situations likely to occur in the patient's life, e.g., refusing drug offers, applying for a job, asking a "straight" woman for a date, etc., were discussed, modeled, and finally rehearsed, role-played, and videotaped by members of a small, ongoing therapy group. Subsequent discussion and practice emphasized improving specific verbal and nonverbal communication styles targeted for each group member.

Reeder (84, 85) assigned heroin addicts in a residential treatment facility to a "video-model" presentation of action-oriented scenarios of coping behavior or content-oriented coping information (video-lecture). Although an impressive amount of pre-, post-, and follow-up data was obtained, the "video-model" group was superior only on follow-up measures at 30, 90, and 180 days posttreatment. Similarly, Tsoi–Hosmand (97) describes a program designed to train addicts in negotiation, vocation, and sensitivity–communication skills, and Ross et al. (83) describe a broad–spectrum behavioral approach for skills training in a curriculum format.

In most of these studies, many of the specific and isolated behaviors associated with drug use were identified and a combination of behavioral techniques applied to modify them. Although the differential effectiveness of each approach is difficult to measure because of the problems inherent in concurrent or overlapping treatments, the use of several treatment methods applied to target behaviors may be most effective in dealing with a clinical problem that includes many different aspects of physiology, personality, and society.

SOME RECOMMENDATIONS FOR FUTURE BEHAVIORAL DRUG TREATMENT RESEARCH

Use Subjects That Are More Representative Of the Drug Abusers Seen in Treatment Programs

For the most part, past investigations did not include subjects that represented good examples of "street addicts" or addicts entering treatment programs by court order. For example, the subjects selected in the case studies by Wolpe, a

31-year-old physician (109), Kraft, a 50-year-old female (53), and Boudin, a female graduate student (8), have very few of the charactristics of the majority of street addicts, e.g., lower socioeconomic status, high school education or less, criminal record (20, 31, 62, 78, 93, 95). It is thus difficult to evaluate how generalizable the results of these studies are. In addition, it is necessary for the future investigator to understand the various "con games" and other manipulatory behavior commonly found when working with drug abusers (86).

It would be helpful for researchers to speculate about how their treatments and procedures would be altered for drug patients with different demographic and behavioral characteristics. Some behavioral treatments may be most effective with a specific drug patient population, but not generally applicable to all addicts. For example, covert methods, requiring honest reports from the patient on his ability to vividly imagine suggested scenes, may be useful with middle-class, college drug users but not with long-term street addicts. Tsoi-Hosmand (97), for example, concluded that her program appeared best suited for younger nonopiate users.

Because the generalizability of treatment results is strongly influenced by a variety of subject variables, future research should include an estimate of the intensity of drug abuse by combining variables such as type of drug used, history of use, typical dose, socioeconomic status, criminal record, and past treatment failures. For example, one category may include chronic, heavy-dose heroin users of low socioeconomic status with a long history of both drug- and nondrug-related criminal arrests. A different category may include younger, more infrequent users of psychedelics and amphetamines of middle to upper socioeconomic status with few criminal arrests. This type of descriptive subject variable may be helpful in obtaining a relative index of motivation and probability of treatment success, and it may enable researchers to determine if specific therapeutic techniques are more effective with one category of drug abusers than with others.

Develop a Larger Variety of Reliable and Representative Dependent Measures

The successful treatment of a drug abuse patient should be assessed by objective evidence which describes variables related to his natural behavior. Several specific target problems can be defined by breaking down *drug abuse* into small behavioral components and identifying the behaviors surrounding the illicit use of drugs. Boudin and Valentine (9) identified and measured many variables they felt covaried with drug taking, e.g., drug urges, frustration ratings, social discomfort ratings, inability to relax, sexual performance, etc. Data were obtained on each of these behaviors and analyzed in an attempt to identify trends. Ross and Jones (82) obtained similar data in addicts describing marijuana use, spontaneous group therapy verbalizations, physical activity, and subjective urges, and intercorrelated these measures to determine which behaviors were most related to drug intake patterns.

In addition to investigating a greater variety of dependent measures related to drug use, future studies in this area could develop two general measurement techniques. The first is measurement *in vivo* of behavior in a variety of natural settings. Although this type of performance measure has traditionally been difficult to develop and obtain, it is of particular importance to isolate and measure drug–related and posttreatment behaviors that occur away from the hospital or clinic in a natural environment. This type of measurement would include assessment of several frequently occurring problem areas like refusing drug offers, meeting nondrug friends, finding and maintaining a job, etc., in these patients.

The second type of measurement needed could be called "ongoing program performance measurement." These include a series of assessments of observable and verifiable performances of tasks while the patient is in treatment, to assess his ability to deal with the difficult problems likely to occur after treatment termination. For example, the use of prearranged situations involving a patient role–playing a difficult situation, such as being offered drugs or being asked to sell drugs, might give the therapist a better assessment of the patient's behavior than would self–report. These performance tasks could be video– or audiotaped, which would allow the researcher to rate reliably verbal and nonverbal performance in both group and single–subject treatment designs. Ongoing behavioral measurement prior to treatment termination has the advantage of allowing the researcher to assess better the possible confounding effects of variables such as maturation and concurrent treatments. Ongoing measurements also tend to be more valid and reliable than self–report. MacDonough (68) recorded the intensity, duration, drug, and specific situation associated with drug cravings in addicts in a residential drug program and compared these data to actual drug use. The finding that the tendency for increased drug use was not related to reports of maximum urges to use drugs points out the poor predictive validity of self–reported urges. Although seldom used, it is also strongly recommended that urine analysis be employed whenever possible to verify both treatment and self–reported data.

Place Greater Emphasis on Quantitative Data Presentation and Analysis

There is a need for more precise quantification of treatment data and a movement away from self–report of outcome. At the simplest level, a graphical analysis of data can be useful in demonstrating that the study assessed some measures of change beyond verbal self–report. At a higher level of quantification, a statistical analysis of data not only demonstrates the direction and magnitude of change, but also makes a comparative statement about the reliability of differences.

One graphical way to present comparative change of behaviors is to compare several dependent measures obtained from a representative subject in group studies, or from the patient himself in case studies, during several different stimulus conditions. This type of analysis, which compares drug use with behaviors predicted to influence drug use, has three advantages. First, it forces the researcher to assess many of the antecedent and consequent conditions surrounding the target behaviors. Second, a functional analysis clarifies the reasons for a particular behavioral treatment approach. Finally, this type of analysis provides an organized way to evaluate a patient's performance in a particular treatment program.

Boudin and Valentine (9) provide an example of a functional analysis of drug use and the behaviors predicted to influence drug use. They used a graphical analyis of several dependent measures to illustrate many inverse and converse functional relationships between drug use and important situational and emotional events. For group research designs, a statistical analysis helps determine the direction, magnitude, and reliability of behavior changes. Because research approaches begin on a small scale, statistical techniques that do not depend on large sample sizes are suggested.

Use Procedures to Ensure Greater Experimental Control

Most research has emphasized the description of treatment approaches rather than how data were obtained and experimental control ensured. The need for controlled large–group designs has not yet surpassed the need for well–controlled single–subject and small–group studies. Several recommendations for increasing experimental control in single–subject and small–group treatment research can be made. First, accurate and stable baseline data should be obtained for all dependent measures prior to starting treatment. In addition, an accurate history should be obtained from the drug user and, if possible, from one or more persons familiar with his drug intake. For drug–related behaviors, self–ratings or behavioral observations should be made to ensure stable baseline performance. These data are particularly important when research is done in institutional or private inpatient drug programs in order to demonstrate that the drug user had adapted to his new environmental setting.

Whenever possible, case studies should employ some form of reversal or multiple baseline design. Investigators should attempt to test their treatment programs by either replicating pretreatment baseline conditions after a suitable treatment period (reversal design) or by recording baseline data on several problem behaviors simultaneously, then treating one behavior at a time (multiple baseline design). The two case studies reported by Ross and Jones (82) are good examples of reversal and multiple baseline designs in drug treatment research. In small–group treatment research, future studies should include at least one control group of patients matched with the experimental treatment group. Callner and Ross (13) and O'Brien et al. (74) use experimental and control subjects in a small–group design to gain a more comparative assessment of the treatment intervention. Because small–group research is applicable to subpopulations within large inpatient drug programs, a discussion of the other treatments existing in the program and speculation about interaction with the experimental treatment approach would be useful in evaluating the possible confounding effects of concurrent treatments.

Finally, all information pertaining to the description, duration, sequence, and timing of the treatment approaches should be included so that changes in performance can accurately be related to treatment interventions. This is particularly important in the case of inpatient drug treatment programs in order to identify which treatment intervention, if any, was associated with behavioral performance. The descriptions reported by Sammons (86) and Wisocki (107), for example, provide useful information on how the treatment, sequencing, duration, and timing of treatment affected performance measures.

Develop Better Procedures for Obtaining Accurate And Representative Measures of Posttreatment Follow–Up

With drug–abuse patients, the most meaningful estimate of treatment effectiveness is obtained by accurate and reliable follow–up assessment. Although the majority of behavioral drug treatment studies to date have not concentrated on follow–up data, the research in the last two years has tended to move in this direction. Several changes could be made in follow–up studies. First, more reliable and realistic measures than self–report at follow–up are needed. People knowledgeable about the patient's behavior should be sought as rigorously as data are sought from the patient himself. For example, if informal reports or behavioral checklist data could be obtained from the patient's employers, family members, and peers, a more representative appraisal of posttreatment success could be made, and the reliability of the patient's self–reports could be checked. O'Brien et al. (75) provide a good example of reports obtained from others which describe the patient's posttreatment progress. The validity of the patient's self–reported drug use should, of course, be checked by urine analysis.

In vivo performance is probably the best follow–up assessment of treatment and outcome. Although difficult to obtain, a technology could be developed to evaluate the drug abuser in natural or contrived situations, e.g., confederate offering drugs to the patient, thus enabling a more realistic assessment of the patient's posttreatment performance than self-report.

The dependent measures at follow–up assessment should be similar to those used during treatment to allow the researcher to assess the progress of the patient at various times and in various settings. This procedure will also enable the researcher to assess how effectively his treatment measures predict posttreatment performance.

Finally, follow–up assessments should be made frequently after treatment termination to detect early relapse trends or problems, and less frequently as the patient becomes more successful in his responses to problems. If early follow–up detects problems or relapse, appropriate "booster treatments" should be included in the treatment program. These treatments may be particularly important when counterconditioning techniques are used to treat drug abuse to minimize extinction to the conditioned aversion. It is also important to obtain follow–up data after more extended posttreatment periods with patients that show initial therapy success. Of interest is the ten–year follow–up by Lesser (61) of his original 1967 case study of the successful treatment of a student morphine user.

More Detailed Discussion of Variables Affecting Both Treatment Success as Well as Failure Is Necessary

Because the research in behavioral drug treatment is still in the early developmental stages, it is particularly important to assess critically each variable associated with treatment objectives and outcomes. Two general recommendations will increase our knowledge of the variables affecting drug treatment effectiveness. First, journal editors should encourage reports of controlled treatments that do not necessarily have successful results. At this stage of development, it may be more important to isolate and discuss an ineffective treatment carried out in a well–controlled study than to demonstrate success without controls. Because of the complexity and variability of drug abuser's problems, replication research should also be encouraged. Secondly, researchers should suggest future research based on the refinement, elaboration, or replication of their own work. This will help void the accumulation of a heterogeneous body of literature which replicates poor studies with replicating methodological errors, e.g., poor measures, unrepresentative subjects, confounding variables, etc. Steinfeld et al. (92) made some suggestions about what directions they intend to take in future study of covert sensitization approaches to drug abuse.

Greater Awareness of the Biochemical and Pharmacological Aspects of Drugs Should be Sought by Behavioral Drug Treatment Researchers

Researchers looking at both the treatment of drug abusers and the evaluation of treatment techniques should remain aware of current research trends in the biochemical and pharmacological study of drug abuse. Behavioral researchers should consider the usefulness of various pharmacological agents when designing their treatment programs. Drugs such as tranquilizers, narcotic antagonists, and methadone are frequently encountered when treating drug abusers and can often be used to supplement behavioral approaches (e.g., Liebson and Bigelow, 64). The work of Altman et al. (1) and Jones and Prada (46) illustrates the use of pharmacological agents to influence drug–taking behavior. It is necessary to understand the biochemistry and physiology of commonly abused drugs in order to better understand their behavioral pharmacology. The combined use of antagonistic pharmacological agents with behavioral technology suggested by Wikler (105) presumes a basic understanding of the organism and its reaction to physiological change.

Animal research in drug abuse should not be ignored. Within the last two years, there has been a great deal of effort towards identifying the complex variables affecting drug–taking behavior in both man and animals. For example, the "Symposium on Control of Drug Taking Behavior by Schedules of Reinforcement" (49) included many studies designed to test drug interactions, schedule effects, and dose–response relationships. Although it is beyond the scope of this review even to summarize this research, it emphasizes the multitude of variables which effect drug–related behaviors in animals. For example, Downs and Woods (30) showed that contingent naloxone administration can function as either a positive or a negative reinforcer in both narcotic–dependent and nondependent monkeys, depending on the temporal relationships, the dose, and the degree of previous training. Careful study of the conditions surrounding withdrawal, relapse, and addiction is necessary before all of the possible treatment variables can be understood. Copeman (23) and Copeman and Shaw (25), for example, have begun to speculate about the treatment of drug abusers after reviewing the animal literature describing tolerance, abstinence, and relapse.

Although this review has primarily addressed itself to the evaluation of treatment research, several brief recommendations about the general field of drug treatment can also be made. First, large–scale drug treatment programs should include individualized therapy specifically tailored to the individual drug patient. Programs addressed to each individual's historical development, problems, and goals may help augment the general principles taught within the larger drug program. The poor follow–up results commonly found may indicate the inability of treatment contingencies to remain intact in posttreatment settings. Treatment programs should be designed to utilize the events and occurrences within the patient's natural environment. Research in other addictive behaviors (smoking, alcoholism, obesity) may be applicable to drug–abuse research and treatment. For example, MacDonough (67) compared drug abusers and alcoholics on their response to a broad–spectrum behavior modification program. This type of program will be essential to future combined clinical populations.

Finally, it is recommended that therapists employ a variety of techniques aimed at preparing the drug patient to face the many problems of maintaining a drug–free life, for example, learning how to turn down drug offers, to control drug urges, to interview for a job, and to interact successfully with nondrug users. In this way, the patient may be more completely prepared for his posttreatment environment.

Although behaviorally oriented treatment programs often represent the most efficient and successful treatment approach to several problem behaviors, only carefully planned treatment research utilizing techniques to ensure control, representativeness, and accuracy of inference will determine the usefulness of these treatment approaches to drug abuse. Only after steps are taken to ensure that more valid and reliable data are collected can the specific behavioral treatment approaches be evaluated and their differential effectiveness determined.

REFERENCES

1. Altman, J.L., Meyer, R.E., Mirin, S.M., McHomes, H.B., and McDougle, M. Opiate antagonists and the modification of heroin self–administration behavior in man: An experimental study. *Intern. J. Add.* 11:485–499, 1976.
2. Anant, S.S. Treatment of alcoholics and drug addicts by verbal aversion techniques. *Int. J. Add.* 3:381–388, 1968.
3. Bandura, A. *Principles of Behavior Modification.* New York: Holt, Rinehart and Winston, 1969.
4. Beatty, J.D. Jr. *The effect of contingency behavioral contracting with heroin addicts.* Ph.D. dissertation, Rutgers University, 1975.
5. Bernstein, D.A. Modification of smoking behavior: An evaluative review. *Psychol. Bull.* 71:418–440, 1969.
6. Blachly, P.H. An "electric needle" for aversive conditioning of the needle ritual. *Int. J. Add.* 6:327–328, 1971.
7. Blake, B.G. The application of behavior therapy to treatment of alcoholism. *Behav. Res. and Ther.* 3:75–85, 1965.
8. Boudin, H.M. Contingency contracting as a therapeutic tool in the deceleration of amphetamine use. *Behav. Ther.* 3:604–608, 1972.
9. Boudin, H.M., and Valentine, V.E. *Behavioral techniques as an alternative to methadone maintenance.* Unpublished manuscript, University of Florida, 1973.
10. Brecher, E.M., and Editors of *Consumer Reports. Licit and Illicit Drugs.* Mt. Vernon, N.Y.: Consumers Union, 1972.

11. Cahoon, D.D., and Crosby, C.C. A learning approach to chronic drug use: Sources of reinforcement. *Behav. Ther.* 3:64–71, 1972.

12. Callner, D.A. Behavioral treatment of drug abuse: A critical review of the research. *Psychol. Bull.* 82:143–164, 1975.

13. Callner, D.A., and Ross, S.M. The reliability and validity of three measures of assertion in a drug addiction population. *Behav. Ther.* 7:659–667, 1976.

14. Callner, D.A., and Ross, S.M. The assessment and training of assertion skills with drug addicts: A preliminary study. *Int. J. Add.* 13:227–239, 1978.

15. Cautela, J.R. Treatment of compulsive behavior by covert sensitization. *Psychol. Rec.* 16:33–41, 1966.

16. Cautela, J.R. Covert sensitization. *Psychol. Rep.* 20:459–468, 1967.

17. Cautela, J.R. Covert reinforcement. *Behav. Ther.* 1:33–50, 1970.

18. Cautela, J.R. Covert process and behavior modification. *J. Nerv. Ment. Dis.* 157:27–36, 1973.

19. Chappel, J.N., Senay, E.C., and Jaffee, J.H. Cyclazocine in a multimodality treatment program: Comparative results. *Int. J. Add.* 6:509–523, 1971.

20. Chein, I. Psychological, social, and epidemiological factors in drug addiction. *Rehabil. Narc. Add.* Washington, D.C.: Vocational Rehabilitation Administration, 1966.

21. Chein, I., Gerard, L., Lee, S., and Rosenfeld, E. *The Road to H.* New York: Basic Books, 1964.

22. Clausen, J.A. Social and psychological factors in narcotic addiction. *Law Contemp. Prob.* 22:34–51, 1957.

23. Copeman, C.D. Drug addiction: I. A theoretical framework for behavior therapy. *Psychol. Rep.* 37:947–958, 1975.

24. Copeman, C.D. Drug addiction: II. An aversive counterconditioning technique for treatment. *Psychol. Rep.* 38:1271–1281, 1976.

25. Copeman, C.D., and Shaw, P.L. Effects of contingent management of addicts expecting commitment to a community based treatment program. *Br. J. Add.* 71:187–191, 1976.

26. Crowley, T.J. The reinforcers for drug abuse: Why people take drugs. *Comp. Psychiatry.* 13:51–62, 1972.

27. Dole, V.P., and Nyswander, M. A medical treatment for diacetylmorphine (Heroin) addiction. *JAMA* 193:646–650, 1965.

28. Dole, V.P., and Nyswander, M. Rehabilitation of heroin addicts after blockade with methadone. *NY State J. Med.* 66:2011–2017, 1966.

29. Dole, V.P., and Nyswander, M. Heroin addiction: A metabolic disease. *Arch. Intern. Med.* 120:19–24, 1967.

30. Downs, D.A., and Woods, J.H. Naloxone as a negative reinforcer in rhesus monkeys: Effects of dose, schedule, and narcotic regimen. *Pharm. Rev.* 27:397–406, 1976.

31. Feldman, H.W. Ideological supports to becoming and remaining a heroin addict. *J. Health Soc. Behav.* 9:131–139, 1968.

32. Fink, M., Zahs, A.M., and Freedman, A.M. Clinical trial of Cyclazocine in depression, in *Narcotic Antagonists* (Rep. Ser. 25, No. 1). Washington, D.C.: National Clearinghouse for Drug Information, 1973.

33. Fischmann, V.S. Drug addicts in a therapeutic community. *Int. J. Add.* 3:351–359, 1968.

34. Fort, J.P. The psychodynamics of drug addiction and group psychotherapy. *Int. J. Group Psychother.* 5:150–156, 1955.

35. Franks, C.M. Alcohol, alcoholism, and conditioning. *J. Ment. Sci.* 104:14–33, 1958.

36. Franks, C.M. Behavior therapy, the principles of conditioning and the treatment of the alcoholic. *Q. J. Stud. Alcohol.* 25:511–529, 1963.

37. Glasscote, R.M. *The Treatment of Drug Abuse.* Washington, D.C.: Joint Information

Service of the American Psychiatric Association and the National Association for Mental Health, 1971.

38. Glicksman, M., Ottomanelli, G., and Cutler, R. The earn–your–way credit system: Use of a token economy in narcotic rehabilitation. *Int. J. Add.* 6:525–531, 1971.

39. Glover, G. *On the Early Development of Mind.* New York: International Universities Press, 1956.

40. Grafton, S. (ed.). *Addiction and Drug Abuse Report* 2:2, 1971.

41. Hoffman, M. Drug addiction and "Hypersexuality": Related modes of mastery. *Compar. Psychiatry* 5:262–270, 1964.

42. Homme, L. *How to Use Contingency Contracting in the Classroom.* Champaign, Ill.: Research Press, 1969.

43. Hsu, J. Electroconditioning therapy of alcoholics: A preliminary report. *Q. J. Stud. Alcohol.* 26:449–459, 1965.

44. Isbell, H. Perspectives in research of opiate addiction, in D.M. Wilmer and G.G. Kassenbaum (eds.), *Narcotics.* New York: McGraw–Hill, 1965.

45. Jaffe, J.H. Drug addiction and drug abuse, in L.s. Goodman and A. Gilman (eds.), *The Pharmacological Basis of Therapeutics,* 4th ed. London: Collier–Macmillan, 1970.

46. Jones, B.E., and Prada, J.A. Drug–seeking behavior during methadone maintenance. *Psychopharmacologia* 41:7–10, 1975.

47. Jones, M. *The Therapeutic Community.* New York: Basic Books, 1953.

48. Jones, M. *Beyond the Therapeutic Community.* New Haven: Yale University Press, 1968.

49. Kelleher, R.T., and Goldberg, S.R. (chairpersons). Symposium on control of drug taking behavior by schedules of reinforcement, Part I. *Pharmacol. Rev.* 27, 291–299, 1975.

50. Knox, D. *Marriage Happiness.* Champaign, Ill.: Research Press, 1972.

51. Kraft, T. Social anxiety and drug addiction. *Br. J. Soc. Psychiatry* 2:192–195, 1968.

52. Kraft, T. Successful treatment of a case of Drinamyl addiction. *Br. J. Psychiatry* 114:1363–1364, 1968.

53. Kraft, T. Successful treatment of a case of chronic barbiturate addiction. *Br. J. Add.* 64:115–120, 1969.

54. Kraft, T. Treatment of Drinamyl addiction. *Int. J. Add.* 4:59–64, 1969.

55. Kraft, T. Successful treatment of "Drinamyl" addicts and associated personality changes. *Can. Psychiatric Assoc. J.* 15:223–227, 1970.

56. Kraft, T. Treatment of Drinamyl addiction. *J. Nerv. Ment. Dis.* 150:138–144, 1970.

57. Krasnegor, N.A., and Boudin, H.M. Behavior modification and drug addiction: The state of the art. *Proceedings of the 81st Annual Convention of the American Psychol. Association* 8:913–914, 1973.

58. Kurland, A.A., McCabe, L., and Hanlon, J. Contingent naloxone treatment of the narcotic addict: A pilot study. *Int. J. Add.* 11:131–142, 1976.

59. Laskowitz, D., Wilbur, M., and Zucker, A. Problems in the group treatment of drug addicts in the community: Observations on the formation of a group. *Int. J. Add.* 3:361–379, 1968.

60. Lesser, E. Behavior therapy with a narcotics user: A case report. *Behav. Res. and Ther.* 5:251–252, 1967.

61. Lesser, E. Behavior therapy with a narcotics user. A case report. Ten–year follow–up. *Behav. Res. and Ther.* 14:381, 1976.

62. Levine, S., and Stephens, R. Games addicts play. *Psychiatric Q.* 45:582–592, 1971.

63. Liberman, R. Aversive conditioning of drug addicts: A pilot study. *Behav. Res. and Ther.* 6:229–231, 1968.

64. Liebson, I., and Bigelow, G. A behavioral–pharmacological treatment of dually addicted patients. *Behav. Res. and Ther.* 10:403–405, 1972.

65. Lynch, J.J., Fertizer, A.P., Teitelbaum, H.A., Cullen, J.W., and Gantt, W.H. Pavlovian conditioning of drug reactions: Some implications for problems of drug addiction. *Cond. Reflex.* 9:1–18, 1973.

66. MacCulloch, M.J., Feldman, M.P., Orford, J.F., and MacCulloch, M.L. Anticipatory avoidance learning in the treatment of alcoholism: A record of therapeutic failure. *Behav. Res. and Ther.* 4:187–196, 1966.

67. MacDonough, T.S. The relative effectiveness of a medical hospitalization program vs. a feedback–behavior modification program in treating alcohol and drug abusers. *Int. J. Add.* 11:269–282, 1976.

68. MacDonough, T.S. The validity of self–recording reports made by drug and alcohol abusers in a residential setting. *Int. J. Add.* 11:447–466, 1976.

69. Marston, A.R., and McFall, R.M. Comparisons of behavior modification approaches to smoking reduction. *J. Consult. Clin. Psychol.* 36:153–162, 1971.

70. McGuire, R.M., and Vallance, M. Aversion therapy by electric shock: A simple technique. *Br. Med. J.* 1:151–153, 1964.

71. Nash, G. *The sociology of Phoenix House—A therapeutic community for the resocialization of narcotic addicts.* Unpublished paper, Columbia University, 1969.

72. Nash, G., Waldorf, D., Foster, K., and Kyllingstad, A. *The Phoenix House program: The results of a two–year follow–up.* Unpublished Manuscript, 1971.

73. O'Brien, J.S., and Raynes, A.E. Treatment of heroin addiction with behavioral therapy, in W. Keup (ed.), *Drug Abuse: Current Concepts and Research.* Springfield, Ill.: Charles C. Thomas, 1972.

74. O'Brien, J.S. Raynes, A.E., and Patch, V.D. An operant reinforcement system to improve ward behavior in in–patient drug addicts. *J. Behav. Ther. Exper. Psychiatry* 2:239–242, 1971.

75. O'Brien, J.S., Raynes, A.E., and Patch, F.D. Treatment of heroin addiction with aversion therapy, relaxation training, and systematic desensitization. *Behav. Res. and Ther.* 10:77–80, 1972.

76. Ottomanelli, G.A. Follow–up of a token economy applied to civilly committed narcotic addicts. *Int. J. Add.* 11:793–806, 1976.

77. Paul, G. Outcome of systematic desensitization I II, in C. Franks (ed.), *Behavior Therapy: Appraisal and Status.* New York: McGraw–Hill, 1969.

78. Preble, E., and Casey, J.J., Jr. Taking care of business—The heroin user's life in the streets. *Int. J. Add.* 4:1–24, 1969.

79. Premack, D. Toward empirical behavior laws: I. Positive reinforcement. *Psychol. Rev.* 66:219–233, 1959.

80. Rado, S. The psychoanalysis of pharmacothymia (drug addictio). *Psychoanaly. Q.* 2:1–23, 1933.

81. Raymond, M.J. The treatment of addiction by aversion conditioning with apomorphine. *Behav. Res. and Ther.* 1:287–291, 1964.

82. Ross, S.M., and Jones, C.G. Contingency contracting with drug abusers, in D. Cannon (chair.), *Social Skills Training in a Drug Rehabilitation Program.* Symposium presented at the meeting of the American Psychol. Association, Montreal, 1973.

83. Ross, S.M., Lantinga, L.J., Homer, A.L., and Malee, J. *Behavioral treatment of addictions: I. A curriculum approach for skills training.* Paper presented at the fourth annual National Drug Abuse Conference, San Francisco, 1977.

84. Reeder, C.W. *Effects of videotaped models upon heroin addicts' acquisition of drug–abstinence behavior.* Ph.D. dissertation, University of Missouri, 1974.

85. Reeder, C.W., and Kunce, J.T. Modeling techniques, drug–abstinence behavior and heroin addicts: A pilot study. *J. Counseling Psychol.* 23:560–562, 1976.

86. Sammons, R.A. *Contingency management in a drug treatment program.* Paper presented at the first annual Rocky Mountain Conference on Behavior Modification, Denver, 1972.

87. Siegler, M., and Osmond, H. Models of drug addiction. *Int. J. Add.* 3:3–24, 1968.

88. Snowden, L.R. Jr. *Heroin abuse modification through covert sensitization tailored to locus of control.* Ph.D. dissertation, Wayne State University, 1975.

89. Spevack, M., Pihl, R., and Rowan, T. Behavior therapies in the treatment of drug abuse: Some case studies. *Psychol. Rec.* 23:179–184, 1973.

90. Steinfeld, G.J. The use of covert sensitization with institutionalized narcotic addicts. *Int. J. Add.* 5:225–232, 1970.

91. Steinfeld, G.J., Rautio, E.A., Rice, H.H., and Egan, M.J. Group covert sensitization with narcotic addicts: Further comments. *Int. J. Add.* 9:447–464, 1974.

92. Steinfeld, G.J., Rice, A., Rautio, E.M., and Egan, M. *The Use of Covert Sensitization with Narcotic Addicts (Further Comments).* Danbury, Conn: Federal Correctional Institution, Narcotic Unit, 1973.

93. Stephens, R., and Levine, S. The "street addict role": Implications for treatment. *Psychiatry* 34:351–357, 1971.

94. Stuart, R.B. Behavioral contracting within the families of delinquents. *J. Behav. Ther. Exper. Psychiatry* 2:1–11, 1971.

95. Sutter, A.G. The world of the righteous dope fiend. *Issues in Criminology* 2:177–222, 1966.

96. Thomson, I.G., and Rathod, N.H. Aversion therapy for heroin dependence. *Lancet* 2:382–384, 1968.

97. Tsoi-Hosmand, L. Behavioral competence training: A model of rehabilitation. *Int. J. Add.* 11:709–718, 1976.

98. Voegtlin, W.L., and Lemere, F. The treatment of alcohol addiction: A review of the literature. *Q. J. Stud. Alcohol.* 2:717–803, 1942.

99. Waldorf, D. Social control in therapeutic communities for the treatment of drug addicts. *Int. J. Add.* 6:29–43, 1971.

100. Wallerstein, R.S., et al. *Hospital Treatment of Alcoholism.* New York: Imago Press, 1957.

101. Wikler, A. A psychodynamic study of a patient during self-regulated re-addiction to morphine. *Psychiatric Q.* 26:270–293, 1952.

102. Wikler, A. Conditioning factors in opiate addiction and relapse. *Narcotics.* New York: McGraw-Hill, 1965.

103. Wikler, A. Some implications of conditioning theory for problems of drug abuse. *Behav. Sci.* 16:92–97, 1971.

104. Wikler, A. Dynamics of drug dependence. *Arch. Gen. Psychiatry* 28:611–616, 1973.

105. Wikler, A. Sources of reinforcement for drug-using behavior—A theoretical formulation. *Pharmacology and the Future of Man: Proceedings of the 5th International Congress on Pharmacology.* Basel: Karger, 1973.

106. Wikler, A., and Rasor, R.W. Psychiatric aspects of drug addiction. *Am. J. Med.* 14:556–570, 1953.

107. Wisocki, P.A. The successful treatment of a heroin addict by covert conditioning techniques. *J. Behav. Exper. Psychiatry* 4:55–61, 1973.

108. Wolpe, J. *Psychotherapy by Reciprocal Inhibition.* Stanford: Stanford University Press, 1958.

109. Wolpe, J. Conditioned inhibition of craving in drug addiction: A pilot experiment. *Behav. Res. and Ther.* 2:285–287, 1965.

110. Yablonsky, L. *Synanon: The Tunnel Back.* Baltimore: Penguin Books, 1967.

111. Yates, A.J. *Behavior Therapy.* New York: Wiley, 1970.

CHAPTER 12

Strategies for the Modification of Smoking Behavior: Treatment and Prevention

Terry F. Pechacek
Alfred L. McAlister

INTRODUCTION

Cigarette smoking has been characterized as "the most addictive and dependence producing form of object specific self–administered gratification known to man" (241). Conceptually it can be viewed as a multidetermined and tenacious habit involving a complex interplay of social, psychological, and pharmacological factors (87, 206, 219). Therefore, the modification of cigarette smoking offers a problem area well suited to the multidisciplinary blend of expertise and skills found within the emerging field of behavioral medicine (166, 252, 253). Indeed, the lack of such integration of expertise and skills appears to be one factor that has delayed progress toward the prevention and modification of smoking behavior.

In order to facilitate continued progress in research and intervention efforts focusing on cigarette smoking, this review will attempt to fulfill several goals: a) provide a general overview of the problem area, b) summarize the current status of adult intervention strategies, c) briefly review the state–of–the–art in early prevention, and d) provide general guidelines for intervention at various levels. In the process, this review will attempt to maintain a broad and multidisciplinary perspective on the problem so that the outcome data on specific treatment approaches can be viewed more objectively.

GENERAL PERSPECTIVE ON THE PROBLEM

Magnitude of the Problem

Smokers have become a "troubled minority" in this country (285). Since the 1964 Surgeon General's Report (280) and the U.S. Public Health Service campaigns have made the health risks of smoking more widely known, surveys of U.S. adult smoking behavior have documented a pattern of steady decline in the proportion of smokers (281, 282, 283, 287). As Figure 1 indicates, these declines are most apparent in men, among whom the smoking proportion has dropped from 52% to 39%. Moreover, these broad behavioral changes have been accompanied or possibly precipitated by generalized changes in public attitudes, even among the smokers, favoring stronger action against smoking (281, 282, 283). The continuing smoker is faced with risking concern from their families and friends regarding the effects of smoking on their health (285) and, not surprisingly in light of this pressure, about 90% of current cigarette smokers have tried or want to quit smoking completely (85, 283).

ADULT SMOKERS - 1964-1975

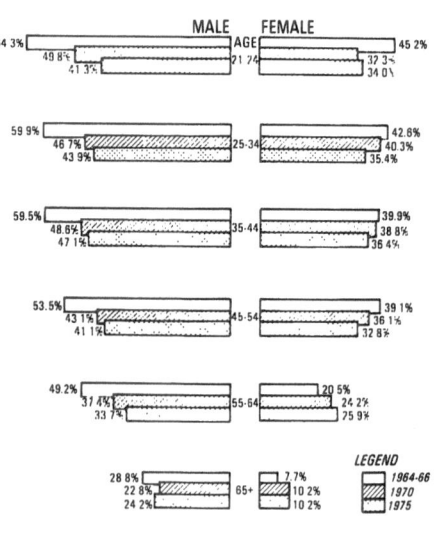

(PERCENT IN EACH CATEGORY WHO ARE SMOKERS)

Fig. 1. From: *The Smoking Digest* (285).

Most people point to these encouraging data as a symbol of the positive effects of the continuing efforts to educate the general public regarding the health risks of cigarette smoking. However, the situation is not as positive as it may first appear. Actually, due to population increases, the *number* of smokers has scarcely declined since the late 1960's and remains in excess of 50 million (229, 283). While the number of former smokers has swelled to over 30 million, active recruitment of new teenage and preteen smokers keeps the *number* of smokers at high levels (229, 284, 286, 289). As is detailed in Table 1, this pattern is especially evident among women, where the *number* of smokers has actually been on the *increase*. Despite a growing and almost uniform awareness of the health risks of smoking among children and young adults (284, 286), the prevalence of smoking among teenage females has almost reached parity with that of males, among whom the rate has remained basically unchanged in recent years. Equally ominous is the fact that recent surveys of adult smokers reveal that from 60-80% of the current smokers report having tried unsuccessfully to quit smoking.

These facts concerning the proportions and numbers of young and adult smokers and the documented tenacity of the habit emphasize that cigarette smoking remains a significant medical problem. Research has continued to clarify the etiological role of smoking in cardiovascular diseases, chronic-obstructive-broncho-pulmonary diseases, and a variety of cancers, especially of the lungs, throat, and mouth (55, 239, 250, 280, 288, 289). In light of these data and the large number of smokers, it is easy to recognize why smoking has been characterized as the largest preventable cause of premature death, illness, and disability in developed nations (55, 215, 250, 289). The magnitude of smoking impact on the U.S. Health Care System is staggering. It is estimated that over 37 million Americans (at a rate of about 325,000 per year) will die years prematurely from cigarette smoking (215, 289). The estimated economic impact of smoking (including both direct and indirect health-care costs) is astonishing—almost $26 billion a year, or about 11.3% of the economic cost of all disease (100, 142). When the cost of tobacco products is included, the drain of smoking on this nation's resources escalates to about $4.5 billion, or approximately 2.5% of the GNP.

Thus, cigarette smoking has been identified as a major contributing factor in the United States' Health Care crisis (1, 100, 142, 215, 239). While there has been significant progress over the last 15 years in combating this problem, the technology for both preventing the onset of smoking and modifying the established patterns remains basically in its infancy. Despite the fact that smokers are becoming a "troubled minority" aware of their health risks, many are unable to quit on their own. Finally, young adults, especially women, are continuing to replenish the ranks of smokers as rapidly as older smokers quit.

Table 1. Estimates of Cigarette Smokers in the United States in 1955, 1965, and 1975 Among Teenagers (Ages 13–19) and Adults (Ages 20 and Over) and Separately for Males and Females

Both Sexes Combined: Numbers in Millions

		Total Population	Current Cigarette Smokers	Former Smokers	Never Smoked	I Smokers	Quit Rate
Teenagers	1955	16.0	2.2	0.2	13.6	14	8%
13–19	1965	24.4	3.5	1.4	19.5	14	29%
	1975	29.5	6.0	3.1	20.4	20	34%
Adults	1955	104.8	39.6	7.5	57.6	38	16%
20 & Over	1965	118.0	49.7	17.8	50.5	42	26%
	1975	138.6	46.9	29.5	62.4	34	39%
All Persons	1955	120.7	41.8	7.7	71.2	35	16%
Aged 13 &	1965	142.4	53.2	19.2	70.0	37	27%
Over	1975	168.3	52.9	32.6	82.8	31	38%
MALES							
Teenagers	1955	7.6	1.5	0.1	6.0	20	6%
(Boys)	1965	12.4	2.3	0.9	9.1	19	29%
13–19	1975	15.0	3.1	1.6	10.3	21	34%
Adults (Men)	1955	50.9	26.5	5.5	18.9	52	17%
20 & Over	1965	56.8	30.0	12.7	14.2	53	30%
	1975	66.1	25.9	19.0	21.2	39	42%
All Males	1955	58.5	28.0	5.6	24.9	48	17%
Aged 13 &	1965	69.2	32.3	13.6	23.3	47	30%
Over	1975	81.1	29.0	20.6	31.5	36	42%
FEMALES							
Teenagers	1955	8.0	0.7	0.1	7.2	9	10%
(Girls)	1965	12.0	1.2	0.5	10.4	10	28%
13–19	1975	14.5	2.9	1.5	10.1	20	35%
Adults	1965	53.9	13.1	2.0	38.7	24	13%
(Women)	1965	61.2	19.7	5.1	36.3	32	21%
20 & Over	1975	72.7	21.0	10.5	41.2	29	33%
Females	1955	61.8	13.8	2.1	45.9	22	13%
Aged 13 &	1965	73.2	20.9	5.6	46.7	29	21%
Over	1975	87.2	23.9	12.0	51.3	27	33%

1. These data, provided by Dr. Daniel Horn, Director, National Clearinghouse for Smoking and Health, Center for Disease Control, Public Health Service, were included in a statement to the Commission on Smoking Policy of the American Cancer Society, Los Angeles, California, March 22, 1977.

From: Reeder, "Sociocultural Factors in the Etiology of Smoking Behavior: An Assessment," (185).

Understanding Current Smoking Behavior

Consistent with its multidetermined nature, smoking has been the subject of study by numerous investigators from a variety of perspectives. However, from an intervention perspective, we still have little definitive data about what is the most effective method to either prevent the onset of smoking or encourage its cessation (203). Hence, before considering intervention strategies, the sociological, psychological, and pharmacological aspects of smoking need to be briefly considered.

To begin with, the factors controlling smoking behavior appear to change as the smoker progresses from initiation to cessation (30, 113, 152, 217, 219, 240). Analyses of factors associated with experimentation and initiation of regular smoking indicate that sociocultural influences and peer–group dynamics seem to predominate (2, 16, 30, 56, 65, 67, 68, 174, 177, 183, 229, 284, 301). Surveys clearly indicate that youth are almost uniformly aware of the health consequences of smoking (284, 286). Thus, even though most young people report negative attitudes toward smoking, experimentation with cigarettes is embedded in a complex milieu of social forces which often overwhelm educated rationality (174, 177).

Data clearly indicate that smoking onset rates significantly increase when adolescents have parents and/or older sibling smoking models (284, 286, 301). If an older sibling and both parents smoke, the child is *four* times as likely to begin smoking as is a child with no smoking models in the family (284). Furthermore, some data suggest that parental ambivalence or acceptance of smoking experimentation also plays an important role in the establishment of regular smoking (30, 67, 68, 177, 240, 301).

However, the major factor that students themselves report as influencing their decision to experiment with tobacco is *peer pressure* (30, 120, 174, 177, 186, 195, 196, 301). Data on "best friends" smoking behavior (284, 286, 301) clearly indicate the powerful influences of group conformity pressures. The first cigarette rarely is reported to be enjoyable and commonly is smoked with an older friend or close peer (16, 67, 68, 120, 174, 177).

During the critical period of adolescent development, cigarette smoking has retained its traditional role as a means of expresing independence from adult authority and as a sign of social or sexual precocity (16, 17, 30, 31, 49, 56, 94, 120, 152, 174, 177, 183, 255, 273, 286, 301). Theories of socialization and adolescent personality development (4, 5, 64, 68, 108, 130, 158, 262, 306) clarify the process by which group norms and values supporting curiosity–seeking, risk–taking, and precocious striving for adulthood can make the use of cigarettes a sign of autonomy and maturity. Early smokers among a peer group may be influenced by older sibling, parental, or attractive adult smoking models (4, 5, 174, 177). While there is no solid evidence that tobacco advertising exerts a direct influence in the smoking adoption process, the common themes of smokers looking "tough" and "cool" or women as "liberated" and "adventurous" at least support other factors encouraging smoking onset (65, 67, 68, 174, 177).

The correlation between smoking onset and socioeconomic status (SES) (16, 30, 31, 68, 103, 201, 229, 284, 301) may possibly be explained by the greater pressure on the poor or educationally deprived to show independence or maturity (174, 177). Furthermore, the onset of smoking may integrate with cognitive development from the moralistic absolutism of childhood to the questioning and more tolerant thinking of adolescence (177, 251). While the association between smoking and various personality "traits" such as rebellious-ness (2, 30, 49, 56, 120, 255), risk-taking (30, 49, 201, 255, 294), precociousness (16, 17, 30, 49, 255), or delinquency (30, 31) should be viewed with caution (188, 189), psychosocial theories of modeling (4, 5), socialization (108, 262, 306), and personality development (64, 130, 158) clarify why smoking has retained a degree of attractiveness and social utility among groups of adolescents displaying such general characteristics.

The recent and dramatic increase in smoking among young women seems to reflect additional socialization forces, including the dramatic changes in psychosexual role definitions in recent years (273, 286, 303). While the factors influencing male smoking onset seem to have remained relatively stable (286), females appear additionally influenced by the need to express a liberated or more autonomous image (49, 286). Male smoking experimentation continues to be characterized by social uneasiness and the need to prove masculinity, but teenage girl smokers tend to be more self-confident and socially sophisticated than their nonsmoking peers (286). Thus, the changing image of the smoking women may be encouraging teenage females to seek equality with their young male peers in smoking rates as well as other activities.

Once regular smoking behavior has become established, the mechanisms controlling the maintenance of the pattern appear to shift away from the broad social-psychological factors which more strongly influence smoking onset. However, certain general psychosocial influences appear to remain important in the maintenance of adult smoking behavior also. As noted earlier in Figure 1 and Table 1, there are a number of significant gender differences with respect to percent smoking and cyclic changes in the behavior. Table 2 summarizes a number of other differences between men and women and highlights several unusual phenomena. Most Americans (74%) were currently married at the time of the 1975 survey of adult smoking behavior (283); however, those who were currently divorced or separated (5.7% of the males and 7.7% of the females) were found to have markedly higher smoking rates. The impact of educational level on smoking was also consistent across the genders; however, family income and respondent's occupation revealed inverse patterns for the men and women. Additionally, in a more specific survey of young women (aged 18–35), smoking

**Table 2. Smoking Rates by Gender, Marital
Status, Education, Income, and Occupation
among Adults in 1970 & 1975**

	MALES		FEMALES	
	1970	1975	1970	1975
ALL PERSONS	42.2%	39.3%	30.5%	28.9%
BY MARITAL STATUS				
Single (never married)	56%	38%	36%	31%
Married (currently)	40%	38%	32%	28%
Divorced or Separated (currently)	76%	60%	44%	50%
BY EDUCATION				
High School	49%	46%	33%	32%
Some College	37%	36%	36%	32%
College Graduates	31%	28%	26%	21%
BY ANNUAL FAMILY INCOME				
Less than $10,000	43.2%	45.6%	27.9%	27.3%
$10,000 to $19,999	43.9%	39.1%	37.3%	31.3%
More than $20,000	31.2%	35.0%	39.4%	34.0%
BY OCCUPATION				
Blue Collar	51%	47%		
White Collar	37%	36%		

From: USDHEW, PHS, CDC, NCSH. *Adult Use of Tobacco, 1*

rates were not found to significantly differ between working women and housewives; but the smoking housewives reported being heavier smokers and expressed less interest in cessation (286). Therefore, the sociology of adult smoking is complex, especially among the women. However, it does appear that among the more affluent women and among women in the white–collar professions, smoking parity with their male counterparts is being maintained (54, 70, 86) and may reflect the general trend toward equality in virtually all domains of social and economic life (229, 273).

While social factors influence adult smoking behavior, the maintenance of regular smoking can best be explained by psychological and pharmacological models. Initial attempts to characterize smoking tended to represent the behavior within a general psychological theory (107). Tomkins (276) proposed that smoking is maintained by its role in managing affect (enhancing the positive and reducing the negative). Horn (111) further delineated this model and recently has focused more on the rewarding aspects of smoking (112) and the decision–making process at the various stages of the habit (113). This latter conceptualization outlined how cost/benefit appraisal at initiation, establishment, and maintenance support smoking, while the appraisal prior to cessation finally shifts toward nonsmoking. However, such broad psychosocial interpretations of smoking have tended to have little validating data and limited heuristic value (161, 206).

As Bernstein (10) and Keutzer, Lichtenstein, and Mees (136) predicted, learning theory conceptualizations of smoking gained popularity during the 1970's due to their more concise definitions and general heuristic nature. These models viewed smoking as a learned response established under massed trials in diverse stimulus conditions and under partial reinforcement schedules (116, 117). Therefore, the tenacity and resistance to extinction of the smoking response could be easily predicted by theories of learning (116, 117).

A variety of research resulted from the learning theory model of smoking; however, the results generally failed to fulfill the promise of increased efficacy (159, 179, 304). More recently, theorists have considered these data and suggested that the basic model may still have merit, since almost all studies failed to apply a complete learning theory analysis to the problem (63, 160).

As the preceeding models failed to produce successful treatments, analyses of the possible role of pharmacological factors increased (59, 242). Unfortunately, the biochemistry of nicotine and other tobacco compounds is such that pharmacologists have not been able to unravel the possible mechanisms of chemical dependency (127). While it is generally agreed that nicotine is the most likely chemical involved (127, 242), traditional drug research has not defined exactly how it may be reinforcing (127). Russell (242) has presented a persuasive argument supporting the role of nicotine in tobacco dependency (240, 241), and Schachter and associates (247, 248) have presented some provocative data; however, experimental attempts to evaluate the effects of intravenously presented nicotine on *ad libitum* smoking has raised doubts about the strength of the role of nicotine in tobacco dependency (23, 143).

Independent of these former models, a variety of social–psychological research was continuing related to smoking behavior. Leventhal (154, 155, 156, 157), Rogers (235, 236), and Mausner and Platt (170) have outlined various expectancy models of smoking cessation. However, most of the research that has arisen from these models has sought to answer theoretical questions rather than generate specific interventions. Several recent models have attempted to integrate this line of research with the learning theory and pharmacological models of smoking. Glad, Tyre, and Adesso (87) have provided a multidimensional model integrating a diversity of theoretical perspectives. Similarly, Pechacek and Danaher (206) have conceptualized smoking cessation within a cognitive–behavioral framework. Finally, Pomerleau (219) has attempted to formulate an integrated perspective on the smoking problem. Each of these later formulations appears to have sufficient specificity to stimulate additional research on the smoking problem. Additionally, new research on specific aspects of the problem is expanding our understanding of the situational aspects of smoking (14, 37, 62, 78, 81). Therefore, new treatments based on these new models may benefit from the increased integration across past data bases.

REVIEW OF INTENSIVE INTERVENTION

Overview

Since the health risks of smoking have become more widely known, there has been a rapid proliferation in efforts to both prevent smoking and encourage cessation. A wide variety of strategies has been tried; however, the social relevancy of the problem has guided most of the effort toward unevaluated cessation programs rather than formal evaluations and careful research (203). Unevaluated interventions have been especially evident in the area of early prevention (67, 68, 275) and large-scale media campaigns (203). Nevertheless, a wealth of data does exist on the relative efficacy of strategies, and these data present a surprisingly uniform picture. With regard to prevention, almost all strategies appear to produce attitude changes consistent with nonsmoking, but almost all programs have failed to actually deter smoking behavior (67, 68, 177, 275).

The cessation research has been extensively reviewed and categorized (10, 11, 13, 19, 63, 118, 136, 159, 161, 172, 180, 203, 204, 206, 254, 261, 275) and presents a similarly disappointing picture. Namely, almost any sensible strategy or technique will produce initial and dramatic reductions in smoking behavior, but almost none has been able to demonstrate success rates consistently higher than the commonly cited pattern shown in Figure 2. In general, only 20–30% of the subjects who are abstinent at treatment termination remain nonsmokers during long-term follow-ups (118, 119). This pattern of initial success followed by rapid relapse has made the interpretation of relative efficacy difficult, since few projects have collected complete follow-up data or included adequate control groups needed for accurate evaluations (10, 203, 254, 261).

But even if follow-up data are available, recent findings suggest that the validity of self-report data may be questionable. Several reports have now documented that up to 20% of the subjects claiming to be abstinent may in fact be smoking (24, 51, 76, 124, 198, 265). Since almost all research to date has been evaluated based on self-reported smoking behavior, the potential invalidity of this type of dependent variable raises serious problems (76). This problem is especially acute in prevention programs with children, where the social climate and demand characteristics inhibit the reporting of smoking behavior (66, 120, 174, 177).

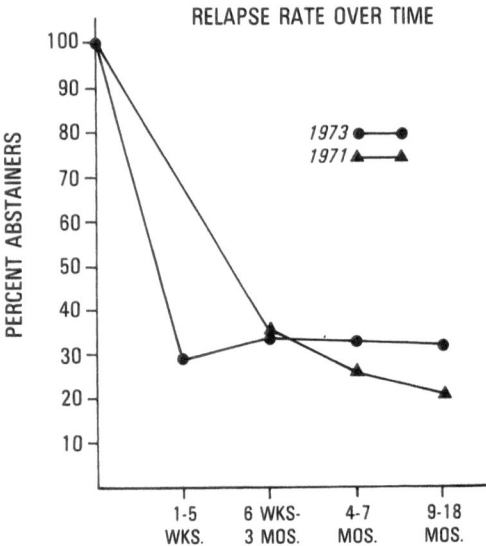

Fig. 2. From: Hunt and Bespalec, "An evaluation of current methods of modifying smoking behavior" (118).

Thus, the evaluation of research data in the area of both prevention of smoking onset and cessation strategies is difficult. Most programs have not been adequately evaluated, and many claim encouraging success rates without providing the type of follow-up data needed for objective analysis. Even when data are available from controlled studies, the potential invalidity of self-report data makes conclusions tentative at best.

Prevention Programs

Until very recently, little progress has been made in the quality of intervention programs to deter the onset of smoking (67, 68, 177, 275). As discussed above, experimentation occurs within a complex social milieu, and the instilling of information and attitudes counter to smoking may be insufficient to deter smoking. Horn and associates (114) demonstrated the pattern of results that are still common; namely, a variety of success in changing attitudes and beliefs regarding smoking but little success in depressing the rate of smoking onset. Evans (67, 68) and Thompson (275) have recently reviewed the wide array of school campaigns which have almost uniformly failed to achieve any degree of long-term success. Even well-conceived and evaluated programs like the

Saskatoon smoking study (212, 213, 214) have displayed no significant differences in smoking rates between students exposed to student–directed education programs versus those provided with no antismoking treatment.

These findings have led many health and medical professionals to adopt a very pessimistic attitude toward smoking prevention programs; however, behavioral and social scientists trained in the complexities of adolescent socialization and personality development view the problem with more optimism (65, 67, 68, 174, 177). The theoretical models of social learning (4, 5), adolescent personality (64, 130, 158), persuasive communication (137, 154, 155, 156, 169, 182, 235), and group dynamics (158, 262, 306) provide the foundation for a social–psychological strategy for countering the complex forces encouraging smoking onset during teenage years (65).

Evans and his students and colleagues at the University of Houston and Baylor School of Medicine (65, 69, 191) pioneered in the development and testing of a social–psychological smoking prevention program to deal with the problem. The treatment model incorporated a variety of psychological principles including "psychological inoculation" (i.e., skills to counter common pressures to smoke) (182), and communication theory (154, 155, 156, 169) and capitalized on immediate negative effects (elevated carbon monoxide level, bad breath, and the like). Furthermore, Evan's group recognized the need to improve the validity of self-report data by means of physiological monitoring (66).

The University of Houston treatment (65, 69) involved film programs with nonsmoking peers presenting persuasive communication regarding immediate negative effects of smoking and inoculation against peer pressures and media models. This program, along with saliva monitoring (66), was tested in the seventh grade versus monitoring–only and questionnaire–only control. While the monitoring appeared to reduce the onset of smoking versus the questionnaire-only school, the complete program did not produce any additional effect (69).

Research adapting the University of Houstin model (65) in other centers has been successful, however (74). Studies at Stanford University School of Medicine and Harvard School of Public Health have expanded upon the basic inoculation and persuasive communication model presented by Evans (66, 69). The distinctive features of these new studies are: (a) utilization of slightly older peers (peer leaders) as the primary agents delivering the program; and (b) active role–playing to enhance the learning of the pressure resistance skills. These latter adaptions stem from social learning theory (4, 5) and have been suggested by recent publications (104, 290). A seven-session program involving slide presentations and group discussions led by a high school student who is adventurous and unconventional but a nonsmoker has been tested in pilot experiment near San Jose, California (177). One school served as control while the other received the program. Self-report data validated by random samplings of exhaled breath tests for carbon monoxide level revealed that smoking levels in the treatment school increased to 5.6% during the treatment year, while the control school increased to 9.9% (p <0.5) (177).

A program at the University of Minnesota (120, 167) has attempted to combine both the Evans model and features of the Stanford program. Film messages almost identical to those used in Houston were made with local seventh graders as actors; two peer opinion leaders from each class worked with college–aged group leaders in conducting role–playing sessions like those used in the Stanford model. The program was tested among 1530 seventh graders from four suburban junior high schools. Self-report measures of smoking were collected at all four schools on three occasions. Three schools additionally received saliva thiocyanate monitoring to increase validity of self-report data. Two schools received three videotape films and two group discussions. The actors for the films were drawn from one school while the other school received unpersonalized films like those used in Houston.

Treatment results from the University of Minnesota program have been very encouraging (120, 167, 193a). The number of students reporting smoking a "few cigarettes a month or more" at the end of the school term increased by 132% in the control school receiving monitoring only, by 48% in the school viewing the nonpersonalized film, and by 20% in the school with class peer leaders serving as actors and group leaders. Continued follow-up of these treatment groups has revealed that the effects have been maintained into the eighth grade (193a). Results from saliva samples, collected from all students for analysis of thiocyanate levels, have paralleled the self-report data (167).

Thus, initial results suggest that elements from both the Houston and Stanford programs can be successfully adapted. While all of these results are tentative and must be considered as pilot tests, the basic model appears to hold great promise (174, 177). Additional studies at Harvard, Stanford, University of Minnesota, and American Health Foundation are underway and long-term follow-ups are being conducted. If these initial encouraging findings continue, a major step toward effective prevention will have been made.

Adult Programs

General Populations

A vast number of different strategies and techniques has been attempted to aid smokers in quitting their habit. Many of these programs have focused on this goal exclusively rather than on the testing of specific strategies. Such nonspecific interventions have resulted in a vast amount of well–meaning effort lacking outcome data needed for critical appraisal. Nevertheless, a great store of data on cessation strategies has been accumulated. In fact, the number of studies is so extensive that it is beyond the scope of this chapter to review all of the data. Fortunately, the difficult task of evaluating the relative efficacy of various treatments and strategies has been very adequately done in past and more recent reviews (10, 11, 13, 19, 63, 118, 136, 159, 161, 172, 180, 203, 204, 254, 261, 275). Therefore, this chapter will utilize those reviews as a point of departure so that critical issues and recent developments can be emphasized.

The most common form of smoking treatment has been cessation clinics offering encouragement advice, and other nonspecific techniques (10, 203, 261). Public service and proprietary programs have proliferated since 1964 but most have been intermittent and rarely evaluated (254, 261). However, the programs of the American Cancer Society and the Five–Day Plans of the Church of the Seventh Day Adventists have probably treated more smokers than any other organized efforts (172). Unfortunately, when these programs have been evaluated adequately, their group–treatment approaches appear to produce the commonly cited (see Figure 2) pattern of 20–25% long–term abstinence (96, 97, 226, 274). Other clinics that have similar or more elaborate formats have reported fairly equivalent outcome data (257, 258, 263, 264, 300).

In light of these data on public–service and research clinics, the claims of impressive results made by proprietary programs must be viewed with some skepticism (172, 261). What published outcome data that does exist suggest that initial success rates are encouraging but that relapse deteriorates even the best programs down to 30–40% long–term success rates (261). However, there is some data that such clinics may have higher success rates for males than for females (131).

In view of these data, Bernstein's (10) conclusion would still seem valid that clinics can serve a useful purpose only when more effective modification strategies have been developed. The striking finding is that almost any type of treatment or control condition offered under the guise of a group cessation clinic will produce from 15–25% long–term abstinence (96, 97, 257, 258). Thus, this rate provides a good estimate of the "placebo" effect of any strategy.

With the failure of the clinic model, pharmacologically based treatments developed. Early results were almost uniformly discouraging (95, 203), especially attempts to substitute Lobeline for smoking (48). More recently, a nicotine chewing gum has been developed and tested with some limited success (20, 72). In a well–conceived double–blind study, Russell and associates (245) demonstrated some success in controlling smoking rate and withdrawal symptoms with the nicotine chewing gum, but its effects appeared to be a small component in the overall cessation rate. Therefore, current data suggest that the usefulness of pharmacological cessation aids has yet to be demonstrated (95, 203) and that they would need to be combined within a broader cessation program in order to produce either initial or long–term abstinence.

Hypnosis has been another intervention with widespread claims of efficacy but little objective outcome data for evaluation. Clinicians claim success rates up to 86% at 6- to 12-month follow–ups (203, 261). Unfortunately, these claims have not been substantiated by comparative research. Recent studies support the conclusions of both Johnson and Donahue (128) and Orne (199) that no research data have documented hypnotherapy as an effective strategy for the elimination of smoking behavior. Studies by Pederson and associates (208), Shewchuk and associates (264), and Barkley and associates (8) all found that hypnosis did not differ either from control conditions or exceed the often–noted 20–25% long–term success rates of almost any treatment (see Figure 2).

Social Learning and Behavior Modification Approaches

The most prolific research has been based on the experimental and social–learning theories of smoking. While these studies have many of the common methodological flaws, the research based on learning theories has generally been improving (11, 13, 160, 203). Unfortunately, many studies have adapted the generally successful techniques of behavior modification to smoking without sufficient analysis of the problem (63, 160). Moreover, many researchers have focused more on initial reductions than on long–term change (203, 261). Hence, the literature is replete with studies demonstrating temporary success but minimal or no long–term results (203, 261). Therefore, the wealth of articles in this area will be briefly discussed with special emphasis on those research trends that have demonstrated more consistent findings. More detailed discussions of the literature are presented in various past reviews (10, 11, 13, 19, 63, 118, 136, 159, 161, 172, 180, 203, 204, 254, 261, 275).

The research in this area can be roughly dichotomized into two categories: a) behavioral self–control strategies utilizing high participant involvement, and b) aversion strategies designed to reduce the probability of the smoking response (161). However, the most effective programs have tended to be multicomponent interventions combining certain strategies from both categories (11, 13, 203, 204).

Self–Control Strategies

Subject awareness on controlling stimuli is basic to this type of approach; therefore, self–monitoring of smoking behavior has been a fundamental element in all treatments. Since treatments are based on learning–theory formulations, subjects are taught to reduce the strength and range of controlling cues. While such a process should theoretically make cessation easier, with some exceptions most smokers seem to reach a floor effect at about 10–12 cigarettes per day (75, 157). Many programs have displayed initial suppression of smoking rates followed by rapid relapse (11, 13, 161, 178, 179, 203); however, a few programs developed by systematic research have been able to demonstrate some more encouraging findings (21, 22, 220).

One specific technique which has shown some recent encouraging data has been contingency contracting. While early research was equivocal several studies have produced impressive results (13, 1611, 203). In combination with other self–control strategies it appears both to initiate change and to help maintain success during follow–up (145, 146).

Other techniques, such as systematic desensitization, have not faired as well. In general, this technique produced equivocal and unimpressive long–term results (11, 13, 161, 203). Similarly covert strategies have demonstrated only temporary treatment effects (11, 13, 161, 203).

Therefore, the literature on self–control strategies has been generally discouraging. Even when applied in more complex, multicomponent formats, treatment results have been only moderately encouraging (25, 133, 181). While some success have been noted by Brengelmann (21, 22) and Pomerleau (220), most studies have not demonstrated results superior to the generally expected rates of 20–30% abstinence during follow–up (see Figure 2).

Aversion Strategies

Interventions designed to reduce the probability of smoking by pairing it with some aversive stimuli have been commonly utilized. The most common aversive stimuli have been electric shock, covert images, and cigarette smoke itself. More recently, these aversion strategies have been included into multicomponent packages that include self–control techniques as well. However, the research on aversive conditioning approaches has generally been inconsistent, with initially impressive results failing to be replicated. Nevertheless, aversion strategies have produced some of the most encouraging data of any behavioral approach.

Electric shock has almost always failed to produce impressive long–term results in controled research (11, 161, 203) or even superiority over attention–placebo controls (161, 203). Moreover, the recent report by Russell and associates (243) suggested that "traditional conditioning processes do not contribute significantly to the clinical response of human subjects to electric aversion therapy for cigarette smoking" (p. 108). However, both Chapman and associates (34) and Dericco and associates (53) have produced impressive long–term results when shock is combined with other strategies and maintained over extended periods. Thus, the data suggest that as a sole treatment, electric shock fails because the treatment effects do not generalize well outside the lab, but when combined with other procedures such as self–management training an effective treatment package can be produced (161, 203).

Covert sensitization has often been discussed as a mechanism for generalizing treatment effects outside the lab (33); however, as a primary treatment for smoking, the procedure has failed to produce meaningful or encouraging levels of long–term abstinence (11, 161, 203). However, recent reports suggest that the procedure may be an effective maintenance aid and can be effectively combined within multicomponent treatments (13).

The most effective aversion strategies have utilized some form of smoke aversion. It has been suggested that cigarette smoke is a particularly appropriate aversive stimulus, since it effects many of the endogenous cues that characterized smoking (161). Three main versions of smoke aversion have been used: a) satiation—doubling or tripling daily consumption prior to abstinence; b) warm, stale smoke blown into the smoker's face; or c) rapid smoking—inhaling every six seconds until unable to continue. While the data on smoke aversion techniques have been inconsistent and often mixed, continued research has produced some promising results.

Early research on the warm smoking air procedure produced minimal or no long–term success (161); however, Lichtenstein and associates (249) continued to refine the procedure and produced impressive results of 60% abstinence at six–month follow–up. Subsequent replications (161, 164) relative to control conditions established that both the rapid smoking and the warm smoky air procedures seem equally effective. Since the rapid smoking procedure was simpler and more convenient, it became increasingly popular (43, 161). However, subsequent data became more mixed (43, 165). Many studies failed to replicate the 60% long–term success rates, and some obtained almost no effect (43). However, Danaher (43) has attempted to clarify these data by highlighting the departures from the original treatment procedures which could have accounted for these nonreplications. Thus, it appears that the rapid smoking procedure can be potentially effective, but a warm personal client–therapist relationship, flexible or individualized treatment scheduling, and continuation of treatment until abstinence is attained all may be important (43, 202, 203). Finally, however, numerous nonreplications and one direct test (197) have demonstrated that the production of definite physiological aversion and conditioning effects alone are insufficient to produce long–term abstinence.

The final smoke aversion strategy is satiation. Early research on this method of self–imposed aversion produced a reported success rate of 63% at four–month follow–up (232, 233); however, the weight of evidence on the procedure since then has been negative (11, 161, 203). Controlled studies have been unable to replicate the initial success or even demonstrate superiority versus control conditions (35, 147). Nevertheless, some very impressive results have been produced with satiation combined within a multicomponent treatment package. Best and associates (13, 15) and Delahunt and Curran (50) both have demonstrated that satiation plus behavioral self–control training are superior to attention placebo conditions. Best and associates produced 35-55% success at six months with a take-home version of their treatment package (13, 15), while Delahunt and Curran (50) observed 56% abstinence at six months.

Both Elliott (61) and McAlister (173) also found encouraging results with programs combining rapid smoking and self-control techniques. However, other studies have not found that self-control techniques enhanced the efficacy of the rapid smoking procedure (42, 89, 138, 153, 202). Thus, the positive results for combinations of self-control and aversion strategies must still be viewed with caution. The study by Flaxman (75) of several combinations of self-control and aversion strategies highlights the complexity of the problems, since males responded differently than females and gradual reduction strategies seem to hamper success with or without aversion techniques.

As the smoke aversion strategies were gaining in popularity, concerns were raised regarding their safety. Since the techniques induce aversion by means of the physiological discomforts of excessive smoking, the cardiopulmonary stress of increased nicotine and carbon-monoxide intake has been noted with concern (105, 109, 110). A number of studies have been undertaken to quantify the impact of the most extreme of these procedures, rapid smoking, on the cardiovascular system (101, 163, 190, 246). Much of this data has been summarized by Lichtenstein and Glasgow (163), and recent studies by Hall and associates (101, 246) and Miller and associates (190) have documented that rapid smoking does produce acute and dramatic effects upon the cardiopulmonary system. Thus, the procedure appears to be contraindicated for individuals with possible cardiovascular diseases, and adequate medical screening of potential treatment participants has been strongly encouraged (101, 163, 190, 246). Data have yet to be published on the relative risks of the other smoke aversion procedures, but the doubling or tripling of smoking consumption during the satiation procedure may induce significant effects also. Nevertheless, it should be noted that in excess of 35,000 participants have been exposed to some form of rapid smoking with informally reported morbidity rate from nonspecific complications (such as fainting or heart problems) of about 0.023% and no reported deaths (163). But until the relative risks of the procedures have been more completely defined, all smoke aversion procedures should be used with appropriate screening and monitoring (101, 163, 190, 246).

Due to the relative risks of existing smoke aversion strategies, several less stressful alternatives have been experimented with. Several pilot studies utilizing normal-paced smoke aversion procedures combined with behavioral self–control packages have produced encouraging results (98, 99). A controlled test of rapid puffing (every three seconds) without inhaling showed less optimistic findings, however (202). Finally, a recent report by Tori (277) demonstrated that a taste-aversion technique involving holding the smoke in the mouth without inhaling was as effective as rapid smoking, with 68% abstinence at six-month follow-up versus 60% for rapid smoking. Unfortunately the study lacked experimental controls; thus, the issue of less stressful alternatives requires additional testing.

While the research data on behavioral treatments has yet to produce a clearly superior treatment strategy, multicomponent treatments appear to be the most encouraging. Those packages utilizing some combination of behavioral self-control techniques and integrating aversive control procedures can be effective. However, it appears that they are most effective when refined by systematic developmental research and applied by treatment teams sensitive to the complexity of the smoking problem (203). Thus, while there have been several notably successful programs (15, 34, 50, 53, 61, 173, 271), others with similar treatment elements have been markedly less effective (38, 42, 46, 89, 138, 202). Therefore, the manner in which the procedures are individualized to the participants' needs appears to be a critical variable (43, 161).

Finally, the best of the behavioral technology has now been reduced to self-study (44, 45) and take-home (15, 90) versions. This broadening of the service delivery mode is encouraging. Smokers continued to report interest in such self-help methods (84, 256), but until very recently no effective materials have been available. The initial test of the self-study approach to smoking cessation aids has been mixed (89, 90, 202), but the results presented by Best and associates (15) are encouraging. Clearly this is a line of research which merits additional attention.

Controlled Smoking

As many smokers find that they are unable to quit completely despite several attempts, they have become more interested in ways to reduce their risks without quitting (85, 283, 285). There has been a dramatic shift in the types of cigarettes consumed, with filtered and lower tar/nicotine cigarettes becoming the norm (26, 102, 200). Despite this obvious interest, little research has been conducted to develop strategies to aid smokers in this process of reducing risks. However, Fredricksen and associates (77, 78, 79, 80, 81, 82) have systematically been investigating the components of the smoking topography which produce risk. They have demonstrated that modifying the topography, including changing how much smoke is inhaled and how many puffs per cigarette are taken as well as the strength and type of cigarette smoked, produces measurable changes in exposure (81, 82). While the technology is still in the developmental stage, it is clearly important. In addition to continuing smokers who need to reduce their exposure, cigarette smokers who shift to cigars or pipes also need assistance. Data suggest that many such individuals continue to unconsciously inhale and expose themselves to even higher levels of toxics from the stronger smoke (80,

279). Similarly, smokers who simply shift to a lower tar/nicotine cigarette may compensate by inhaling deeper and similarly be exposing themselves to high levels of carbon monoxide or other gases (244, 278). Thus, the controlled smoking technology is needed for many smokers in order to control their exposure from either cigarettes or their substitutes.

Maintenance of Nonsmoking

The data on all interventions (see Figure 2) clearly indicate that initial high rates of success often deteriorate over time. Therefore, all major reviews of the smoking literature have continued to stress the need for more effective maintenance strategies (11, 13, 118, 161, 172, 203, 204, 261). However, the continuing problem of identifying clearly effective *cessation* strategies has kept most of the energies of research focused on this phase of treatment. Little new data has been produced regarding maintenance programming, but what has been shown is encouraging. Dubren (58) reported some optimistic finding utilizing a simple tape–recorded telephone reinforcement method. Also, Lando has been finding that contingency contracting enhanced the long–term results of a broad–spectrum, aversive smoking program with 76% abstinence with contract– ing versus 35% with treatment only at six–month follow–up (146). Case study data are also supportive of this concept (203).

Therefore, some progress is being made in the development of techniques to prevent the common pattern of relapse after treatment. Nevertheless, many smokers continue to relapse. Therefore, this issue is beginning to receive direct attention by several researchers (13, 141, 146, 205, 218, 231). Hopefully, there will be continued interest in identifying the types of situations and patterns of behavior which make the ex–smoker more vulnerable to relapse. With such data, the developing technology of maintenance programming can be enhanced.

Special Populations

Almost all research on cessation strategies has been conducted upon volunteer populations without restriction regarding medical conditions or motivations. However, several types of clinical or experimental investigations have focused more exclusively on specific groups of smokers who are at higher risks; namely, smokers already displaying heart or lung diseases or smokers identified at high risk for such diseases. The results from such populations indicate that treatment can be clearly more effective than the results found in the general population. The most dramatic example of this has been the success rates with the postmyocardial infarction (MI) patients. Men who have survived a MI have been found to quit smoking in large proportions (30–50%) after only minimal counseling and to maintain these changes for several years (28, 40, 106, 237, 299). When specific treatment was introduced, even more encouraging results were produced (28). Burt and associates (28) reported 63% abstinence in a post–MI group which received counseling versus only 27% for the standard treatment condition.

These types of findings have also been found with other symptomatic smokers (27, 129, 206). In fact, Jones (129) has noted that quitting smoking is often a very good indicator of increased respiratory symptoms and, thus, can serve as a good diagnostic cue. Moreover, surveys of ex–smokers have consistently revealed that a primary motivation in self–initiated cessation continues to be an increase in symptoms (cough, breathlessness, or the like) that are identified with smoking (93, 206, 266).

Likewise, men who have been made aware of their elevated cardiovascular risk status also seem to respond well to smoking intervention, even if it is brief (125, 230, 302). Several studies have documented that large changes can be produced when risk–factor screening is followed by some systematic counseling which clearly links smoking to increased risks for heart disease (125, 230, 237). Rose (237) and Lichtenstein and Danaher (162) have reviewed the data on physician counseling and have offered sound advice about what to expect and how to effectively treat smoking in an office practice.

The Multiple Risk Factor Intervention Trial (MRFIT) is one of the largest and most ambitious of the multicomponent efforts to influence cigarette smoking, along with other CHD risk factors, among middle–aged men (192, 193, 272). Over 6000 men, aged 35–57, have been taking part in a six–year coronary prevention program which is attempting to reduce blood pressure and serum cholesterol levels as well as encourage smoking cessation. Initial eight– to ten–week intensive interventions focusing on dietary and smoking changes to reduce CHD risk have been followed by monthly or bimonthly maintenance contacts (193). Initial results reveal that approximately 43% of the smokers were abstinent at the first annual visit (approximately eight months after the end of the intensive interventions). Most importantly, the data reveal that almost 80% of the successful quitters were produced in the intensive intervention with subsequent cessation being sporadic and subject to higher relapse (193). Thus, the data is similar to the post–MI data noted above; namely, once subjects are convinced concerning the smoking–heart disease link, dramatic changes in behavior are possible while later changes are more subject to relapse.

In an attempt to further evaluate the process and techniques of MRFIT, a small trial labeled the Heart Attack Risk Reduction Trial (HARRT) has been conducted on 63 smokers with elevated serum cholesterols (125). Physician counseling similar to that used in MRFIT was compared to self–directed group therapy and repeated risk–factor screenings. Initial results suggested that the physician counseling was significantly more effective; however, by the one–year follow–up all intervention modes had very similar cessation rates of about 20% (125). Thus, the long–term results of the MRFIT trial appear to reflect both notable initial results and effective maintenance programming.

The fact that the data that does exist on physician counseling is generally positive and that smokers continue to look to the medical profession for advice regarding smoking (83, 237, 283) suggests that more emphasis needs to be placed on the development of more effective techniques that can be distributed by health–care professionals (162, 237). Furthermore, Raw (227) has demonstrated that health–care workers besides physicians can also be important in encouraging cessation. Therefore, additional research is needed to evaluate the best techniques derived from behavioral research which are translated into formats applicable for use in medical settings (162, 216, 221, 237).

MODIFICATION OF GENERAL POPULATIONS

Cessation Efforts

Mediated interventions to reach broader population groups are now beginning. Several studies have now demonstrated that moderate but encouraging results can be obtained with minimal or no personal contact. One demonstration in New York produced small absolute changes (about 8% cessation rate) with a televised cessation clinic, but they seem to maintain well during follow–up (57, 58).

Most encouraging results were obtained by Best in a recent televised cessation clinic (12). Among the 1400 subscribed viewers who sent in for a program guide, postclinic abstinence was reported in 11.5%; however, the success rate climbed during follow–up to 14.7% at three months and 17.6% at six months postclinic. Thus, the results were moderate but clearly cost–effective, especially in view of the fact that upwards of 20,000 other nonenrolled viewers also may have benefited (12).

Community Programs

Programs aimed at total communities have also produced encouraging data. During the peak of the antismoking campaign in the late 1960's, Greenfield, Iowa participated in a unique effort encouraging cessation (59). Thirty–seven percent of the adults signed to try quitting and 14.2% of the males and 3.9% of the females were still reporting abstinence seven months later, with the higher socioeconomic groups being more successful.

Communitywide coronary prevention programs have offered additional results on the potentials of treating large groups of smokers. The North Karelia Project (140, 224, 225) has been providing a comprehensive coronary prevention program since 1972 to reduce blood pressure and serum cholesterol levels and encourage smoking cessation. By the end of the first year of intensive intervention, the proportion of 25–59–year–old smokers had decreased from 54% to 43% in the North Karelia province but had changed little in the reference counties in western Finland. These dramatic changes in smoking have been maintained for over five years, with the final survey revealing 42% smoking in the males. Little change was noted in female smoking, since the rate was always low—about 11–13%.

Even more specific data are available on the communitywide coronary prevention program conducted by Stanford Heart Disease Prevention Program from 1972–75 (71, 168, 176, 187). An extensive two–year mass–media campaign focusing on general CHD risk–factor change was presented to two California communities while a third community served as control (71, 168). Face–to–face behavioral counseling (71, 175) was offered to two–thirds of the high–risk members (upper 20% on a CHD risk score) in one of the media communities. Three years after the program started, the proportion of smokers had decreased by only 3% in the control community and 8% in the media–only community, but by 24% in the media–plus–counseling community (71, 168). Additionally, 50% of the high–risk smokers receiving face–to–face counseling quit versus only 11% in the media–only community (71, 176).

Thus, the moderate changes produced by media education regarding the rationale and techniques of risk–factor (including smoking cessation) change can be amplified by some form of more personal contact. McAlister has demonstrated that cessation techniques can be effectively disseminated by video but peer–group support may be needed (173). Communitywide cessation programs presented by television may be more effective if supplemented by support groups who watch the programs together. This format has received initial testing in Finland and merits additional demonstration.

RECOMMENDATIONS FOR FUTURE RESEARCH AND TREATMENT

Methological Issues

Any reviewer of the literature on smoking prevention or modification is faced with an almost impossible task of sorting through outcome data permeated with methodological flaws. The most pervasive problem is the validity of the data. Almost all programs, clinics, or research studies have relied primarily on unverified self–report data as their critical dependent measure. However, when physiological monitoring of smoking has been done, misrepresentation has been common both in children (66, 120, 167) and among adults completing a cessation program (24, 76, 124, 198, 265). Additionally, self-reported levels of smoking are subject to error due to digit bias in reporting and underreporting due to nonspecific demand characteristics (76, 296). Moreover, self-reports were found to have questionable reliability when assessed on the same day (291).

Many studies are beginning to utilize some form of self-monitoring to improve the quality of the data; however, the technique is reactive (178) and is still subject to the demand characteristics. Therefore, biochemical measures of smoking are clearly desirable.

Among children, the very act of monitoring appears to both enhance the validity of self-report and inhibit smoking (66, 120). Similarly, among adults confronted with biochemical data in conflict with their self-report (e.g., contradicting self-reports of abstinence), many report "occasional" cigarettes, or pipe/cigar smoking (24, 51, 198). Thus, researchers should be aware that uncorroborated self-reports may lead to an overestimation of success.

Several biochemical measures are available for monitoring smoking. Carbon monoxide level in expired air can be measured easily and inexpensively (36, 144, 228, 234). However, CO has a short half-life (two to six hours) (268), is affected by environmental sources (268, 295), and shows high diurnal variability (185). Cotinine or nicotine levels can be measured in urine, saliva, or serum (151); however, nicotine has a very short half-life (30 minutes) (123), and both cotinine and nicotine are relatively difficult to measure (73, 115, 149, 150, 298, 305).

Thiocyanate levels in urine, saliva, or serum have been recommended as a preferable biochemical measure of smoking due to their 10–14-day half-life (29, 209). A variety of data is available on the method and on distributions among smokers and nonsmokers (9, 18, 29, 41, 47, 52, 148, 171, 209, 210). Unfortunately, thiocyanate can also be confounded by nonsmoking sources, especially dietary sources of cyanide and thiocyanate (148, 207). However, when thiocyanate is combined with carbon monoxide (291, 292, 293), the discrimination power of the two measures is greatly enhanced.

In addition to the serious problem with data of questionable validity, attributions of causality of outcome results to independent treatment factors are almost impossible without adequate designs and controls. This is an especially difficult problem in smoking prevention studies where entire schools must be treated as units of observation. Techniques of quasi-experimental design are commonly utilized (32, 88, 134, 135, 267); however, such approaches may yield questionable results due to the nonindependence of the subjects (39, 174, 177). Thus, it is preferable to match schools on important variables and then randomly assign them to treatment conditions (174, 177).

Adult cessation studies generally do not face the same design problems as prevention studies; however, as has been commonly noted in the past (10, 254), cessation studies often lack adequate controls, especially attention–placebo controls. Given the commonly noted quit rate of 15–20% even in untreated or minimally treated control groups (203, 261), a credible and appropriate control group should be included in all studies of smoking cessation.

Finally, all field studies should strive for comprehensive follow–ups. Guidelines for such follow–ups have been given (194, 261), and follow–up results based only on participants who respond or who are readily available are especially suspect. Helpful suggestions, such as obtaining the name of a contact person who will know the future whereabouts of the participant, have been offered (165).

Research Needs

In the area of smoking prevention, initial and encouraging data are beginning to emerge (120, 167, 177); however, the basic model (65, 69) needs to be clarified and components tested. Critical issues regarding the optimal time for intervention and the lasting effects of early intervention need to be addressed in prospective and longitudinal studies. Furthermore, the role of classroom teachers who express interest in smoking prevention (3) needs to be evaluated within the basic social–psychological model (65, 69, 177).

Among adult smokers, the pattern of unaided cessation outside of formal programs suggests that smokers can quit on their own (85, 283). It has been estimated that 95% of the 29 million smokers who have quit since 1964 have done so on their own (285); however, little is known about how to maximize this process (223). Existing survey data (84, 256) suggest that most smokers are not interested in attending formal cessation clinics; rather, they want some form of do–it–yourself treatment (256). Even when smokers express an interest in a treatment group, most do not attend (84, 132).

Little is known about what types of self–help programs smokers view as credible or attractive (121, 122). Initial attempts have been made to translate the existing behavioral technology into self–help and self–study formats (15, 45, 90, 222); but more evaluations of this type of program are needed.

The continuation of various public–service clinics suggests that this mode of service delivery also needs to be upgraded and evaluated more completely. Continuing research is needed to refine behavioral strategies that are applicable to clinic administration. However, the often–cited pattern of high relapse rates (see Figure 2) clearly indicates that more research is needed on strategies to ensure maintenance of the behavior changes. Thus, while procedures and programs to aid smokers to quit smoking need to be refined, effective maintenance procedures need to be developed and integrated into the treatment program.

Several reviewers of the smoking problem (63, 81, 203) have suggested that additional progress both in the refinement of cessation procedures and the development of maintenance strategies requires more basic research on the topography of smoking. Specific smoking topography variables, including where and when cigarettes are smoked and how cigarettes are integrated into specific problem–solving and coping strategies, are probably very important both in guiding initial treatment and defining the types of special behavioral skills and social supports needed to maintain abstinence (37, 60, 62, 78, 81).

Treatment Recommendations

Intensive Treatments

The research literature clearly indicates that certain types of treatments are more encouraging than others. In general, well–conceived behavioral treatments can be effective if offered by a treatment team knowledgeable in the complex problems of smoking cessation (172, 206). However, consideration needs to be given to the manner in which the techniques are presented (139, 206). Most smokers attend treatment programs looking for certain forms of assistance. Treatments should be multifocused and structured so that the individual needs of the smoker can be met. Data from the rapid smoking procedure seem to indicate that even this relatively effective technique can be deemed ineffective if it is offered in a rigid and inflexible manner, without the warm supportive atmosphere which encourages optimism. Thus, reliance upon a single technique will generally fail.

Additional assistance may be needed to help some smokers in dealing with specal problems such as withdrawal syndromes (7, 95) or negative affect (126, 205, 220, 259, 260). Multicomponent treatments can help in personalizing the program to the individual smoker's needs. Additionally, care needs to be taken so that the smoker attains abstinence and a sense of success rapidly enough so that the initial motivations to quit can be capitalized upon (206). Initial successes need to be channeled toward amplification of self–efficacy, and cognitive skills in problem–solving and maintenance planning need to be encouraged early (6, 206). Care should be taken to identify the potential problem areas early so that skills training and rehearsals of coping strategies can be accomplished while the smoker is still in treatment (206). The data on maintenance aids clearly indicate that waiting upon after–treatment termination generally produces little utiliza- tion of additional assistance (13, 218). Contingency contracting seems to be one specific technique which can be effectively utilized to aid the smoker through the initial period of nonsmoking.

Finally, more consideration needs to be given to training the smoker both in the immediate negative physiological aspects of smoking (carbon–monoxide levels, decreased resistance to lung infections, decreased exercise tolerance) and the physiology of withdrawal from smoking (rapid lung clearance of sputum, decreased heart rate, weight gains, readjustments in catecholamine stimulation) (91, 289). Some data suggest that smokers are more receptive to information on the negative effects of smoking, especially those that they can escape, during the period of initial cessation (218, 220). Thus, smokers need specific information about the realistic problems of cessation as well as the immediate benefits of quitting.

Mediated Treatments

The survey data clearly indicate that smokers are almost uniformly aware of the fact that smoking is harmful to their health (84, 283, 289); however, smokers generally are not aware of how various immediate and common aspects of smoking (e.g., chronic cough) are related to these long–term effects. Additionally, many smokers are not clear how smoking effects the cardiovascular system. Moreover, health consequences are often only one of the major motivations that finally persuade the smoker to consider cessation (206). Other socially relevant aspects of smoking, such as self–image and self–concept (e.g., view of self as hooked on a drug and out of control), can also be very important in making smoking sufficiently negative so that the constant reinforcements of the habit are countered (206). Hence, the initial motivation–enhancing messages need to be diverse enough so that most smokers will appraise their smoking behavior as less attractive and more expendable (5, 156).

Once this change is encouraged, specific skills need to be presented to operationalize the initial behavioral intentions (5, 175). Several programs have successfully translated multicomponent behavioral programs into mediated and printed formats (45, 90, 173, 222). The specifics of procedures recommended under intensive interventions also apply here; namely, presenting multicomponent treatments in a manner such that individual needs can be fulfilled as well as special needs of some participants for assistance with difficult problems. The maintenance of positive self–appraisals during cessation and the development of negative images of smoking supportive of continued nonsmoking are also important (6). Finally, a problem–solving model of dealing with potentially difficult situations during maintenance needs to be demonstrated as a part of treatment. Recent ex–smokers need special assistance in developing the cognitive and social supports needed to maintain the fledgling nonsmoking alternative behaviors until they are integrated into the ex–smokers' life style. Hence, while mediated treatments tend to be brief and time limited, the format needs to be such that the treatment effects persist well beyond the formal presentations.

Table 3. Cumulative Quit Rates by Age and
Sex in 1964, 1966, 1970, & 1975[a]

	MALES				FEMALES			
AGES	1964	·1966	1970	1975	1964	1966	1970	1975
21–24	12%	10%	29%	28%	15%	14%	29%	23%
25–34	23%	25%	37%	34%	19%	21%	32%	32%
35–44	28%	27%	39%	35%	19%	21%	29%	33%
45–54	32%	33%	44%	47%	16%	19%	30%	32%
55–64	33%	39%	53%	54%	25%	34%	40%	37%
65+	47%	51%	66%	60%	30%	41%	44%	51%
Total	30%	31%	44%	43%	19%	22%	33%	33%

Sources: USDHEW, PHS, CDC, NCSH. *Use of Tobacco: Practices, Attitudes, Knowledge, and Beliefs, Fall 1964 and Spring* 1966 (227); *Adult Use of Tobacco, 1970* (282); and *Adult Use of Tobacco, 1975* (283).

[a]QUIT RATES are computed by dividing the number of former smokers by the number of ever smokers in each cohort (see original references for definitions of categories). Due to the higher death rates among smokers, this method may slightly underestimate the actual quit rates in older age cohorts.

CONCLUSIONS

Dramatic changes have been occurring in smoking behavior, especially among middle-aged males (see Table 3); however, a very significant problem remains. Most smokers want to quit, but they are generally unsuccessful in their initial self-help attempts. Too often smoking persists until the symptoms of chronic lung or cardiovascular diseases become obvious enough to demand change. However,.when the smoker turns to the medical and behavioral scientists for assistance, interventions of proven efficacy are not available.

The technology of smoking cessation is still in its infancy. Models to guide the development of more effective treatments are still lacking, since our understanding of the social, behavioral, and pharmacological aspects of smoking is still very imperfect. Therefore, basic research is needed to clarify this problem area and to guide more effective treatment. The multidisciplinary areas of behavioral medicine would seem to be well suited to such continuing research and refinement of cessation techniques. The complex nature of the smoking problem requires that a variety of disciplines bring to bear their expertise so that the problem can be successfully addressed.

Moreover, the continuing problem with adolescent onset of smoking indicates that more effort needs to be focused on the development of multidisciplinary programs that can counter the persuasive forces which continue to encourage smoking experimentation. More research is needed both on the physiology of early smoking and on the immediate effects that can be demonstrated to children. Such medical and scientific information can then be translated into persuasive behavioral programs to combat the atmosphere on smoking onset.

Hence, the smoking problem continues to offer a unique challenge to the varied disciplines of behavioral medicine. It is an aspect of personal life style with many sociological and behavioral facets which produces a wide array of physical and medical complications. Thus, the solutions to this challenge will require continued integration across disciplines.

ACKNOWLEDGMENTS

Preparation of this chapter was supported in part by NHLBI Training Grant Number 5–T32–H607036–02 and NHLBI Grant Number HL21287–01.

REFERENCES

1. Abelson, P. Cost–effective health care: Editorial. *Science* 192:862, 1976.
2. Allegrante, J.P., O'Rourke, T.W., and Tuncalp, S. A multivariate analysis of selected psychosocial variables on the development of subsequent youth smoking behavior. *J. Drug Ed.* 7:237–248, 1978.
3. American Cancer Society. *A Study of Public School Teachers' Cigarette Smoking Attitudes and Habits and Their Role in Smoking Education.* New York: American Cancer Society, 1976.
4. Bandura, A. *Principles of Behavior Modification.* new York: Holt, Rinehart and Winston, 1969.
5. Bandura, A. *Social Learning Theory.* Englewood Cliffs, N.J.: Prentice–Hall, 1977.
6. Bandura, A. Self–efficacy: Toward a unifying theory of behavioral change. *Psychol. Bull.* 84:191–215, 1977.
7. Barefoot, J.C., and Girodo, M. The misattribution of smoking cessation symptoms. *Can. J. Behav. Sci.* 4:359–363, 1972.
8. Barkley, R.A., Hastings, J.E., and Jackson, T.L. The effects of rapid smoking and hypnosis in the treatment of smoking behavior. *Int. J. Cl. Exp. Hyp.* 25:7–17, 1977.
9. Barylko–Pikielna, N., and Pangborn, R.M. Effect of cigarette smoking on urinary and salivary thiocyanates. *Arch. Environ. Hlth.* 17:739–745, 1968.
10. Bernstein, D.A. Modification of smoking behavior: An evaluative review. *Psych. Bull.* 71:418–440, 1969.
11. Bernstein, D.A., and McAlister, A. The modification of smoking behavior: Progress and problems. *Addic. Behav.* 1:89–102, 1976.
12. Best, J.A. Final report: *Effectiveness of self–help mass media clinics for smoking cessation.* Ottawa, Canada: Department of National Health and Welfare, 1978.
13. Best, J.A. and Bloch, M. On improving compliance: Cigarette smoking, in R.B. Haynes and D.L. Sackett (eds.), *Compliance.* Baltimore: Johns Hopkins University Press, 1979.
14. Best, J.A., and Hakstian, A.R. A situation–specific model for smoking behavior. *Addict. Behav.* 3:79–92, 1978.

15. Best, J.A., Owen, L.E., and Trentadue, L. Comparison of satiation and rapid smoking in self-managed smoking cessation. *Addic. Behav.* 3:71-78, 1978.

16. Bewley, B.R., Bland, J.M., and Harris, R. Factors associated with the starting of cigarette smoking by primary school children. *Br. J. Prev. Soc. Med.* 28:37-44, 1974.

17. Bland, J.M., Bewley, B.R., and Day, I. Primary schoolboys: Image of self and smoker. *Br. J. Prev. Soc. Med.* 29:262-266, 1975.

18. Boxer, G.E., and Rickards, J.C. Studies on the metabolism of the carbon of cyanide and thiocyanate. *Arch. Biochem.* 39:7-26, 1952.

19. Bradshaw, P.W. The problem of cigarette smoking and its control. *Int. J. Addict.* 8:353-371, 1973.

20. Brantmark, B., Ohlin, P., and Westling, H. Nicotine-containing chewing gum as an anti-smoking aid. *Psychopharm.* 31:191-200, 1973.

21. Brengelmann, J.C., and Sedlmayr, E. *Experimente sur Behandlung des Rauchens.* Koln: Bundeszentrale fur gesundheitliche aufklarung, 1976.

22. Brengelmann, J.C., and Dedlmayr, E. Experiments in the reduction of smoking behavior, in J. Steinfeld et al. (eds.), *Health Consequences, Education, Cessation Activities, and Governmental Action,* Volume II. Proceedings of the Third World Conference on Smoking and Health, New York, June 2-5, 1975. DHEW Publication No. (NIH) 77-1413, 1977.

23. British Medical Journal. Do people smoke for nicotine? *Br. Med. J.* 2:1041-1042, 1977.

24. Brockway, B.S. Chemical validation of self-reported smoking rates. *Behav. Ther.,* 9:685-686, 1978.

25. Brockway, B.S., Kleinmann, G., Edleson, J., and Gruenewald, K. Nonaversive procedures and their effect on cigarette smoking. *Addic. Behav.* 2:121-128, 1977.

26. Bross, I.D.J. Less harmful way of smoking, in E.L. Wynder et al. (eds.), *Modifying the Risk for the Smoker,* Volume I. Proceedings of the Third World Conference on Smoking and Health, New York, June 2-5, 1975. DHEW Publication No. (NIH) 76-1221, 1976.

27. Burns, B.H. Chronic chest disease, personality, and success in stopping cigarette moking. *Br. J. Prev. Soc. Med.* 23:23-27, 1969.

28. Burt, A., Thornley, P., Illingworth, D., White, P., Shaw, T.R.D., and Turner, R. Stopping smoking after myocardial infarction. *Lancet* 1:304-306, 1974.

29. Butts, W.C., Kuehneman, M., and Widdowson, G.M. Automated method for determining serum thiocyanate to distinguish smokers from nonsmokers. *Clin. Chem.* 20:1344-1348, 1974.

30. Bynner, J.M. *The Young Smoker.* London, H.M.S.O.: Government Social Survey, 1969.

31. Bynner, J.M. Behavioral research into children's smoking. *Roy. Soc. Hlth. J.* 90:159-163, 1970.

32. Campbell, D.T., and Stanley, J.C. *Experimental and Quasi-experimental Designs for Research.* Chicago: Rand McNally & Co., 1966.

33. Cautela, J.R. Treatment of smoking by covert sensitization. *Psych. Rep.* 26:415-420, 1970.

34. Chapman, R.F., Smith, J.W., and Layden, T.A. Elimination of cigarette smoking by punishment and self-management training. *Behav. Res. and Ther.* 9:255-264, 1971.

35. Claiborn, W.L., Lewis, P. and Humble, S. Stimulus satiation and smoking: A revisit. *J. Clin. Psychol.* 28:416-419, 1972.

36. Cohen, S.I., Perkins, N.M., Ury, H.K., and Goldsmith, J.R. Carbon monoxide uptake and cigarette smoking. *Arch. Environ. Hlth.* 22:55-60, 1971.

37. Collins, F.L. Jr., and Epstein, L.H. Temporal analysis of cigarette smoking. *Addic. Behav.* 3:93-97, 1978.

38. Conway, J.B. Behavioral self-control of smoking through aversive conditioning and

self–management. *J. Consult. Clin. Psychol.* 45:348–357, 1977.

39. Cronbach, L.J., et al. *Analysis of covariance in nonrandomized experiments: parameters affecting bias.* Stanford Evaluation Consortium, Stanford University, 1978.

40. Croog, S.H., and Richards, N.P. Health beliefs and smoking patterns in heart patients and their wives: A longitudinal study. *Am. J. Publ. Hlth.* 67:921–929, 1977.

41. Dacre, J.C., and Tabershaw, I.R. Thiocyanate in saliva and sputum: Relationship to smoking and industrial exposures. *Arch. Environ. Hlth.* 21:47–49, 1970.

42. Danaher, B.G. Rapid smoking and self–control in the modification of smoking behavior. *J. Consult. Clin. Psychol.* 45:1068–1075, 1977.

43. Danaher, B.G. Research on rapid smoking: Interim summary and recommendations. *Addic. Behav.* 2:151–166, 1977.

44. Danaher, B.G. *Innovative directions for smoking research: Expanding the boundaries of behavioral medicine.* Paper presented at Association for Advancement of Behavioral Medicine, Atlanta, December 1977.

45. Danaher, B.G., and Lichtenstein, E. *Become an Ex–smoker.* Englewood Cliffs, N.J.: Prentice–Hall, 1978.

46. Danaher, B.G., Shisslak, C.M., Thompson, C.B., and Ford, J.D. A smoking cessation program for pregnant women: An exploratory study. *Am. J. Publ. Hlth.* 68:896–898, 1978.

47. Dastur, D.K., Quadros, E.V., Wadia, N.H., Desai, M.M., and Bharucha, E.P. Effect of vegetarianism and smoking on vitamin B_{12}, thiocyanate, and folate levels in the blood of normal subjects. *Br. Med. J.* 3:260–263, 1972.

48. Davison, G.C. and Rosen, R.C. Lobeline and reduction of cigarette smoking. *Psychol. Rep.* 31:443–456, 1972.

49. Dekker, E. Youth culture and influences on the smoking behavior of young people, in J. Steinfeld, et al. (eds.), *Health Consequences, Education, Cessation Activities, and Governmental Action,* Volume II. Proceedings of the Third World Conference on Smoking and Health, New York, June 2-5, 1975. DHEW Publication No. (NIH) 77-1413, 1977.

50. Dalahunt, J., and Curran, J.P. Effectiveness of negative practice and self–control techniques in the reduction of smoking behavior. *J. Consult. Clin. Psychol.* 44:1002–1007, 1976.

51. Delarue, N.C. A study of smoking withdrawal. *Can. J. Publ. Hlth.* 64:S5–S19, 1973.

52. Densen, P.M., Davidow, B., Bass, H.E., and Jones, E.W. A chemical test for smoking exposure. *Arch. Environ. Hlth.* 14:865–874, 1967.

53. Dericco, D.A., Brigham, T.A., and Garlington, W.K. Development and evaluation of treatment paradigms for the suppression of smoking behavior. *J. Appl. Behav. Anal.* 10:173–181, 1977.

54. Dickens, C., and Bryson, R. Psychology in action: The smoking of psychology. *Amer. Psychol.* 33:504–507, 1978.

55. Doll, R. Smoking and disease: Prospects for control. *Roy. Soc. Hlth. J.* 97:167–176, 1977.

56. Downey, A.M., and O'Rourke, T.W. The utilization of attitudes and beliefs as indicators of future smoking behavior. *J. Drug Ed.* 6:283–295, 1976.

57. Dubren, R. Evaluation of a televised stop–smoking clinic. *Publ. Hlth. Rep.* 92:81–84, 1977.

58. Dubren, R. Self–reinforcement by recorded telephone messages to maintain nonsmoking behavior. *J. Consult. Clin. psychol.* 45:358–360, 1977.

59. Dunn, W.L. (ed.). *Smoking Behavior: Motives and Incentives.* Washington, D.C.: Winston & Sons, 1973.

60. Eiser, J.R., and Sutton, S.R. Smoking as a subjectively rational choice. *Addic. Behav.*

2:129-134, 1977.

61. Elliott, C.H. A multiple component treatment approach to smoking behavior. Doctoral dissertation, University of Kansas, 1976. *Dissertation Abs. Int.* 38:893B-894B, 1977.

62. Epstein, L.H., and Collins, F.L. The measurement of situational influences on smoking. *Addic. Behav.* 2:47-53, 1977.

63. Epstein, L.H., and McCoy, J.F. Issues in smoking control. *Addic. Behav.* 1:65-82, 1975.

64. Erikson, E. *Childhood and Society.* New York: Norton, 1950.

65. Evans, R.I. Smoking in children: Developing a social psychological strategy of deterrence. *Prev. Med.* 5:122-127, 1976.

66. Evans, R.I., Hansen, W.B., and Mittelmark, M.B. Increasing the validity of self-reports of smoking behavior in children. *J. Appl. Psychol.* 62:521-523, 1977.

67. Evans, R.I., Henderson, A.H., Hill, P.C., and Raines, B.E. Current behavioral research in control and prevention of smoking. *Atherosclerosis Reviews,* 1979, in press.

68. Evans, R.I., Henderson, A.H., Hill, P.C., and Raines, B.E. Smoking in Children and Adolescents: Psychosocial determinants and prevention strategies. In U.S.D.H.E.W., Smoking and Health: A report of the Surgeon General. Washington, D.C.: U.S.G.P.O., 1979.

69. Evans, R.I., Rozelle, R.M., Mittelmark, M.B., Hansen, W.B., Bane, A.L., and Havis, J. Deterring the onset of smoking in children: Knowledge of immediate physiological effects and coping with peer pressure, media pressure, and parent modeling. *J. Appl. Soc. Psychol.,* 8:126-135, 1978.

70. Eyres, S.J. Report of the 1972 APHA smoking survey. *Amer. J. Publ. Hlth.* 63:846-852, 1973.

71. Farquhar, J.W., Maccoby, N., Wood, P.D., Alexander, J.K., Breitrose, H., Brown, B.W. Jr., Haskell, W.L., McAlister, A.L., Meyer, A.J., Nash, J.D., and Stern, M.P. Community education for cardiovascular health. *Lancet* 1:1192-1195, 1977.

72. Fernoe, O. The development of a chewing gum containing nicotine and some comments on the role played by nicotine in the smoking habit, in J. Steinfeld, et al. (eds.), *Health Consequences, Education, Cessation Activities, and Governmental Action,* Volume II. Proceedings of the Third World Conference on Smoking and Health, New York, June 2-5, 1975. DHEW Publication No. (NIH) 77-1413, 1977.

73. Feyerabend, C.T., Russell, M.A.H. Improved gas-chromatographic method and micro-extraction technique for the measurement of nicotine in biologic fluids. *J. Pharm. Pharmacol.* 31:73-76, 1979.

74. Fisher, L. These students helped design their own smoking education programs. *Amer. Lung Assoc. Bull.* 63(5):2-9, 1977.

75. Flaxman, J. Quitting smoking now or later: Gradual, abrupt, immediate, and delayed quitting. *Behav. Ther.* 9:260-270, 1978.

76. Fox, B.H. Discussant for section on epidemiology, in Jarvik, M.E., et al. (eds.), *Research on Smoking Behavior,* NIDA Monograph 17. Washington, D.C.: U.S.G.P.O., 1977. DHEW Publication No. (ADM) 78-581, 1977.

77. Frederiksen, L.W. Single-case designs in the modification of smoking. *Addic. Behav.* 1:311-319, 1976.

78. Frederiksen, L.W. Temporal distribution of smoking. *Addic. Behav.* 2:178-192, 1977.

79. Frederiksen, L.W., Epstein, L.H., and Kosevsky, B.P. Reliability and controlling effects of three procedures for self-monitoring smoking. *Psychol. Record* 25:255-264, 1975.

80. Frederiksen, L.W., and Martin, J.E. Carbon monoxide and smoking behavior. *Addic. Behav.* 4:21-30, 1979.

81. Frederiksen, L.W., Miller, P.M., and Peterson, G.L. Topographical components of smoking behavior. *Addic. Behav.* 2:55-61, 1977.

82. Frederiksen, L.W., and Peterson, G.L. Controlled smoking: Development and maintenance. *Addic. Behav.* 1:193–196, 1976.
83. Fredrickson, D.T. Cigarette smoking: Questions patients ask doctors. *Chest* 58:147–151, 369–372, 1970.
84. Gallup Opinion Index. *Public puffs on after ten years of warnings.* Gallup Opinion Index (Report No. 108):20–21, June 1974.
85. Gallup Opinion Index. *Smoking in America: Public attitudes and behavior.* Gallup Opinion Index (Report No. 155):1–26, June 1978.
86. Garkinkel, L. Cigarette smoking among physicians and other health professionals, 1959–1972. *CA—Cancer J. Clin.* 26:373–375, 1976.
87. Glad, W.R., Tyre, T.E., and Adesso, V.J. A multidimensional model of cigarette smoking. *Am. J. Clin. Hyp.* 19:82–90, 1976.
88. Gilbert, J.P., Light, R.J., and Mosteller, F. Assessing social innovations, in C.A. Bennet and A.A. Lumsdaine (eds.), *Evaluation and Experiment.* New York: Academic Press, 1975.
89. Glasgow, R.E. Effects of self-control manual, rapid smoking, and amount of therapist contact on smoking reduction. *J. Consult. Clin. Psychol.,* in press.
90. Glasgow, R.E., and Rosen, G.M. Behavioral bibliotherapy: A review of self-help behavior therapy manuals. *Psychol. Bull.* 85:1–23, 1978.
91. Gordon, T., Kannel, W.B., Dawber, T.R., and McGee, D. Changes associated with quitting cigarette smoking: The Framingham Study. *Am. Heart J.* 90:322–328, 1975.
92. Gould, L.C., Berberian, R.M., Kasl, S.V., Thompson, W.D., and Kleber, H.D. Sequential patterns of multiple-drug use among high school students. *Arch. Gen. Psychiatry* 34:216–222, 1977.
93. Graham, S., and Gibson, R.W. Cessation of patterned behavior: Withdrawal from smoking. *Soc. Sci. Med.* 5:319–337, 1971.
94. Gritz, E.R. Smoking: The prevention of onset, in M.E. Jarvik et al. (eds.), *Research on Smoking Behavior,* NIDA Monograph 17. Wasington, D.C.: U.S.G.P.O., 1977. DHEW Publication No. (ADM) 78–581, 1977.
95. Gritz, E.R., and Jarvik, M.E. Pharmacological aids for the cessation of smoking, in J. Steinfeld, et al. (eds.), *Health Consequences, Education, Cessation Activities, and Governmental Action,* Volume II. Proceedings of the Third World Conference on Smoking and Health, New York, June 2–5, 1975. DHEW Publication No. (NIH) 77–1413, 1977.
96. Guilford, J.S. Sex differences between successful and unsuccessful abstainers from smoking, in S.V. Zagona (ed.), *Studies and Issues in Smoking Behavior.* Tucson: University of Arizona Press, 1967.
97. Guilford, J.S. Group treatment versus individual initiative in the cessation of smoking. *J. Appl. Psychol.* 56:162–167, 1972.
98. Hackett, G., and Horan, J.J. Behavioral control of cigarette smoking: A comprehensive program. *J. Drug Ed.* 7:71–79, 1977.
99. Hackett, G., Horan, J.J., Stone, C.I., Linberg, S.E., Nicholas, W.C., and Lukaski, H.C. Further outcomes and tentative predictor variables from an evolving comprehensive program for the behavioral control of smoking. *J. Drug Ed.* 7:225–229, 1977.
100. Haggerty, R.J. Changing lifestyles to improve health. *Prev. Med.* 6:276–289, 1977.
101. Hall, R.G., Sachs, D.P.L., and Hall, S.M. Medical risk and therapeutic effectiveness of rapid smoking. *Behav. Ther.,* 10:249–259, 1979.
102. Hammond, E.C., Garfinkel, L., Seidman, H., and Lew, E.A. "Tar" and nicotine content of cigarette smoke in relation to death rates. *Environ. Hlth.* 12:263–274, 1976.

103. Hanley, J.A., and Robinson, J.C. Cigarette smoking and the young: A national survey. *Can. Med. Assoc. J.* 114:511–517, 1976.
104. Hartup, W., and Louge, R. Peers as models. *School Psychology Digest* 4:11–21, 1975.
105. Hauser, R. Rapid smoking as a technique of behavior modification: Caution in selection of subjects. *J. Consult. Clin. Psychol.* 42:625, 1974.
106. Hay, D.R., and Turbott, S. Changes in smoking habits in men under 65 years after myocardial infarction and coronary insufficiency. *Br. Heart J.* 32:738–740, 1970.
107. Hochbaum, G.M. Psychosocial aspects of smoking with special reference to cessation. *Am. J. Publ. Hlth.* 55:692–697, 1965.
108. Hollander, E.P. *Principles and Methods of Social Psychology,* 3rd ed. New York: Oxford University Press, 1976.
109. Horan, J.J., Hackett, G., Nicholas, W.C., Linberg, S.E., Stone, C.I., and Lukaski, H.C. Rapid smoking: A cautionary note. *J. Consult. Clin. Psychol.* 45:341–343, 1977.
110. Horan, J.J., Linberg, S.E., and Hackett, G. Nicotine poisoning and rapid smoking. *J. Consult. Clin. Psychol.* 45:344–347, 1977.
111. Horn, D. Some factors in smoking and its cessation, in E.F. Borgatta and R.R. Evans (eds.), *Smoking, Health, and Behavior.* Chicago: Aldine, 1968.
112. Horn, D. Man, cigarettes, and the abuse of gratification. *Arch. Environ. Hlth.* 20:88–92, 1970.
113. Horn, D. A model for the study of personal choice health behavior. *Int. J. Hlth. Ed.* 19:89–98, 1976.
114. Horn, D., Courts, F.A., Taylor, R.M., and Solomon, E.S. Cigarette smoking among high school students. *Am. J. Publ. Hlth.* 49:1497–1511, 1959.
115. Horning, E.E., Horning, M.G., Carroll, D.I., Stillwell, R.N., and Dzidic, I. Nicotine in smokers, nonsmokers, and room air. *Life Sciences* 13:1331, 1973.
116. Hunt, W.A. (ed.). *Learning Mechanisms in Smoking.* Chicago: Aldine, 1970.
117. Hunt, W.A. (ed.). New approaches to behavioral research on smoking. *J. Abnorm. Psychol.* 81:107–198, 1973.
118. Hunt, W.A., and Bespalec, D.A. An evaluation of current methods of modifying smoking behavior. *J. Clin. Psychol.* 30:431–438, 1974.
119. Hunt, W.A., Barnett, W., and Branch, L.G. Relapse rates in addiction programs. *J. Clin. Psychol.* 27:455–456, 1971.
120. Hurd, P.D., Johnson, C.A., Pechacek, T., Bast, L.P., Jacobs, D.R., and Luepker, R. Prevention of cigarette smoking in 7th-grade students. *J. Behav. Med.,* in press.
121. Hynd, G.W., Chambers, C., Stratton, T.T., and Moan, W. Credibility of smoking control strategies in non-smokers: Implications for clinicians. *Psychol. Rep.* 41:503–506, 1977.
122. Hynd, G.W., Stratton, T.T., and Severson, H.H. Smoking treatment strategies, expectancy outcomes, credibility in attention–placebo control conditions. *J. Clin. Psychol.* 34:182–186, 1978.
123. Isaac, P.F., and Rand, M.J. Cigarette smoking and plasma levels of nicotine. *Nature* 236:308–310, 1972.
124. Isacsson, S.O., and Janzon, L. Results of a quit–smoking research project in a randomly selected population. *Scand. J. Soc. Med.* 4:25–29, 1976.
125. Jacobs, D., Grimm, R.H. Jr., Mills, D., Olson, M., Robitaille, M., Gorder, D., George, V., and Blackburn, H. *Heart Attack Risk Reduction Trial (HARRT): Behavioral methods for cigarette smoking cessation and serum cholesterol lowering.* Unpublished manuscript, University of Minnesota, 1978.
126. Jacobs, M.A., Spilken, A.Z., Norman, M.M., Wohlberg, G.W., and Knapp, P.H. Interaction of personality and treatment conditions associated with success in a smoking

control program. *Psychosom. Med.* 33:545–556, 1971.

127. Jarvik, M.E. Biological factors underlying the smoking habit, in M.E. Jarvik, et al. (eds.), *Research on Smoking Behavior,* NIDA Monograph 17. Washington, D.C.: U.S.G.P.O., 1977. DHEW Publication No. (ADM) 78–581.

128. Johnson, E., and Donoghue, J.R. Hypnosis and smoking: A review of the literature. *Am. J. Clin. Hyp.* 13:265–272, 1971.

129. Jones, J.S. Cigarette abandonment: Its significance. *Br. J. Dis. Chest* 71:285–288, 1977.

130. Kagan, J., and Coles, R. *Twelve to Sixteen: Early Adolescence.* New York: Norton, 1972.

131. Kanzler, M., Jaffe, J.H., and Zeidenberg, P. Long- and short-term effectiveness of a large-scale proprietary smoking cessation program—A four-year follow-up of Smok-Enders participants. *J. Clin. Psychol.* 32:661–669, 1976.

132. Kanzler, M., Zeidenberg, P., and Jaffe, J.H. Response of medical personnel to an on-site smoking cessation program. *J. Clin. Psychol.* 32:670–674, 1976.

133. Katz, R.C., Heiman, M., and Gordon, S. Effects of two self-management approaches on cigarette smoking. *Addic. Behav.* 2:113–119, 1977.

134. Kenny, D.A. A quasi-experimental approach to assessing treatment effects in the nonequivalent control group design. *Psychol. Bull.* 82:345–362, 1975.

135. Kenny, D.A. *Correlational Inference.* New York: Wiley, 1978.

136. Keutzer, C.S., and Lichtenstein, E. Modification of smoking behavior: A review. *Psychol. Bull.* 70:520–533, 1968.

137. Kiesler, C.A., Collins, B.A., and Miller, N. *Attitude Change: A Critical Analysis of Theoretical Approaches.* New York: Wiley, 1969.

138. Kopel, S.A. The effects of self-control, booster sessions, and cognitive factors on the maintenance of smoking reduction. Doctoral dissertation, University of Oregon, 1974. *Dissertation Abs. Int.* 35:4182B–4183B, 1975.

139. Kopel, S.A., and Arkowitz, H. The role of attribution and self-perception in behavior change: Implications for behavior therapy. *Genetic Psychol. Monog.* 92:175–212, 1975.

140. Koskela, K., Puska, P., and Tuomilehto, J. The North Karelia Project: A first evaluation. *Int. J. Hlth. Ed.* 19:59–66, 1976.

141. Kreitler, S., Shaher, A., and Kreitler, H. Cognitive orientation, type of smokers, and behavior therapy of smoking. *Br. J. Med. Psychol.* 49:167–175, 1976.

142. Kristein, M.M. Economic issues in prevention. *Prev. Med.* 6:252–264, 1977.

143. Lader, M. Nicotine and smoking behavior. *Br. J. Clin. Pharmacol.* 5:289–292, 1978.

144. Lando, H.A. An objective check upon self-reported smoking levels: A preliminary report. *Behav. Ther.* 6:547–549, 1975.

145. Lando, H.A. Aversive conditioning and contingency management in the treatment of smoking. *J. Consult. Clin. Psychol.* 44:312, 1976.

146. Lando, H.A. Successful treatment of smokers with a broad spectrum behavioral approach. *J. Consult. Clin. Psychol.* 45:361–366, 1977.

147. Lando, H.A., and Davison, G.C. Cognitive dissonance as a modifier of chronic smoking behavior: A serendipitous finding. *J. Consult. Clin. Psychol.* 43:750, 1975.

148. Langer, P., and Greer, M.A. *Antithyroid Substances and Naturally Occurring Goitrogens.* New York: S. Karger-Basel, 1977.

149. Langone, J.J., Gjika, H.B., and Van Vunakis, H.: Nicotine and its metabolites, radioimmunoassays for nicotine and cotinine. *Biochemistry* 12:5025–5030, 1973.

150. Langone, J.J., Van Vunakis, H., and Hill, P. Quantitation of cotinine in sera of smokers. *Res. Commun. Chem. Pathol. Pharmacol.* 10:21–28, 1975.

151. Larson, P.S., and Silvette, H. *Tobacco: Experimental and Clinical Studies,* Supplements I, II, III. Baltimore: Williams & Wilkins, 1961, 1968, 1971, 1975.

152. Laughlin, T.J., and Wake, F.R. Socio-psychological aspects of cigarette smoking. *Can. J.*

Publ. Hlth. 61:301-312, 1970.
153. Levenberg, S.B., and Wagner, M.K. Smoking cessation: Long-term irrelevance of mode of treatment. *J. Behav. Ther. Exper. Psychiat.* 7:93-95, 1976.
154. Leventhal, H. Experimental studies of anti-smoking communications, in E.F. Borgatta and R.R. Evans (eds.), *Smoking, Health, and Behavior.* Chicago: Aldine, 1968.
155. Leventhal, H. Fear appeals and persuasion: The differentiation of a motivational construct. *Amer. J. Publ. Hlth* 61:1208-1224, 1971.
156. Leventhal, H. Changing attitudes and habits to reduce risk factors in chronic disease. *Am. J. Cardiol.* 31:571-580, 1973.
157. Levinson, B.L., Shapiro, D., Schwartz, G.E., and Tursky, B. Smoking elimination by gradual reduction. *Behav. Ther.* 2:477-487, 1971.
158. Lewin, K. The field theory approach to adolescence, in J.M. Seidman (ed.), *The Adolescent: A Book of Readings.* New York: Holt, Rinehart and Winston, 1953.
159. Lichtenstein, E. Modification of smoking behavior: Good designs—ineffective treatments. *J. Consult. Clin. Psychol.* 36:163-166, 1971.
160. Lichtenstein, E. Social learning, in M.E. Jarvik, et al. (eds.), *Research on Smoking Behavior,* NIDA Monograph 17. Washington, D.C.: U.S.G.P.O., 1977. DHEW Publication No. (ADM) 78-581.
161. Lichtenstein, E., and Danaher, B.G. Modification of smoking behavior: A critical analysis of theory, research, and practice, in M. Hersen, et al. (eds.), *Progress in Behavior Modification,* vol. 3. New York: Academic Press, 1976.
162. Lichtenstein, E., and Danaher, B.G. What can the physician do to assist the patient to stop smoking, in R.E. Brashear and M.L. Rhodes (eds.), *Chronic Obstructive Lung Disease: Clinical Treatment and Management.* St. Louis: Mosby, 1978.
163. Lichtenstein, E., and Glasgow, R.E. Rapid smoking: Side effects and safeguards. *J. Consult. Clin. Psychol.* 45:815-821, 1977.
164. Lichtenstein, E., Harris, D.E., Birchler, G.R., Wahl, J.M., and Schmahl, D.P. Comparison of rapid smoking, warm, smoky air, and attention placebo in the modification of smoking behavior. *J. Consult. Clin. Psychol.* 40:92-98, 1973.
165. Lichtenstein, E., and Rodrigues, M.P. Long-term effects of rapid smoking treatment for dependent cigarette smokers. *Addic. Behav.* 2:109-112, 1977.
166. Lipowski, Z.J. Psychosomatic medicine in the seventies: An overview. *Am. J. Psychiatry* 134:233-244, 1977.
167. Luepker, R.V., Pechacek, T., Murray, D.M., Johnson, C.A., Hurd, P., and Jacobs, D.R. Saliva thiocyanate: a chemical indicator of cigarette smoking in adolescents. Unpublished manuscript, University of Minnesota, 1979.
168. Maccoby, N., Farguhar, J.W., Wood, P.D., and Alexander, J. Reducing the risk of cardiovascular disease: Effects of a community-based campaign on knowledge and behavior. *J. Comm. Hlth.* 3:100-114, 1977.
169. Maccoby, N., and Roberts, D. Information processing and persuasion, in R. Kline and P. Clarke (eds.), *Sage Communication Research Annuals,* vol. 2. New York: Sage, 1974.
170. Mausner, B., and Platt, E.S. *Smoking: A Behavioral Analysis.* New York: Pergamon Press, 1971.
171. Maliszewski, T.F., and Bass, D.E. "True" and "Apparent" Thiocyanate in body fluids of smokers and nonsmokers. *J. Appl. Physiol.* 8:289-296, 1955.
172. McAlister, A. Helping people quit smoking: Current progress, in A.J. Enelow and J.B. Henderson (eds.), *Applying Behavioral Science to Cardiovascular Risk.* Proceedings of a conference, Seattle, Washington, June 17-19, 1974. New York: American Heart Association, 1975.
173. McAlister, A. Toward the mass communication of behavioral counseling: A preliminary

experimental study of a televised program to assist in smoking cessation. Doctoral dissertation, Stanford University, 1976. *Dissertation Abs. Int.* 37:5330B, 1977.

174. McAlister, A. Tobacco, alcohol, and drug abuse: Onset and prevention, in National Institute of Medicine (ed.), *Surgeon General Report on Prevention.* Washington, D.C.: U.S.G.P.O., in press.

175. McAlister, A., Farguhar, J.W., Thoresen, C.E., and Maccoby, N. Behavioral science applied to cardiovascular health: Progress and research needs in the modification of risk-taking habits in adult populations. *Hlth. Ed. Monog.* 4:45–74, 1976.

176. McAlister, A., Meyer, A.J., and Maccoby, N. Long-term results of education to reduce smoking: Stanford Three Community Study. *Circulation* 54 (Supp..2):226, 1976 (abstract).

177. McAlister, A., Perry, C., and Maccoby, N. Adolescent smoking: Onset and prevention. *Pediatrics,* 63:650–658, 1979.

178. McFall, F.M. Effects of self-monitoring on normal smoking behavior. *J. Consult. Clin. Psychol.* 35:135–142, 1970.

179. McFall, R.M., and Hammen, C.L. Motivation, structure, and self-monitoring: Role of nonspecific factors in smoking reduction. *J. Consult. Clin. Psychol.* 37:80–86, 1971.

180. McFall, R.M. Smoking cessation research. *J. Consult. Clin. Psychol.* 46:703–712, 1978.

181. McGrath, M.J., and Hall, S.M. Self-management treatment of smoking behavior. *Addic. Behav.* 1:287–292, 1976.

182. McGuire, W.J. Persuasion, resistance, and attitude change, in I. de Sola Pool, et al. (eds.), *Handbook of Communication.* Chicago: Rand McNally, 1973.

183. McKennel, A.C. Implications for health of social influences on smoking. *Am. J. Publ. Hlth.* 59:1998–2004, 1969.

184. McRae, C.F., and Nelson, D.M. Youth to youth communication on smoking and health. *J. School Hlth.* 51:445–447, 1971.

185. Meade, T.W., and Wald, N.J. Cigarette smoking patterns during the working day. *Br. J. Prev. Soc. Med.* 31:25–29, 1977.

186. Mettlin, C. Peer and other influences on smoking behavior. *J. School Hlth.* 46:529–536, 1976.

187. Meyer, A.J., McAlister, A., Nash, J., Maccoby, N., and Farquhar, J.W. Maintenance of cardiovascular risk reduction: Results in high risk subjects. *Circulation* 54(Supp. 2):226, 1976 (abstract).

188. Mischel, W. *Introduction to Personality,* 2nd ed. New York: Holt, Rinehart and Winston, 1976.

189. Mischel, W. *Personality and Assessment.* New York: Wiley, 1968.

190. Miller, L.C., Schilling, A.F., Logan, D.L., and Johnson, R.L. Potential hazards of rapid smoking as a technic for the modification of smoking behavior. *New Engl. J. Med.* 297:590–592, 1977.

191. Mittelmark, M.B. *Information on imminent versus long-term health consequences: Impact on children's smoking behavior, intentions, and knowledge.* Doctoral dissertation, University of Houston, 1978.

192. Multiple Risk Factor Intervention Trial Group. The Multiple Risk Factor Intervention Trial (MRFIT): A national study of primary prevention of coronary heart disease. *JAMA* 235:825–828, 1976.

193. Multiple Risk Factor Intervention Trial Group (J. Ockene). Multiple Risk Factor Intervention Trial (MRFIT): Smoking cessation procedures and recidivism patterns for a large cohort, in J.L. Schwartz (eds.), *Progress in Smoking Cessation.* Proceedings of the International Conference on Smoking Cessation, New York, June 21–23, 1978. New York: American Cancer Society, in press.

193a. Murray, D.M. Luepker, R.V., Johnson, C.A., Pechacek, T.F., and Jacobs, D.M. *Prevention of cigarette smoking in teenagers*. Unpublished manuscript, University of Minnesota, 1979.

194. National Interagency Council on Smoking and Health. *Guidelines for research on the effectiveness of smoking cessation programs:* A Committee report. New York: National Interagency Council on Smoking and Health, 1974.

195. Newman, I.M. Peer pressure hypothesis for adolescent cigarette smoking. *School Hlth. Rev.* 1:15–18, 1970.

196. Newman, I.M. Status configurations and cigarette smoking in a junior high school. *J. School Hlth.* 40:23–31, 1970.

197. Norton, G.R., and Barske, B. The role of aversion in the rapid smoking treatment procedure. *Addic. Behav.* 2:21–25, 1977.

198. Ohlin, P., Lundh, B., and Westling, H. Carbon monoxide blood levels and reported cessation of smoking. *Psychopharm.* 49:263–265, 1976.

199. Orne, M.T. Hypnosis in the treatment of smoking, in J. Steinfeld, et al. (eds.), *Health Consequences, Education, Cessation Activities, and Governmental Action*, vol. 2. Proceedings of the Third World Conference on Smoking and Health, New York, June 2–5, 1975. DHEW Publication No. (NIH) 77–1413.

200. Owen, T.B. Tar and nicotine from U.S. cigarettes: Trends over the past twenty years, in E.L. Wynder, et al. (eds.), *Modifying the Risk for the Smoker*, vol. 1. Proceedings of the Third World Conference on Smoking and Health, New York, June 2–5, 1975. DHEW Publication No. (NIH) 76–1221.

201. Palmer, A.B. Some variables contributing to the onset of cigarette smoking among junior high school students. *Soc. Sci. Med.* 4:359–366, 1970.

202. Pechacek, T.F. An evaluation of cessation and maintenance strategies in the modification of smoking behavior. Doctoral dissertation, University of Texas at Austin, 1977. *Dissertations Abs. Int.* 38:2380B, 1977.

203. Pechacek, T.F. Modification of smoking behavior, in U.S.D.H.E.W., *Smoking and Health: A Report of the Surgeon General*. Washington, D.C.: U.S.G.P.O., 1979.

204. Pechacek, T.F. An overview of smoking behavior and its modification, in N. Krasnegor (ed.), *Behavioral Analysis and Treatment of Substance Abuse*. Washington, D.C.: National Institute on Drug Abuse, 1979.

205. Pechacek, T.F. *Anxiety and smoking cessation*. Unpublished manuscript. University of Minnesota, 1979.

206. Pechacek, T.F., and Danaher, B.G. How and why people quit smoking: Cognitive-behavioral implications, in P.C. Kendall, and S.D. Hollon (eds.), *Cognitive–Behavioral Interventions: Theory, Research and Procedures*. New York: Academic Press, 1979.

207. Pechacek, T.F., Luepker, R.V., Jacobs, D.R. Jr., Fraser, G., and Blackburn, H. *Effect of diet and smoking on saliva and serum thiocyanates*. Paper presented at American Heart Association Conference on Cardiovascular Disease Epidemiology, March 1979.

208. Pederson, L.L., Scringeour, W.G., and Lefcoe, N.M. Comparison of hypnosis plus counseling, counseling alone, and hypnosis alone in a community service withdrawal program. *J. Consult. Clin. Psychol.* 43:920, 1975.

209. Pettigrew, A.R., and Fell, G.S. Microdiffusion method for estimation of cyanide in whole blood and its application to the study of conversion of cyanide to thiocyanate. *Clin. Chem.* 19:466–471, 1973.

210. Pettigrew, A.R., and Fell, G.S. Simplified colorimetric determination of thiocyanate in biological fluids and its application to investigation of the toxic amblyopias. *Clin. Chem.* 18:996–1002, 1972.

211. Pincherle, G., and Wright, H.B. Smoking habits of business executives: Doctor

variation in reducing cigarette consumption. *Practitioner* 205:209–212, 1970.

212. Piper, G.W., Jones, J.A., and Matthews, V.L. The Saskatoon smoking project—The model. *Can. J. Publ. Hlth.* 61:503–508, 1970.

213. Piper, G.W., Jones, J.A., and Matthews, V.L. The Saskatoon smoking project—Results of the first year. *Can. J. Publ. Hlth.* 62:432–441, 1971.

214. Piper, G.W., Jones, J.A., and Matthews, V.L. The Saskatoon smoking project—Results of the second year. *Can. J. Publ. Hlth.* 65:127–130, 1974.

215. Pollin, W. Foreword, in M.E. Jarvik, et al. (eds.), *Research on Smoking Behavior*, NIDA Monograph 17. Washington, D.C.: U.S.G.P.O., 1977. DHEW Publication No (ADM) 78–581.

216. Pomerleau, O. You can get patients to change their habits. *Medical Times* 104:149–158, 1976.

217. Pomerleau, O. Why people smoke: Current psychobiological models, in P. Davidson (ed.), *Behavioral Medicine: Changing Health Lifestyles*. New York: Brunner/Mazel, 1979.

218. Pomerleau, O. Strategies for maintenance: The problem of sustaining abstinence from cigarettes, in J.L. Schwartz (ed.), *Progress in Smoking Cessation*. Proceedings of the International Conference on Smoking Cessation, New York, June 21–23, 1978. New York: American Cancer Society, 1979.

219. Pomerleau, O. Behavioral factors in the establishment, maintenance, and cessation of smoking, in U.S.D.H.E.W., *Smoking and Health: A Report of the Surgeon General.* Washington, D.C.: U.S.G.P.O., 1979.

220. Pomerleau, O., Adkins, D.M., and Pertschuk, M. Predictors of outcome and recidivism in smoking cessation treatment. *Addic. Behav.* 3:65–70, 1978.

221. Pomerleau, O. Bass, F., and Crown, V. Role of behavior modification in preventive medicine. *New Engl. J. Med.* 292:1277–1282, 1975.

222. Pomerleau, O., and Pomerleau, C.S. *Break the Smoking Habit.* Champaign, Ill.: Research Press, 1977.

223. Premack, D. Mechanisms of self-control, in W.A. Hunt (eds.), *Learning Mechanisms in Smoking.* Chicago: Aldine, 1970.

224. Puska, P., Koskela, K., Pakarinen, H., Puumalainen, P., Soininen, V́., and Tuomilehto, J. The North Karelia project: A programme for community control of cardiovascular diseases. *Scan. J. Soc. Med.* 4:57–60, 1976.

225. Puska, P. The North Karelia project: An example of health promotion in action, in J.L. Schwartz (ed.), *Progress in Smoking Cessation.* Proceedings of the International Conference on Smoking Cessation, New York, June 21–23, 1978. New York: American Cancer Society, 1979.

226. Pyszka, R.H., Ruggels, W.L., and Janowicz, L.M. *Health Behavior Change: Smoking Cessation.* Menlo Park, Calif.: Stanford Research Institute, 1973.

227. Raw, M. Persuading people to stop smoking. *Behav. Res. and Ther.* 14:97–101, 1976.

228. Rea, J.N., Tyler, P.J., Kasap, H.S., and Beresford, S.A.A. Expired air carbon monoxide, smoking, and other variables: A community study. *Br. J. Prev. Soc. Med.* 27:114–120, 1973.

229. Reeder, L.G. Sociocultural factors in the etiology of smoking behavior: An assessment, in M.E. Jarvik, et al. (eds.), *Research on Smoking Behavior,* NIDA Monograph 17. Washington, D.C.: U.S.G.P.O., 1977. DHEW Publication No. (ADM) 78–581.

230. Reid, D.D., Brett, G.Z., Hamilton, P.J.S., Jarrett, R.J., Keen, H., and Rose, G. Cardiorespiratory disease and diabetes among middle-aged male civil servants. *Lancet* 1:469–473, 1974.

231. Relinger, H., Bornstein, P.H., Bugge, I.D., Carmody, T.P., and Zohn, C.J. Utilization of

adversive smoking in groups: Efficacy of treatment and maintenance procedures. *J. Consult. Clin. Psychol.* 45:245–249, 1977.

232. Resnick, J. The control of smoking behavior by stimulus satiation. *Behav. Res. and Ther.* 6:113–114, 1968.

233. Resnick, J. Effects of stimulus satiation on the overlearned maladaptive response of cigarette smoking. *J. Consult. Clin. Psychol.* 32:501–505, 1968.

234. Ringold, A., Goldsmith, J.R., Helwig, H.L., Finn, R., and Schuette, F. Estimating recent carbon monixide exposures. *Arch. Environ. Hlth.* 5:308–313, 1968.

235. Rogers, R.W. A protection motivation theory of fear appeals and attitude change. *J. Psychol.* 91:93–114, 1975.

236. Rogers, R.W., Deckner, C.W., and Mewborn, C.R. An expectancy–value theory approach to the long–term modification of smoking behavior. *J. Clin. Psychol.* 34:562–566, 1978.

237. Rose, G. Physician counseling and personal intervention, in J. Steinfeld, et al. (eds.), *Health Consequences, Education, Cessation Activities, and Governmental Action,* vol. 2. Proceedings of the Third World Conference on Smoking and Health, New York, June 2–5, 1975. DHEW Publication No. (NIH) 77–1413, 1977.

238. Rosen, G.M., and Lichtenstein, E. An employee incentive program to reduce cigarette smoking. *J. Consult. Clin. Psychol.* 45:957, 1977.

239. Royal College of Physicians. *Smoking or Health: A Report of the Royal College of Physicians.* London: Pitman Medical, 1977.

240. Russell, M.A.H. Cigarette smoking: Natural history of a dependence disorder. *Br. J. Med. Psychol.* 44:1–44, 1971.

241. Russell, M.A.H. The smoking habit and its classification. *Practitioner* 212:791–800, 1974.

242. Russell, M.A.H. Tobacco smoking and nicotine dependence, in R.J. Gibbins, et al. (eds.), *Research Advances in Alcohol and Drug Problems,* vol. 3. New York: Wiley, 1976.

243. Russell, M.A.H., Armstrong, E., and Patel, U.A. Temporal contiguity in electric aversion therapy for cigarette smoking. *Behav. Res. and Ther.* 14:103–123, 1976.

244. Russell, M.A.H., Wilson, C., Patel, U.A., Cole, P.V., and Feyerabend, C. Comparison of effect on tobacco consumption and carbon monoxide absorption of changing to high and low nicotine cigarettes. *Br. Med. J.* 4:512–516, 1973.

245. Russell, M.A.H., Wilson, C., Feyerabend, C., and Cole, P.V. Effect of nicotine chewing gum on smoking behavior and as an aid to cigarette withdrawal. *Br. Med. J.* 2:391–393, 1976.

246. Sachs, D.P.L., Hall, R.G., and Hall, S.M. Effects of rapid smoking: Physiologic evaluation of a smoking–cessation therapy. *Annals Int. Med.* 88:639–641, 1978.

247. Schachter, S. Pharmacological and psychological determinants of smoking. *Annals Int. Med.* 88:104–114, 1978.

248. Schachter, S., Silverstein, B., Kozlowzki, L.T., Perlick, D., Herman, C.P., and Liebling, B. Studies of the interaction of psychological and pharmacological determinants of smoking. *J. Exper. Psychol.* 106:3–40, 1977.

249. Schmahl, D.P., Lichtenstein, E., and Harris, D.E. Successful treatment of habitual smokers with warm, smoky air and rapid smoking. *J. Consult. Clin. Psychol.* 38:105–111, 1972.

250. Schuman, L.M. The benefits of cessation of smoking. *Chest* 59:421–427, 1971.

251. Schneider, F.W., and Vanmastrigt, L.A. Adolescent–preadolescent differences in beliefs and attitudes about cigarette smoking. *J. Psychol.* 87:71–81, 1974.

252. Schwartz, G.E., and Weiss, S.M. What is behavioral medicine? *Psychosom. Med.* 39:377–381, 1977.

253. Schwartz, G.E., and Weiss, S.M. Yale Conference on Behavioral Medicine: A proposed

definition and statement of goals. *J. Behav. Med.* 1:3-12, 1978.

254. Schwartz, J.L. A critical review and evaluation of smoking control methods. *Publ. Hlth. Rep.* 84:483-506, 1969.

255. Schwartz, J.L. Adolescent smoking behavior: Curiosity, conformity and rebellion, in C.E. Bruess, and M.I. Fisher (eds.), *Selected Readings in Health.* New York: Macmillan, 1970.

256. Schwartz, J.L., and Dubitzky, M. Expressed willingness of smokers to try 10 smoking withdrawal methods. *Publ. Hlth. Rep.* 82:855-861, 1967.

257. Schwartz, J.L., and Dubitzky, M. *Psychosocial factors involved in cigarette smoking and cessation.* Final report of the Smoking Control Research Project. Berkeley, Calif.: Institute for Health Research, 1968.

258. Schwartz, J.L., and Dubitzky, M. One-year follow-up results of a smoking cessation program. *Can. J. Publ. Hlth.* 59:161-165, 1968.

259. Schwartz, J.L., and Dubitzky, M. Requisites for success in smoking cessation, in E.F. Borgatta, and R.R. Evans (eds.), *Smoking, Health, and Behavior.* Chicago: Aldine, 1968.

260. Schwartz, J.L., and Dubitzky, M. Changes in anxiety, mood, and self-esteem resulting from an attempt to stop smoking. *Am. J. Psychiatry* 124:138-142, 1968.

261. Schwartz, J.L., and Rider, G. *Smoking Cessation Methods in the United States and Canada: 1969-1976.* Atlanta, Ga.: U.S. Public Health Service, 1979.

262. Sherif, M., and Sherif, C.W. *Reference Groups: Exploration into Conformity and Deviation of Adolescents.* New York: Harper and Row, 1964.

263. Shewchuk, L.A. Special report: Smoking cessation programs of the American Health Foundation. *Prev. Med.* 5:454-474, 1976.

264. Shewchuk, L.A., Dubren, R., Burton, D., Forman, M., Clark, R.R., and Jaffin, A.R. Preliminary observations on an intervention program for heavy smokers. *Int. J. Addic.* 12:323-336, 1977.

265. Sillet, R.W., Wilson, M.B., Malcolm, R.E., and Ball, K.P. Deception among smokers. *Br. Med. J.* 2:1185-1186, 1978.

266. Srole, L., and Fischer, A.K. The social epidemiology of smoking behavior 1953 and 1970: The Midtown Manhattan Study. *Soc. Sci. Med.* 7:341-358, 1973.

267. Stanley, J.C. Designing psychological experiments, in B.B. Wolman (eds.), *Handbook of General Psychology.* Englewood Cliffs, N.J.: Prentice-Hall, 1973.

268. Stewart, R.D. The effect of carbon monoxide on humans. *Ann. Rev. Pharmacol.* 15:409-425, 1975.

269. Suedfeld, P., and Ikard, F.F. Attitude manipulation in restricted environments: IV. Psychologically addicted smokers treated in sensory deprivation. *Br. J. Addic.* 68:170-176, 1973.

270. Suedfeld, P., and Ikard, F.F. Use of sensory deprivation in facilitating the reduction of cigarette smoking. *J. Consult. Clin. Psychol.* 42:888-895, 1974.

271. Suedfeld, P., and Best, J.A. Satiation and sensory deprivation combined in smoking therapy: Some case studies and unexpected side-effects. *Int. J. Addic.* 12:337-359, 1977.

272. Syme, S.L., and Jacobs, M.J. Smoking cessation activities in the Multiple Risk Factor Intervention Trial: A preliminary report, in J. Steinfeld, et al. (eds.), *Health Consequences, Education, Cessation Activities, and Governmental Action,* vol. 2. Proceedings of the Third World Conference on Smoking and Health, New York, June 2-5, 1975. DHEW Publication No. (NIH) 77-1413, 1977.

273. Tamerin, J.S. Recent increase in adolescent cigarette smoking. *Arch. Gen. Psychiatry* 28:116-119, 1973.

274. Thompson, D.S., and Wilson, T.R. Discontinuance of cigarette smoking: "Natural" and with "therapy." *JAMA* 196:1048-1052, 1966.

275. Thompson, E.L. Smoking education programs 1960-1976. *Am. J. Publ. Hlth.* 68:250-

257, 1978.
276. Tomkins, S. A modified model of smoking behaviors, in E.F. Borgatta, and R.R. Evans (eds.), *Smoking, Health, and Behavior*. Chicago: Aldine, 1968.
277. Tori, C.D. A smoking satiation procedure with reduced medical risks. *J. Clin. Psychol.* 34:574–577, 1978.
278. Turner, J.A.M., Sillett, R.W., and Ball, K.P. Some effects of changing to low–tar and low–nicotine cigarettes. *Lancet* 2:737–739, 1974.
279. Turner, J.A.M., Sillett, R.W., and McNicol, M.W. Effect of cigar smoking on carboxyhaemoglobin and plasma nicotine concentrations in primary pipe and cigar smokers and ex–cigarette smokers. *Br. Med. J.* 2:1387–1389, 1977.
280. U.S. Public Health Service. *Smoking and health: Report of the Surgeon General's Advisory Committee*. Washington, D.C.: U.S.G.P.O., 1964. U.S.P.H.S. Publication No. 1103.
281. U.S. Public Health Service. *Use of Tobacco: Practices, attitudes, knowledge, and beliefs—United States, Fall 1964 and Spring 1966*. Washington, D.C.: National Clearinghouse for Smoking and Health, 1969.
282. U.S. Public Health Service. *Adult Use of Tobacco—1970*. Atlanta: National Clearinghouse for Smoking and Health, 1973. DHEW Publication No. (HSM) 73–8727.
283. U.S. Public Health Service. *Adult Use of Tobacco—1975*. Atlanta: National Clearinghouse for Smoking and Health, 1976.
284. U.S. Public Health Service. *Teenage Smoking—National patterns of cigarette smoking, ages 12 through 18, in 1972 and 1974*. Washington, D.C.: U.S.G.P.O., 1976. DHEW Publication No. (NIH) 76–931.
285. U.S. Public Health Service. *The Smoking Digest: Progress report on a nation kicking the habit*. Washington, D.C.: National Cancer Institute, 1977.
286. U.S. Public Health Service. *Cigarette smoking among teenagers and young women*. Washington, D.C.: U.S.G.P.O., 1977. DHEW Publication No. (NIH) 77–1203.
287. U.S. Public Health Service. *Smoking behavior and attitudes: Physicians, dentists, nurses, pharmacists*. Washington, D.C.: Center for Disease Control, 1977.
288. U.S. Public Health Service. *The health consequences of smoking: A reference edition*. Washington, D.C.: Center for Disease Control, 1978. DHEW Publication No. (CDC) 78–8357.
289. U.S. Public Health Service. *Smoking and Health: Report of the Surgeon General*. Washington, D.C.: U.S.G.P.O., 1979. DHEW Publication No. (PHS) 79–50066.
290. Utech, D.A., and Hoving, K.L. Parents and peers as competing influences on the decisions of children of differing ages. *J. Soc. Psychol.* 78:267–274, 1969.
291. Vogt, T.M. Smoking behavioral factors as predictors of risks, in M.E. Jarvik, et al. (eds.), *Research on Smoking Behavior*, NIDA Monograph 17. Washington, D.C.: U.S.G.P.O., 1977. DHEW Publication No. (ADM) 78–581.
292. Vogt, T.M., Selvin, S., Widdowson, G., and Hulley, S.B. Expired carbon monoxide and serum thiocyanate as objective measures of cigarette exposure. *Am. J. Publ. Hlth.* 67:545–549, 1977.
293. Wald, N., Idle, M., and Bailey, A. Carboxyhaemoglobin levels and inhaling habits in cigarette smokers. *Thorax* 33:201–206, 1978.
294. Walker, R.E., Nicolay, R.C., Kluezny, R., and Riedel, R.G. Psychological correlates of smoking. *J. Clin. Psychol.* 25:42–44, 1969.
295. Wallace, N.D., Davis, G.L., Rutledge, R.B., and Kahn, A. Smoking and carboxyhemoglobin in the St. Louis Metropolitan Population. *Arch. Environ. Hlth.* 29:136–142, 1974.
296. Warner, K.E. Possible increases in the underreporting of cigarette consumption. *J. Amer. Stat. Assoc.* 73:314–318, 1978.

297. Waingrow, S., Horn, D., and Ikard, F.F. Dosage patterns of cigarette smoking in American adults. *Am. J. Publ. Hlth.* 58:54–70, 1968.
298. Watson, I.D. Rapid analysis of nicotine and cotinine in the urine of smokers by isocratic high-performance liquid chromatography. *J. Chromatology* 143:203–206, 1977.
299. Weinblatt, E., Shapiro, S., and Frank, C.W. Changes in personal characteristics of men, over five years, following first diagnosis of coronary heart disease. *Am. J. Publ. Hlth.* 61:831–842, 1971.
300. West, D.W., Graham, S., Swanson, M., and Wilkinson, G. Five year follow–up of a smoking withdrawal clinic population. *Am. J. Publ. Hlth.* 67:536–544, 1977.
301. Williams, T.M. *Summary and implications of review of literature relating to adolescent smoking.* Washington, D.C.: Center for Disease Control, 1971.
302. World Health Organization. Working group on methodology of multifactor prevention trials in ischaemic heart disease. *Comm. Hlth.* 5:101–103, 1973.
303. Yankelovich, D. *The New Morality.* New York: McGraw–Hill, 1974.
304. Yates, A.J. *Theory and Practice in Behavior Therapy.* New York: Wiley, 1975.
305. Zeidenberg, P., Jaffe, J.H., Kanzler, M., Levitt, M.D., Langone, J.J., and Van Vunakis, H. Nicotine:Cotinine levels in blood during cessation of smoking. *Comprehensive Psychiatry* 18:93–101, 1977.
306. Zigler, E., and Child, I.L. Socialization, in G. Lindsey and E. Aronson (eds.), *Handbook of Social Psychology,* vol. 3. Reading, Mass.: Addison–Wesley, 1969.

Dentistry: Acquisition of Oral Hygiene Skills

Murray and Epstein point out that dental disease is one of the most prevalent diseases in the United States, and probably in the world. Although many public–health measures have been developed, including water fluoridation, improved diet, and the provision of toothbrushes, toothpaste, and dental floss, these are not used in a way appropriate to maximize dental care. Appropriate oral hygiene skills are easily acquired, and this behavioral model, both for these behaviors and for their effects on dental pathology, is easily assessed. The authors review the assessment literature and the effect of instruction, modeling, and feedback with contingency management on the acquisition and maintenance of oral hygiene skills. They conclude that a program incorporating these factors is effective and that the gains appear to be maintained over time. Although further research should be performed to determine the specific effect of components, it is clear that in this case a behavioral program can make a significant contribution to health care.

CHAPTER 13

Acquisition of Oral Hygiene Skills: An Overview

Jo A. Murray
Leonard H. Epstein

Dental disease is one of the most prevalent diseases in the United States (11, 17). The development of dental disease may be a function of numerous factors, including genetic predisposition; environment—e.g., water fluoridation—and behavior patterns, including poor diet, inadequate toothbrushing and flossing skills. Poor dental habits appear to be a significant factor in the development of dental disease, and their correction may lead to a reduction in the prevalence of dental disease.

This paper is designed to present information on the assessment and modification of two oral hygiene behaviors, toothbrushing and flossing. Representative research on the use of several treatment approaches for modifying brushing and flossing will be presented. An overall review of the social and behavioral aspects in dental disease has recently been presented (12).

ASSESSMENT

Emphasis on the evaluation of procedures for the acquisition of appropriate oral hygiene skills requires easily administered, reliable measurement devices. Several such instruments have been developed. Assessment of dental skills may involve two techniques: Persons interested in assessing dental hygiene may examine the skill itself, such as observing toothbrushing; or they may examine the results of the skill on the actual teeth. The simplest procedures that have been developed measure the amount of plaque left on teeth as a partial assessment of brushing or flossing.

Greene and Vermillion (2) developed the Simplified Oral Hygiene Index, which has two components: The Debris Index and the Calculus Index. Each of these components is based on the quantitative evluation of the amount of debris found on teeth. Six surfaces are examined from four posterior, and two anterior teeth. The selected surfaces are then rated on a scale ranging from zero through three, with a score of zero indicating no debris and a score of three indicating debris covering more than two–thirds of the surface. An oral calculus score, based on the deposit of inorganic salts, is then obtained with the use of an explorer. Again a four–point scale is employed. The indices are calculated by totaling the scores obtained and dividing by the number of surfaces scored. The advantage of these procedures is that they take less than one minute per person; however, they do have some error of underestimation and overestimation.

Another method for evaluating oral hygiene performance was developed by Podshadley and Haley (14), the Patient Hygiene Performance Method. This procedure was developed to obtain a simpler and more sensitive measure than the Oral Hygiene Indices. They use a mouth mirror examination of the buccal surfaces of the maxillary molars, the lingual surfaces of the mandibular molars, and the labial surfaces of the maxillary and mandibular molars after the use of an erythrosin–disclosing wafer. If teeth are missing, alternatives are suggested. Assessment involves the division of each tooth surface to be rated into five sections. Longitudinally, each surface is divided into thirds, and the middle third is divided in half, yielding five sections. Each of the divisions is scored as 1 for the presence of plaque or 70 for the absence of plaque. The debris score is determined by adding the values of the subdivisions. The Patient Hygiene Performance score is calculated by dividing the total sum for six teeth by the number of surfaces examined. The authors noted that the PHP method took approximately half the time of the Greene–Vermillion Index. In addition, examiners considered the technique to be simpler than the Oral Hygiene measures. The PHP has provided consistent results across examiners, with intraexaminer replications of high consistency. An example of the method taken from Martens and Meskin (8) is presented in Figure 1.

TREATMENT

Techniques to teach oral hygiene skills will be presented according to the level of complexity of the intervention. Instructional procedures and modeling procedures will be presented first. Both of these techniques are basically stimulus control manipulations with interventions prior to the response. The use of reinforcement procedures, including feedback and positive reinforcement, is also described.

Ⓐ Five subdivisions of PHP scoring Ⓑ Score of 3
Ⓒ Score of 1 Ⓓ Score of 4
Figure 1. Plaque scoring — the PHP method.

DISTAL   MESIAL

A. Gingival one third of middle area
B. Middle one third of middle area
C. Incisal or occlusal one third of middle area
D. Distal area
E. Mesial area
Figure 2. Plaque scoring — the PHP method, modified.

Name _Example, Imagood_ Index Teeth _3, 6, 12, 19, 22, 28_

III A. Date _11-30-70_

Tooth #	A	B	C	D	E	Total
3	F -	-	-	-	-	5
	L -		-	-	-	3
6	F -	-		-	-	4
	L		-	-	-	2
12	F -	-		-	-	4
	L -		-	-	-	2
19	F -		-	-	-	4
	L -	-	-	-	-	5
22	F -	-		-	-	4
	L -		-	-	-	4
28	F -		-	-	-	3
	L -		-	-	-	3
TOTAL	10	7	2	12	12	43

Remarks: _Initial Examin-_
ation.

III B. Date _11-30-70_

Tooth #	A	B	C	D	E	Total
3	F -	-		-	-	3
	L -		-	-	-	3
6	F			-	-	2
	L		-	-	-	2
12	F -	-		-	-	3
	L		-	-	-	2
19	F -		-	-	-	3
	L -	-		-	-	4
22	F -	-		-	-	3
	L -		-	-	-	4
28	F -		-	-	-	2
	L -		-	-	-	3
TOTAL	8	6	0	12	8	34

Remarks: _Brushed as usual-_
Scored—Toothbrushing
and floss instructions,
Disclosing tablets given.

III C. Date _12-29-70_

Tooth #	A	B	C	D	E	Total
3	F -			-	-	3
	L			-	-	2
6	F			-		1
	L			-		1
12	F					0
	L			-	-	2
19	F					0
	L			-	-	3
22	F			-		1
	L					0
28	F					0
	L					1
TOTAL	2	0	0	8	4	14

Remarks: _Scored before_
operative treatment.
Special instruction for
distal areas and post-
erior teeth.

Fig. 1. Oral hygiene performance evaluation. (Martens and Meskins, 1972. Copyright 1972 by the American Society of Dentistry for Children. Reprinted by permission of the author and publisher).

Instructional Procedures

The effects of attempting to motivate subjects to improve their oral hygiene without direct teaching of skills was presented by Shiller and Dittmer (15). These investigators assessed the effects of a variety of instructional procedures on Greene–Vermillion Index debris scores of 256 subjects. The procedures included a training film on patient responsibility; a training film on oral hygiene; instruction in staining and subsequent removal of stain; a demonstration of brushing techniques; dye demonstrations and technique demonstrations; a lecture on acid theory, a lecture and a film on patient responsibility; and a lecture, a technique demonstration, a dye demonstration, and a movie on patient responsibility. Results indicated no reduction in debris or increases in toothbrushing frequency.

Van Voorde (18) conducted a study to examine a movie versus chairside examination to present preliminary oral hygiene information. One hundred and seventy-five patients participated in one of four groups, including individual chairside instruction and demonstration with study models, followed by reading of the script, viewing the film, no instruction, or a combination of methods in the first group and second group. A mixed multiple-choice/true-false questionnaire was used to assess information acquired. Results indicated that the group given both a demonstration and the film obtained more knowledge than the controls. The absence of measures on actual toothbrushing performance reduces the clinical utility of the study.

Other investigators have assessed the effects of supervised brushing on the acquisition and improvement of oral hygiene. Horowitz, Suomi, Peterson, Vogelsung, and Mathews (4) studied the effect of supervised daily toothbrushing and flossing in school on dental decay and gingival inflammation. Baseline oral examinations were performed on 481 schoolchildren participating in the program by means of an index to evaluate gingivitis, another procedure to quantify cavities, and the PHP index to measure oral hygiene. After baseline examinations, subjects were randomly assigned to either a control or a treatment group. The treatment group participated in ten 30-minute sessions of intensive instruction involving plaque removal. The instructors emphasized the meaning of plaque, how to identify it, and how to remove it with brushing and flossing. Films and demonstration were used as teaching aids; however, one-to-one instruction was the primary medium provided by a dental hygienist. For the rest of the school year, students in the treatment group engaged in supervised daily brushing, 15 minutes per day. Results of the study indicated at first-year follow-up that subjects in supervised daily plaque removal did reduce plaque and gingival inflammation scores in contrast to subjects in the control group, who showed no meaningful change.

The effect of supervised oral hygiene was also studied by Koch and Lindhe (5). Seventy-eight 11- to 12-year-old children were randomly assigned to either an experimental or no-treatment control group. The experimental group was shown a vertical one-way rotating brushing technique with each brushing stroke starting when the nurse indicated. Five strokes were applied to each of 18 regions of the mouth. The study used both a gingival index and the Greene-Vermillion plaque index to assess effects. On the basis of the results, the investigators concluded that thorough daily brushing significantly reduces the severity and prevalence of gingivitis. While no significant reduction in mean PHP score was found, there was a qualitative difference between the experimental group and the control group in measures of plaque.

Modeling

Pinkham and Stacey (13) employed classroom leaders as models to determine if the oral hygiene performance of grammar–school-age classroom leaders, determined by sociometric analysis, would have a significant effect on their classmates' brushing behavior at school. Nine hundered and sixty-five students were assigned to one of two groups: One group included classes in which the sociometrically defined leader was to be the example–setter; and the other group involved using the sociometrically defined nonleader as an example setter. These two groups were further subdivided; in one group example setters were encouraged by their teachers from the first day of the ten–day study. The other group involved a delay until the fourth day for example setting. Standardized scripts were used by the teachers to enlist the aid of example setters. All children were aware that there was a specified period of time in which they could rest, play, or brush their teeth. Example setters were encouraged to brush their teeth during this period of time. Teachers recorded the students who brushed each day, but no attempt at quality or duration measures was made. The findings indicated that most children initiated brushing and maintained this performance throughout the study regardless of the group; thus the choice of model had little effect.

Newcomb (10) examined instruction in oral hygiene with a group of dental students to assess peer effects of oral hygiene. Thirty freshman dental students were assigned to three separate groups. Groups one and two were told that they would be actively involved while the third group was told they would not be participating in the study. Plaque index scores were obtained for groups one and two during the baseline phase. Group one later learned a technique for tooth brushing via one–to–one instruction. Both groups were then evaluated at 7 and 14 days; group one showed a significant improvement in plaque index scores. On day 14, group three subjects were evaluated without notice. At this point, an extra random sample of ten dental students was selected to serve as a control. Several weeks later, groups were examined unexpectedly and the results were presented to the class. When the results were presented, group one's improvement was praised; in addition, members of this group were encouraged to make statements about their improved oral hygiene. The subjects in the other groups who observed these students received no instruction in toothbrushing techniques; however, the technique was mentioned. Findings from the study indicated that the initial group showed improvement and maintenance of their performance; groups two and three, who were exposed to modeling influences, also improved their performance and improvements were maintained. The control group who did not observe the models showed no change in plaque index measures.

Murray and Epstein (9) performed two studies to evaluate the acquisition and durability of toothbrushing skills using a group videotape modeling procedure

Table 1. Toothbrushing Steps

 1. Pick up and hold the toothbrush.
 2. Wet the toothbrush.
 3. Remove the cap from the toothpaste.
 4. Apply the toothpaste to the brush.
 5. Replace the cap on the toothpaste.
 6. Brush the outside surfaces of the teeth.
 7. Brush the biting surfaces of the teeth.
 8. Brush the inside surfaces of the teeth.
 9. Fill the cup with water.
10. Rinse the mouth.
11. Wipe the mouth.
12. Rinse the toothbrush.
13. Rinse the sink.
14. Put the equipment away.
15. Discard the disposables.

Adapted from Horner, R.D., and Kelitz, I., *Journal of Applied Behavior Analysis,* 1975, 8, 301-309.

for the implementation of the Horner and Kelitz (3) toothbrushing package, which had previously been successfully implemented with retarded children on an individual basis. As part of their procedure they have operationally defined the components of toothbrushing. The 15 steps they developed are presented in Table 1.

In the first experiment by Murray and Epstein (9), oral hygiene performance assessed by the PHP method was improved for an experimental group provided with the videotape modeling procedure for a week, as compared to a no-treatment control group. The modeling procedure involved a young adult demonstrating correct toothbrushing using large model teeth and a toothbrush, with time provided after each step for the children to model the component of toothbrushing. Five subjects served in each group. In a second experiment the videotape treatment was then compared to a feedback-reinforcement technique and a no-treatment control group over a one-week baseline, one-week treatment, and six-week follow-up. Ten subjects served in each group. Results presented in Figure 2 suggest that both experimental treatments were superior to the no-treatment control during treatment on the basis of the Patient Hygiene Performance scores, and that the effects of the videotape procedure were more durable than feedback. However, the performance of the videotape group did

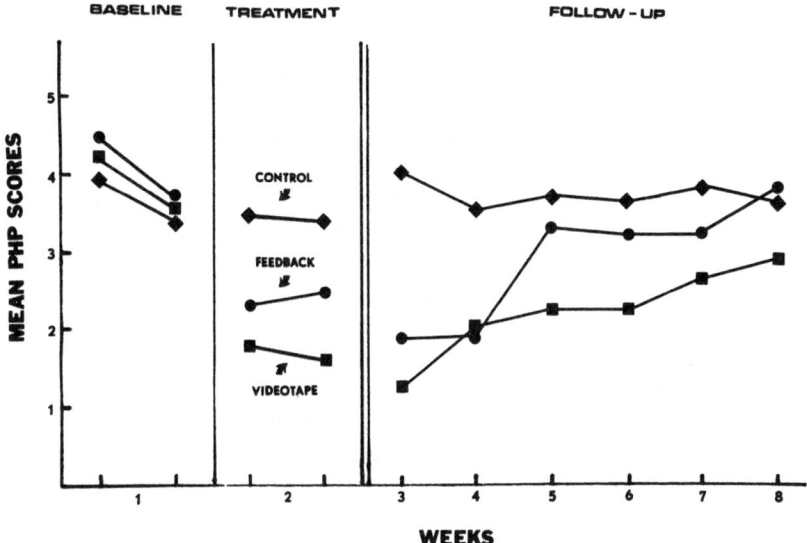

Fig. 2. Mean scores for subjects in the videotape, feedback, and control groups during the baseline, treatment, and follow-up conditions. PHP scores were obtained twice weekly during baseline and treatment, and once per week during follow-up.

decrease by the sixth week of follow-up, suggesting that booster sessions may be needed. One notable aspect of this study was the sizable improvement in oral hygiene produced by a relatively short intervention implemented in a group setting.

Feedback and Contingency Management Studies

Stacey, Abbot, and Jordan (16) assessed improvements in oral hygiene following the administration of information about toothbrushing and social reinforcement for correct brushing. Seventeen residents of a summer camp were recruited as subjects, and the Greene–Vermillion Simplified Debris Index was used to assess the effectiveness of brushing. After an initial assessment of oral hygiene, each child was given a disclosing solution and instructed how to remove the stain from his teeth with a brushing technique. Following this instruction, children were told there would be periodic checks and that they could qualify for prizes of passes for miniature golf each time they achieved the desired level of oral hygiene. Regular periods of nightly supervised brushing were designated for each subject. Expected levels of hygiene were set periodically for each subject based on his dexterity and previous ratings of oral hygiene. Three subsequent ratings of children's teeth were made. These were followed by feedback, reinstruction, and reinforcement when appropriate. Results indicated a slight but increasing improvement in levels of oral hygiene.

Martens, Frazier, Hirt, Meskin, and Proshek (7) attempted to develop brushing performance in second graders, with 169 subjects serving as experimental subjects, and 162 as controls. Controls received no treatment other than the usual instruction in classrooms. The experimental group was exposed to three educational concepts including token rewards as reinforcements for desired behaviors, discovery learning—for example, children could volunteer to participate in projects to gain dental health knowledge—and individual interaction with a hygienist. A baseline screening was done for all children using a variant of the PHP method for assessing oral hygiene. Children were informed of the token rewards they would receive if their hygiene improved, with reinforcement varying according to the level of hygiene attained. Children were examined at four announced times. Results of the study indicate that children in the project group continued to maintain higher levels of oral hygiene than did controls. Though the experimental group performed at a higher level than the control group, the controls also showed a decrease in plaque scores.

Lattal (6) studied contingency management of toothbrushing at a children's summer camp. Eight boys served as subjects with the target behavior being brushing teeth during the daily rest hour immediately following lunch. A baseline frequency of brushing behavior was obtained in morning, afternoon, and evening. Initially students were verbally requested to brush, with low rates observed during baseline and following verbal requests. The contingency management program was instituted and the subjects were initially told that they could go swimming immediately after they had brushed their teeth. After a fairly high rate of toothbrushing during the afternoon was established, an extinction procedure was introduced. The contingent reinforcement produced a high rate of brushing behavior only during the afternoon, and a decline to previous baseline frequencies was observed during extinction. The specificity of control during feedback for only one period of the day indicates that measurement should extend beyond the treatment setting to assess the amount of stimulus control other settings exert over toothbrushing.

An ingenious use of reinforcement contingencies was developed by Clark, Fintz, and Taylor (1). These authors combined numerous instructional aids, including a problem–solving curriculum, a comic book, a teaching film, slides, a work puzzle, and written examinations, with several reinforcement maintenance procedures. During the first week of the program, direct instructions in brushing were given one hour per day in the classroom. During the second week, prompting the technique was performed for ten minutes to half an hour. For the rest of the school year a group motivational procedure was used. Students were paired for hygiene assessment to facilitate peer approval, and the student in the class who had the best plaque record each month became the recorder of a progress chart for each student in the class. In addition, students were prompted to encourage other family members to practice good oral hygiene, and various media presentations on radio and TV were used to encourage family support for good oral hygiene. Control children were given a lecture on the principles of dental health education; however, no information to assist in altering behavior patterns was provided. Results indicated that the 112 children in the experimental group significantly reduced their incidence of dental caries over the 19–month measurement period when compared to the 145 children in the control group. The authors attribute these results to the instructional as well as the motivational variables operating in the experimental group, which could not be separated in this study.

SUMMARY

An overview of the research on the use of behavioral procedures in improving oral hygiene was presented. Oral hygiene is a particularly good target for behavioral procedures because of the obvious implications of toothbrushing and flowing behaviors on oral hygiene. In addition, oral hygiene performance is easily measured. The initial results of training suggest that modeling is an easily implemented technique for improving oral hygiene behaviors in young children. The relatively long–term results presented by Clark et al. (1) show that the gains in hygiene may be maintained. Further research should be performed to determine the specific components that are important to maintenance.

REFERENCES

1. Clark, C.A., Fintz, J.B., and Taylor, R. Effects of the control of plaque on the progression of dental caries: Results after 19 months. *J. Dent. Res.* 53:1468–1473, 1974.
2. Greene, J.C., and Vermillion, J.R. The simplified oral hygiene index. *J. Am. Dent. Assoc.* 68:7–14, 1964.
3. Horner, O.R., and Kelitz, I. Training mentally retarded adolescents to brush their teeth. *J. Appl. Behav. Anal.* 8:301–309, 1975.
4. Horowitz, A.M., Suomi, J.D., Peterson, J.K., Vogelsung, R.H., and Mathews, B.L. Effects of supervised daily dental plaque removal by children: First year results. *J. Public Health Dent.* 36:193–200, 1976.
5. Koch, G. and Lindhe, J. The effect of supervised oral hygiene on the gingiva of children. *Odont. Rev.* 16:327–330, 1965.
6. Lattal, K.A. Contingency management of toothbrushing behavior in a summer camp for children. *J. Appl. Behav. Anal.* 2:195–198, 1969.
7. Martens, L.V., Frazier, P.J., Hirt, K.J., Meskin, L.A., and Proshek, J. Developing

brushing performance in second graders through behavior modification. *Health Serv. Rep.* 88:818–823, 1973.

8. Martens, L.V., and Meskin, L.H. An innovative technique for assessing oral hygiene. *J. Dent. Child.* 39:12–19, 1972.

9. Murray, J.A., and Epstein, L.H. *Videotape modeling in the improvement of oral hygiene skills.* Unpublished manuscript, Auburn University, 1977.

10. Newcomb, G.M. Instruction in oral hygiene for a group of dental students: Its effects on their peers. *J. Public Health Dent.* 34:113–116, 1974.

11. Newman, J.F., and Anderson, O.W. *Patterns of dental service utilization in the U.S.: A nationwide social survey.* Chicago Center for Health Administration Studies, University of Chicago Research Series, 1972.

12. Nikias, M.K. Prevention in oral health problems: Social–behavioral aspects. *Prev. Med.* 5:149–164, 1976.

13. Pinkham, J.R., and Stacey, D.C. Using classroom leaders as models for teaching toothbrushing. *J. Public Health Dent.* 35:91–94, 1975.

14. Podshadley, A.G., and Haley, J.V. A method for evaluating oral hygiene performance. *Public health Rep.* 83:259–267, 1968.

15. Shiller, W.R., and Dittmer, J.C. An evaluation of some current oral hygiene motivation methods. *J. Periodont. Res.* 39:83–93, 1968.

16. Stacey, D.C., Abbot, D.M., and Jordan, R.D. Improvement in oral hygiene as a function of applied principles of behavioral modification. *J. Public Health Dent.* 32:234–242, 1972.

17. U.S. Public Health Service, National Center for Health Statistics. *Dental visits, volume, and interval since last visit.* U.S. Government Printing Office, HEW# (HSM) 72:1066–1081, 1972.

18. Van Voorde, H.E. A movie vs. chairside instruction to present preliminary oral hygiene information. *J. Periodont.* 43:277–280, 1972.

Behavioral Medicine
In the Community

The future of medicine lies in preventing illness, not merely treating it. Unfortunately, the medical-care system has not demonstrated great interest in preventing illness (beyond immunization)—especially in adults—and the system has been even less interested when life-style changes are necessary to reduce or prevent risk from a particular illness.

The Stanford Three Community Study, which forms the basis of this next chapter, demonstrated that life-style can be altered, even on a community-wide basis, and that these changes can translate into risk reduction. This study is a landmark for at least two reasons: (1) health-care education, via media was demonstrated to change knowledge, self-report of behavior and physiology, and associated risk in large populations; and (2) these changes increased with further media exposure. The study was also significant for determining whether intensive instruction in risk reduction, via face-to-face contact for a cohort of individuals with high risk to develop cardiovascular illness, had added advantage over media alone. In the first year, the intensive-instruction group did better than any other—changes maintained to the next year—but did not do significantly better than the media groups, who had continued to improve. As the authors note, "In order to achieve maximum risk reduction, future interventions should use both media methods as well as group process, face-to-face communication, and the networks of interpersonal influence within communities...." The most cost-effective method of achieving these results is unknown, but the Stanford Heart Disease Prevention Program is now studying the effects of similar interventions in even larger communities.

The Comprehensive Handbook of Behavioral Medicine, Volume 3

CHAPTER 14

Applications Of Behavioral Medicine To Disease Prevention In A Total Community Setting: A Review Of The Three Community Study

Joyce D. Nash
John W. Farquhar

It is generally recognized that the current medical care system is based on a medical model that centers on the provision of crisis or illness–oriented treatments by physicians and other health professionals in a medical facility. Little emphasis has been given to the promotion of "wellness" within this traditional medical model. However, primary prevention of chronic disease may very well be an idea whose time has finally come. The escalating costs of health care in the United States during the 1965–75 decade should logically bring national health policy to a turning point. In these ten years, the annual expenditures on national health increased more than 300%, to $118.5 billion (5). Concurrent with this dramatic rise in costs is evidence of a renewed prominence in national health policy for the concepts of disease prevention and health maintenance. In 1975 the Public Health Service (PHS) announced an intention to promote and support an attack on the underlying causes of disease and disability (6). In the "Forward Plan for Health," 1977–81, prevention becomes a prominent feature (6):

> In recent years, it has become clear that only by preventing disease from occurring, rather than treating it later, can we hope to achieve any major improvement in the nation's health. Aside from the possibility of some major research breakthrough, only marginal improvement in longevity, for exampl, can be expected from further expansion of our medical care system (p. 15).

THE CASE OF CARDIOVASCULAR DISEASE

One of the greatest contributors to the spiraling costs of health care is cardiovascular disease, principally fatal and nonfatal episodes of coronary heart disease and stroke. In view of the exceedingly high costs to society of the epidemic of cardiovascular disease (21), it would seem to be a prime target for prevention on a widespread basis. By 1965, it was well established that the United States had one of the highest rates of heart disease in the world; in fact, second only to Finland (23). Fortunately, recent trends indicate that the peak for coronary heart disease was reached in the mid–sixties, and a decline in coronary heart disease has occurred in the past decade, coincident with a similar decrease in animal–fat intake and smoking rates in adults.

As is the case with many chronic illnesses occurring in modern industrialized societies, a number of complex environmental and behavioral factors are implicated in the etiology of cardiovascular disease. Epidemiological studies clearly establish cigarette smoking, high levels of plasma cholesterol, and high blood pressure as principal risk factors for premature cardiovascular disease (1, 3, 18). These factors must be addressed prior to the onset of symptoms if morbidity and mortality are to be greatly reduced. Although there is a genetic component to high plasma cholesterol levels and high blood pressure, both are also strongly influenced by relative body weight (3) and by other variables affected by the environment. It is also clear that these risk factors confer risk throughout a broad range which includes the so–called "normal range" for society, and that behavioral and environmental factors of diet (3), physical activity (8), and maladaptive response to perceived stress, or harmful emotional life styles, are important in determining the level of these risk factors (11, 12).

ORIGINS OF THE THREE COMMUNITY STUDY

Although not all the issues on the status of individual risk factors were as clear in the late sixties as they are today, nor was prevention held in very high esteem, even then it seemed prudent to begin to develop efficient methods for teaching large groups of people about cardiovascular risk factors and how they might be reduced. From this perspective, the Stanford Three Community Study was conceived.

The research of the Stanford Heart Disease Prevention Program stems from the convictions of a group at Stanford University in the late sixties that this problem should be approached through a sustained communitywide educational program designed to gradually change knowledge and attitudes and assist individuals to modify the underlying behaviors associated with an increased risk of cardiovascular disease. Rather than focus on the disease itself, it seemed important to educate the public on ways in which aspects of human behavior are instrumental in influencing overall health and to provide individuals with the necessary skills to successfully make behavioral changes in the recommended directions. These behaviors are often long-engrained, resistant to change, and, if changed, easily reinstated.

However, the Stanford group was convinced then that we as a society were in an era of public health during which behavioral science must become aligned with the traditional biomedical sciences in a multidisciplinary assault to alleviate the human suffering associated with the chronic diseases so prevalent in the U.S. today. Within that context, the Stanford group designed a communitywide public health education study which included elements from both the biomedical and social science traditions. The result was the Three Community Study, in which educational programs were introduced to communities at large to modify knowledge, attitudes, and behaviors associated with cardiovascular disease and to attempt to demonstrate the feasibility of reducing cardiovascular risk for adults in a community setting.

The strategy was to clearly identify the life-style antecedents of cardiovascular disease that were relevant to adults of varying ethnic and occupational groups. Appropriate subpopulations then became the "audiences" to be informed and assist in undertaking long-term modification of their risk-taking behavior. To do this for large groups of individuals, such as total communities, the costs of the risk reduction educational efforts had to be reduced to a practical level.

RATIONALE FOR EDUCATIONAL STRATEGY

If health education to reduce cardiovascular risk is to be widely applied over long periods of time and if it is to be effective in a public health sense, it must reach a satisfactory proportion of the total population in need. This total population in need is depicted in Figure 1 below as the largest circle, 4. The smallest circle, 1, indicates the very small proportion of the total population that would be touched were efforts directed at individuals recruited as volunteers into the existing medical care system. The next larger circle, 2, indicates the estimated scope that could be expected through the use of mass media plus face-to-face contact programs (similar to that actually used in the Stanford Three Community Study). The third larger circle, 3, indicates an even more desirable scope for a community program focused at actively involving a broad application of information and skills training. Even this broad application of a mass media-based information and skills training progrm would fall short of the ideal program which might result if the cooperation of industry and government were added. Important theoretical questions remain before the method is clearly defined on how to achieve this ideal method that would attain the ultimate goal

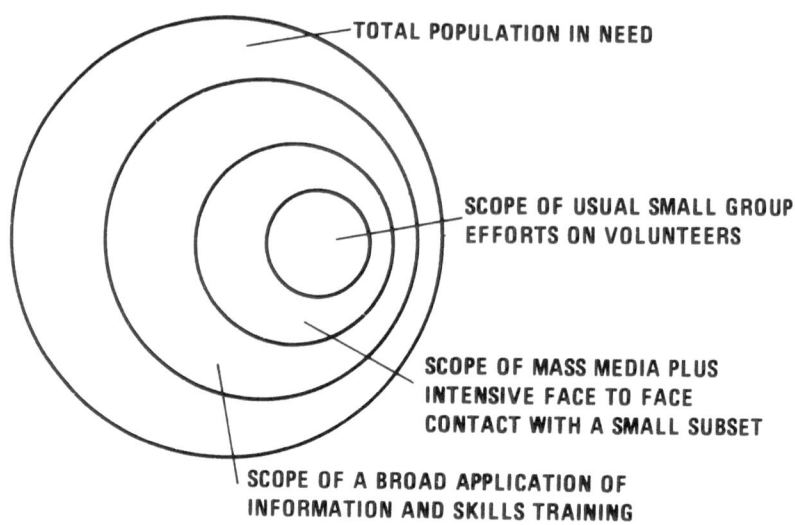

Fig. 1. Scope of Potential Intervention Strategies.

of addressing the entire population in need. However, the Stanford Three Community Study was designed to address many of the necessary precursor stages and to furnish a breadth of involvement of the total population in need sufficient to influence cardiovascular risk within the total community.

Our approach was to convey the risk reduction program, at least in part, through the available channels of the mass media. Mediated risk reduction efforts were one component of an overall educational strategy which also attempted to convey the risk reduction messages through the interpersonal channels of communication, information, and influence that normally form a part of each person's life. The most potentially cost–effective approach, we believed, would be a blending of the mass media, face–to–face instruction, and social or interpersonal networks to provide instruction that is widespread but audience–specific, cost–effective, and successful in assisting individuals to learn new skills to counter disease– or disorder–producing behavior. Understanding the relationship between mediated and face–to–face instruction and its power to evoke diffusion and support through social networks was seen as a central question in the merging understanding of communitywide disease prevention.

COULD IT BE DONE?

The Stanford group was aware that most previous attempts at health education had not been successful in achieving substantial and lasting change in risk behavior (13). In reviewing the literature on the effectiveness of such programs, there was much conflicting evidence regarding the extent to which mass media can bring about important behavior change.

For example, in 1960 Griffiths and Knutson (9) investigated the role of mass media in public health. They concluded that mass media provided at best an information and support function and can achieve but minor shifts in behavior—a view which continues to persist in many quarters still (10). In contrast to the evidence for the effectiveness of print media, Swinehart (20) concluded that television does reach all levels of the population, including the people who need public health information most. More recent evidence suggested that television is a potent source of health information (15, 16). The evidence suggested that simple overt behavior changes, such as purchasing toothpaste or showing up for an immunization shot, stood a good chance of being triggered by mass media, but complex behavior changes such as those required for risk–factor reduction had not yet been demonstrated.

Yet the developing literature on how people learn and change behavior suggested that, with the appropriate use of the tools of mass media and the interpersonal networks that form among people, a health education program did seem to be a reasonable approach. Recent advances in learning theory and in the development of methods of teaching self–directed behavior change (2) led the Stanford group to conclude that previous effectiveness of mass media might be increased if social learning theory and self–help behavior change methods were used in the formation and implementation of a health education campaign. Research evidence was mounting to suggest that self–management behavior therapy was useful in problems such as smoking cessation and weight management. It was the opinion of the Stanford group that complex behavior changes could be engendered if the media were used first to sensitize, increase information levels, and influence opinions, and then were used to support and elaborate self–management skills training.

But even if the methods for a successful health education campaign were available, would the political and economic forces of the social system involved permit such a campaign to be effective? The Stanford group was careful to note the presence of egg and dairy producers in the communities to be studied, though no contacts were made with these groups. Since approximately 15% of the adults in these communities were Spanish–speaking, attempts were made to contact their representatives and opinion leaders to at least ensure their passive support. The Stanford group contacted key political figures, including the mayors of the communities in which it was anticipated the intervention would take place. Formal presentations were made to the county medical societies and to the staffs and task groups of local hospitals. Individual physicians were contacted as well, as were managers and staff of the media serving these communities. It appeared that the political and economic forces in the community were open to the idea of having a coronary heart disease prevention education program undertaken in their communities.

With this, the Stanford group turned to the question of the educational program's content. A sufficient consensus existed in support of the argument that the primary risk factors associated with increased risk of premature heart disease and stroke were cigarette smoking, high blood pressure, and high serum–lipid concentrations. Evidence also existed suggesting that these risk factors could be reduced through changes in life style (14). Consequently, it was decided that the focus of the prevention efforts would be to help people change the quality of their diet to reduce calories, salt, sugar, and saturated fats and cholesterol, to quit smoking, and to increase their levels of physical activity.

THE THREE COMMUNITY STUDY

Although it was established that mass media, together with interpersonal contact to deliver self–management skills, would be used to intervene on specific risk behaviors, a number of problems associated with community selection and design remained to be solved.

Community Selection and Design

The intention of the study was to compare two educational approaches—one community receiving mass media only and a second community receiving mass media plus face–to–face intensive instruction in self–directed change methods—to a nontreated community condition. Because of the nature of a mass–media campaign, it was not possible to assign individuals randomly to conditions. Rather, each community was assigned to an educational condition. Funding and staff limitations allowed the selection and use of only three communities. The alternative of treating a larger number of populations as single units was not feasible, and a quasi–experimental research design had to be adopted (4).

Three semirural communities in California of about 15,000 persons each were selected on the basis of their comparability for media channels and demographic makeup. Watsonville (W) and Gilroy (G) are communities having common television and radio reception but each having a hometown newspaper. They are geographically separated by a range of small mountains. The third community, Tracy (T), was selected as a no–treatment control community because it is geographically remote from the other two and isolated from the media systems serving the other two communities. Gilroy was chosen as the media–only treatment community and Watsonville as the media plus face–to–face intensive instruction community.

A sytematic probability sample of men and women ages 35–59 was drawn from all three communities. To make this sampling, the Polk Directory, in which addresses are organized by street name, was used to generate a random sample for each community. Addresses for business or institutions were first screened out, as were addresses which were outside the city limits. Households were the unit of selection, and anyone residing there became eligible. For multiple-dwelling units, all individuals living there were eligible as well. Using the age distribution for each community as determined from the 1970 census and the known number of residential addresses in each community, the ratio of age–eligibles per household was determined in order to generate a sample containing the desired number of individuals.

Measurement

To assess the effects of the educational program, a baseline survey was conducted in each of the communities prior to the first year of education, and yearly follow–up surveys were done for the next two years. The baseline surveys (S_1) took place in the fall of 1972. The first follow–up survey (S_2) took place in the fall of 1973, and the second follow–up (S_3) was conducted in the fall of 1974. Because such surveys could make the problem more salient to those being measured, thus producing some change by itself, an after–only sample was also made for the S_2 follow–up to measure possible reactivity.

At each survey period, subjects were asked to come into a survey center for a partial medical examination and interview to assess knowledge and attitude and behavior regarding cardiovascular disease risk factors. Demographic character-istics, sample sizes, and response rates for the total participant samples are shown in Table 1.

The medical examination included measures of plasma cholesterol and triglyceride concentrations, blood pressure, relative weight, electrocardiograms, and for a subsample, exercise stress tests. Methods for these measurements have been previously described (7). These data and data on self–reports of smoking were combined into a multiple logistic function of risk based on a procedure developed by Truett, Cornfield, and Kannel in the long–term Framingham study (22). This equation yields a prediction of the probability of a subject's developing coronary heart disease within 12 years.

The interview covered the subject's knowledge and attitudes and self–reported health habits about the risk factors and was developed and used to assess the participants' knowledge of the role of diet, smoking, physical activity, body weight, and general information about heart disease. Self–reports of smoking and smoking cessation were verified with the use of plasma–thiocyanate assays, which indicated only about 4% of those reporting abstinence may have given inaccurate reports (7).

The interview also included a diet history questionnaire, which was developed

TABLE 1. *Demographic Characteristics and Survey Response Rates in Each of Three Communities*

	Watsonville	Gilroy	Tracy
Entire town (1970 census)			
Population (total)	14,569	12,665	14,724
Population (age 35-59)	4,115	3,224	4,283
Mean age of 35-59 year			
old group (yr)	47.6	46.2	47.0
Male/female ratio of			
35-59 year old group	0.86	0.88	0.96
Random sample (age 35-59)			
Original sample	833	659	659
Natural attrition			
(migration or death)	107	79	74
Refusals and dropouts	303	183	201
Participants completing			
all 3 surveys	423	397	384
Percent of potential			
participants (original			
sample less natural			
attrition)	58.3	68.4	65.6
Characteristics of participants			
completing all 3 surveys			
Male/female ratio	0.75	0.78	0.84
Mean age at October,			
1972 (yr)	48.4	45.8	46.9
Spanish speaking (%)	7.8	· 8.3	3.1
Bilingual (%)	9.5	17.9	6.0

in consultation with a professional nutritionist and pretested in a survey conducted in 1971 in Modesto, California—a community similar to the other three. The diet history was designed to characterize the average or usual dietary behavior of the respondents; it concentrated on intake of cholesterol, saturated and polyunsaturated fat, refined sugars, and alcohol. Food models were used to assist in estimating portion sizes. The details of the development and validation of this questionnaire are presented in a prior publication (19).

Two other potentially useful measurements were not incorporated into this study. Although it would have been preferable to have used morbidity and mortality data as end points, resources could not be extended to the selection and monitoring of large enough cities for a sufficiently long period of time to make such analyses possible. In addition, a cost/benefit or cost/effectiveness type analysis would have required additional staff resources and in the end would not have been very meaningful given the prototypic nature of this project. It was decided to forego including such measurements and focus solely on whether or not predicted risk, behavior patterns, and knowledge could be influenced significantly with such an educational program.

Methods

Watsonville was selected to receive both the mass–media campaign and face–to–face intensive instruction and skills training applied to a subset of the surveyed sample. Accordingly, subjects surveyed in Watsonville were given risk scores based on their medical examinations using the multiple logistic of risk formula. The 25% scoring highest, stratified by age–decade, were designated as high–risk subjects. For comparison purposes, similar comparison groups were formed in Gilroy and Tracy, though they received no face–to–face instruction. Within Gilroy and Watsonville, these high–risk subjects had the same mass–media education program as the total sample population. Of the 117 individuals in Watsonville identified as high risk, two–thirds or 77 were randomly assigned to receive face–to–face delivery of behavioral skills training for reducing risk. The remaining third or 40 subjects were no–treatment controls, comparable to the Gilroy meda–only high–risk individuals. All high–risk subjects, including the no–treatment control subjects, were sent letters informing them of their high–risk status. Figure 2 shows the design and time sequence of the various treatment conditions and measurements for each community.

Using the baseline survey (S₁) to formulate campaign objectives, the *media campaign* consisted of public service announcements on radio and television, special programming on radio and television, newspaper columns by a physician and a dietician, direct mailings to individuals in the random sample (participants) of information booklets, cookbooks, and other materials, in both English and Spanish. Table 2 shows the media materials which were produced and used for the campaigns of 1973 and 1974. Altogether, about three hours of television programs and over 50 television spots were produced, as well as about 100 radio spots, several hours of radio programming, weekly newspaper columns, and newspaper advertisements and stories. Printed materials of many kinds were sent via direct mail to the participants, and posters were also used in buses, stores, and work sites. A skilled professional media staff, working with behavioral scientists and medical people as consultants, constantly monitored and revised the ongoing campaigns to adjust for information gain and progress toward achievement of goals.

The *intensive instruction* for skills training took the form of group meetings or at–home instruction. A pretest of the small group intervention for simultaneous modification of diet, weight, smoking, and exercise was designed and conducted in an industry group in a different community (16). The small–group intensive instruction conducted in Watsonville involved analysis of behavior patterns, modeling of new behavior patterns, guided practice in these, and the use of a token reward system. Groups of 12 to 15 persons and the therapists met in local church halls where everyone shared a heart–healthy meal prepared by the dietician, who instructed participants in its virtues and preparation. Participants were taught to use menu plans and to self–observe behavior related to diet and

	1972	1973		1974	1975	
Watsonville (W)	Baseline Survey (S1)	·Media campaign ·(C1) ·Intensive instruction (II) (2/3 of high risk participants)	Second Survey (S2)	·Media campaign (C2) ·Intensive instruction (II) Summer Followup	Third Survey (S3)	·Maintenance (low-level) Media campaign (C3)	Fourth Survey (S4)
Gilroy (G)	Baseline Survey (S1)	·Media campaign	Second Survey (S2)	·Media campaign	Third Survey (S3)	·Maintenance (low-level) Media campaign (C3)	Fourth Survey (S4)
Tracy (T)	Baseline Survey (S1)		Second Survey (S2)		Third Survey (S3)		Fourth Survey (S4)

Fig. 2. The design and sequence of the Stanford Three Community Study.

*Results for 1975 article are not reported in this article.

Table 2. Media Campaign

Media	C₁—1973		C₂—1974	
	English	Spanish	English	Spanish
TV Spots	26 spots 9 months 50-190 times/mo.	12 spots 9 months 20/100 times/mo.	9 spots 7 months 50/260 times/mo.	4 spots 7 months 20-150 times/mo.
TV Programs			Heart Health Test— 60 min. prime time	
Radio Spots	35 scripts to stations	20 scripts to stations 11 spots— Al Corazon	11 musical spots 3 mo. Christmas song	10 musical spots Christmas song
Radio Programs		Succesos— 17 dramas 5 min. 5 months	Sabor Y Salud 30 min. 5 mo. Twice weekly	
Direct Mail	Greeting card Heart of the matter Phone card Cooks Book Give Your Heart A L.	Greeting card Enfermedades D.C. Phone card Dieta Tradicional Dele Vuelo A Su C.	With love—45 rpm./ record. Take care of your heart calendar. Living with your heart	Con Todo C. 45 rpm. Cuide Su Corazon Calendar El Corazon C.C.
Newspaper Columns	31 Dr. Farquhar col. 29 cooking col.	27 Dr. Farquhar col.	19 Dr. Farquhar col.	19 Dr. Farquhar col. 16 Sabor Y Salud col.
Newspaper Ads	Dial A Heart Ads	Succesos Ads	H. Health Test ads.	Sabor Y Salud ads
Newspaper Other	Story on S₂	5 Fotonovella strps. Story on S₂	Story on S₃	Fotonovella insert Story on S₃
Billboards	3 boards 2 months	2 boards 2 months		
Bus Posters			7 posters 3 months	7 posters 3 months
Correspondence	Medical Notice Announcement S₂	Medical Notice Announcement S₂	Medical Notice Announcement S₃	Announcement S₃
Phone-A-Heart	11 Messages 4 mo.			
Other	Schools Kit	Schools Kit	Schools Film	Schools Film

smoking. Points were awarded individually and accumulated by each group according to weight loss, behavior change, and smoking cessation. Friendly competition between groups was encouraged to motivate individual changes. In the first campaign year (C_1) of 1973, intensive instruction consisted of a ten-week program of weekly and then twice-a-month sessions. Of the original 107, 63 took part in small-group meetings held at local churches. These sessions were led by individuals trained in behavior change methods and included the help of a dietician. At-home visits for the remaining 44 intensive-instruction participants were made by the behavior therapists.

The at-home intensive instruction involved training individuals to use menu plans and to analyze behavior patterns. For smokers, a therapist specially trained in smoking cessation techniques made extra calls. Positive reinforcement by the at-home counselor working on a one-to-one basis was an important aspect of this intervention. At-home counselors for Spanish-speaking individuals were themselves Spanish-speaking individuals trained in behavioral counseling techniques.

Of the 169 high-risk subjects identified in Watsonville, 113 were offered treatment originally and 56 were designated no-treatment controls. Of those offered treatment, 107 plus their spouses began treatment. Of these, 77 remained at the first follow-up survey (S_2), the balance having departed due to death, migration, or dropout.

The second campaign year (C_2) of 1974 utilized a somewhat different approach. Intensive at-home counseling for smoking cessation involved the use of aversive imagery and strong positive reinforcement by the therapist for cessation efforts. Guided participation in exercise was conducted, as were small-group sessions focusing on weight control and relaxation therapy. The intensive instruction efforts during C_2 did not reach as many people as those during C_1, partly because of attrition of subjects and partly as a result of designing a less ambitious instruction component intended primarily to facilitate maintenance.

Results

Altogether 12 partially overlapping comparison groups were formed for purposes of evaluation. In each of the three communities, groups of individuals were defined as "total participants," "high-risk subjects," and "after-only subjects" (these drawn only at S_2). Within the Watsonville high-risk group, two more groups were defined: "Intensive instruction subjects" or W-I.I., and "randomized controls" or W-R.C. For purposes of analysis, a twelfth group was constructed in order to provide a measure of the effects of mass media alone in Watsonville. This theoretical sample, which is called Watsonville "reconstituted"

Table 3. Composition of 12 Participant Groups
in Three Communities

	Total Participants	High Risk[a]	After Only (S₁)
Watsonville	423[b]		100
W-I.I.		77[c]	
W-R.C.		40[d]	
W-I.I. Spouses		34[f]	
W-R	423[e]		
Gilroy (G)	397	94	102
Tracy (T)	384	95	107

a. Participants in the baseline survey (S₁) whose examination results placed them in the top quartile of risk of cardiovascular disease, according to a multiple logistic function of risk.

b. Of the 423 total participants, 312 received all three surveys plus media campaign; 77 of the high-risk participants and their 34 spouses also received the intensive instruction program and are included within the total participant group.

c. Two thirds of high-risk group randomly assigned to receive intensive instruction.

d. One third of high-risk group randomly assigned not to receive intensive instruction. W-R.C. = Watsonville Randomized Control.

e. Weighted probability sample reconstituted to the original total participant group with I.I. group replaced by an expanded media-only high-risk group. W-R-Watsonville Reconstituted.

f. Spouses of W-I.I. included in treatment.

or W-R, was created as follows: The intensively instructed, high-risk individuals and the intensively instructed nonhigh-risk spouses were removed from the Watsonville sample, and the sex-specific data from the remaining high-risk and nonhigh-risk individuals were weighted; the former in proportion to the ratio of the total number of high-risk individuals originally present in the sample to the number of high-risk intensive instructees removed, and the latter in proportion to the ratio of the total number of nonhigh-risk individuals originally present in the sample to the number of nonhigh-risk intensively instructed spouses removed. The ratio of high- to nonhigh-risk subjects in the sample was thus preserved, while the effects of intensive instruction were removed. The composition of these 12 groups is shown in Table 3.

Figure 3 shows the percentage change in selected variables after two years. The After-Only and Watsonville Intensive-Instruction-Spouses (W-I.I. Spouses) groups are not included. Baseline values (not shown), were remarkably uniform

Table 4. Changes from Baseline in Egg Consumption per Day After One and Two Years of Risk-Reduction Campaign.

	Total Community Participant Samples*			
	T	G	W-R	W
Baseline mean:†	0.76	0.84	0.79	0.78
Percentage change				
Year 1	-14.9	-27.5‡	-37.1‡	-41.8‡§
Year 2	-15.9	-33.3‡	-42.2‡	-44.4‡

	High-Risk Participant Samples*			
	T	G	W-RC	W-II
Baseline mean:†	0.88	0.93	0.74	0.70
Percentage change				
Year 1	-15.7	-34.5‡	-43.3‡	-61.9‡
Year 2	-19.3	-24.5	-49.3‡	-60.3‡

*See Table 3 for definitions of participant samples.
†Baseline mean is expressed as the number of eggs consumed per day.
‡Indicates a statistically significant difference ($p < 0.05$) for percent change values at Tracy (control) versus Gilroy, or versus Watsonville, study groups. Total participant groups (upper table) are compared with Tracy total participants as control; high-risk groups (lower table) are compared with Tracy high-risk participants as control. A one-trailed test was used to compare percent change values.

§Indicates a statistically significant difference ($p < 0.05$) for percent change values at Gilroy versus Watsonville total participants, or versus the Watsonville reconstituted groups (upper table).

||Indicates a statistically significant difference ($p < 0.05$) for percent change values for Watsonville intensive-instruction group (W-I.I.) versus Watsonville randomized control (W-RC) (lower table).

between groups. After two years of the intervention campaign, both treatment conditions, media–only (G and WR) and media plus face–to–face intensive instruction (W-I.I.), had significant positive effects on all variables except relative weight. Only the Watsonville Intensive Instruction (W-I.I.) group showed significantly lower relative weight at the end of the first year. For all other individual variables, there were slight–to–moderate changes in the expected direction. Incorporating cigarette use, plasma–cholesterol, and systolic blood pressure into the formula for the multiple logistic function of risk, the net difference in estimated total risk between control and treatment samples was 23–30%. A large part of this difference can be attributed to individuals achieving changes in plasma–cholesterol and blood pressure. Watsonville Intensive-Instruction subjects showed increased knowledge gain and significant reduction

PERCENT CHANGE FROM BASELINE
AFTER 2 YEARS

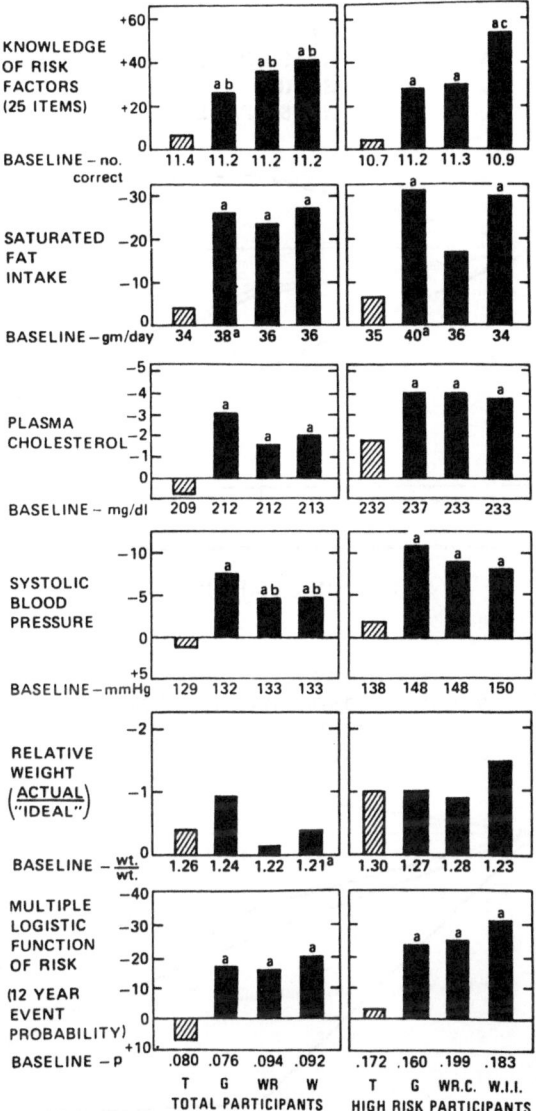

Fig. 3. Absolute baseline values and percentage change in selected variables after two years in control (shaded) or treatment (dark) groups.

See Table 3 for definition of groups. a = p < 0.05 for baseline or differences in percentage change of control versus treatment. b = p < 0.05 for differences in percentage change within treatment G versus W (total) or WR. c = p < 0.05 for differences in percentage change within treatment W–R.C. versus W–I.I.

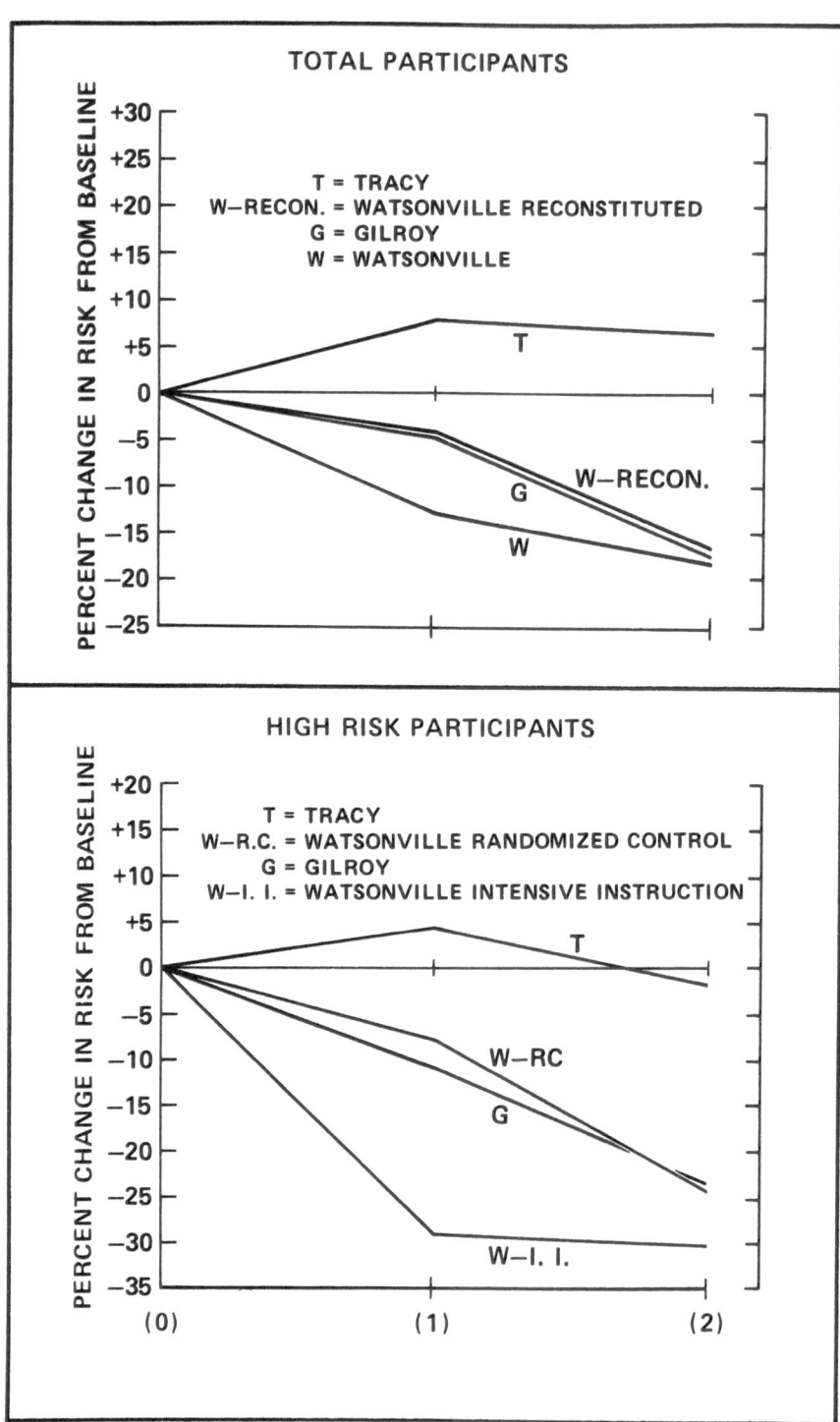

Fig. 4. Percentage change from baseline (0) in risk of coronary heart–disease after 1 and 2 years of health education among participants from three communities.

Groups are defined in Table 2. Cardiovascular risk is measured by a multiple logistic function of risk factors.

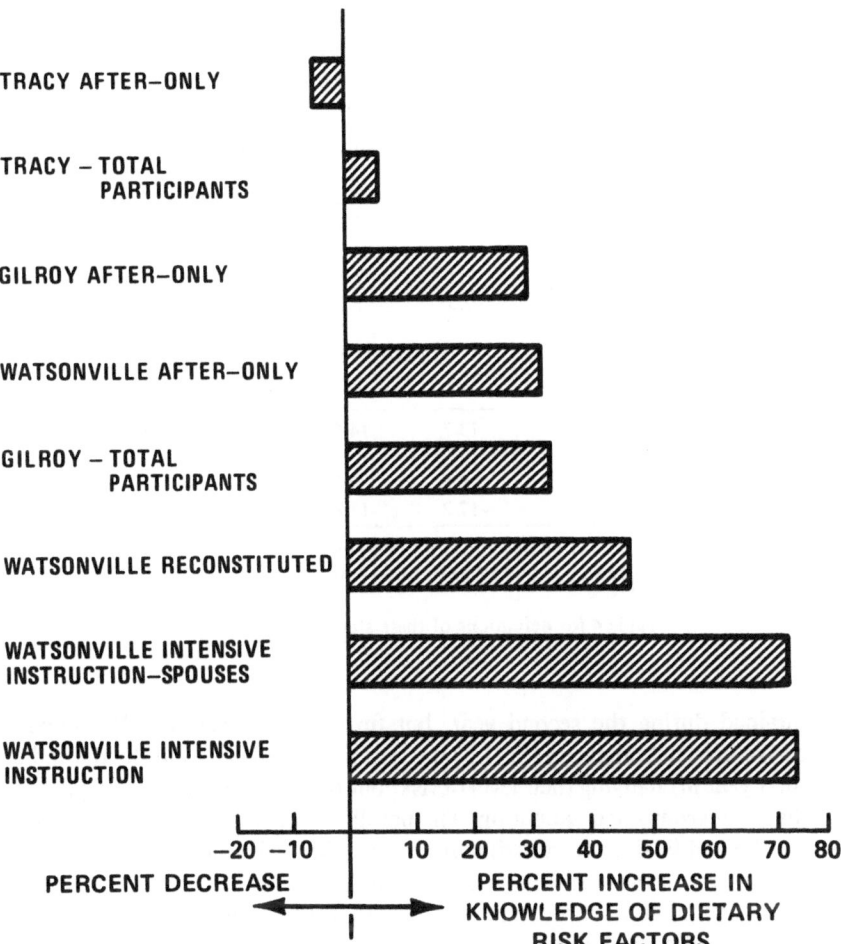

Fig. 5. Percentage of change from the first to the second survey in participants' knowledge about dietary risk factors. The groups are ranked according to an estimation of the increasing intensity of the educational input. Groups are defined in Table 3.

of smoking over other comparison groups. Blood pressure changes were probably the result of interaction between weight loss, salt restriction, and better adherence to antihypertensive medications, the latter being an unintended consequence of exposure to the campaign intervention (7).

Changes in cardiovascular risk scores for the various comparison groups are shown in Figure 4. Changes made by the end of the first year were not only

**Table 5. Changes from Baseline in the Number
of Cigarettes Smoked per Day After One
and Two Years of Risk-Reduction Campaign**

	Total Community Participant Samples*			
	T	G	W-R	W
Baseline mean:†	6.9	6.8	6.8	7.2
Percentage change				
Year 1	-1.1	-2.3	-6.9	-18.9**
Year 2	-2.5	-7.3	-13.7**	-24.1**

	High-Risk Participant Samples*			
	T	G	W-RC	W-II
Baseline mean:†	13.7	14.6	14.2	14.4
Percentage change				
Year 1	-8.5	-9.8	-5.8	-36.3**
Year 2	-17.2	-13.8	-15.1	-42.3**

*See Table 3 for definitions of participant samples.
†Baseline mean is expressed as the total number of cigarettes smoked per day.
**See Table 4 for definitions of these statistical symbols.

maintained during the second year, but further improved. The Watsonville Intensive–Instruction group (W–I.I.) did better than other groups by the end of the first year in changing their level of risk, but by the end of the second year the media–only groups had caught up. The parallel relation of the two media–only groups (G and W–Reconstituted) indicates that the media campaigns had similar effects on risk in the two treatment communities.

Closer examination of measures indicates that the various comparison groups can be ranked according to the intensity of treatment received. As predicted, there appeared to be some effect resulting from surveying, and the cohorts followed did show some improvement over the after–only samples. Figure 5 shows that knowledge about risk factors changed relative to the intensity of treatment, with Tracy After–Only showing decrease from baseline in knowledge and Watsonville Intensive–Instruction (W–I.I.) showing the most increase in knowledge.

Changes in dietary and plasma lipids is presented elsewhere (19), and these substantiate the self–report measures of egg consumption shown in Table 4. The yolks of eggs are very high in cholesterol, and curtailment of their consumption was an important part of the campagin. Although Table 4 indicates that there is a significant secular trend operating in the nonintervention community as well, reductions in the number of eggs eaten are very much greater in the intervention groups.

Likewise, Table 5 shows that the Watsonville Intensive–Instruction group achieved a substantial reduction in the mean number of cigarettes smoked per day compared with the nonintervention community. This difference is maintained the second year.

Finally, Figure 6 presents the results of an analysis of the interrelationship between changes in total risk based on medical factors, changes in knowledge of risk factors, and changes in behavior at the end of two years for the various comparison groups. Apparently the more the participants learned, the more they changed their behavior, and thus their physiological risk of disease decreased. Only the no–treatment control group (T) increased in risk, and they showed essentially no changes in knowledge or behavior. At the other extreme, the greatest reduction in risk, a decrease of 30%, occurred in the Watsonville Intensive–Instruction cohort. Other groups changed within the midrange on these dimensions. It is interesting that spouses of the high–risk participants who received intensive instruction achieved less behavior change, although they showed a comparable knowledge gain. This suggests that having been identified as being at high risk is an important motivator for changing behavior.

SUMMARY AND DISCUSSION

In 1972 the Stanford Heart Disease Prevention Program launched a heart disease prevention education campaign in three communities in California. With this Three Community Study considerable success was achieved in changing selected risk–factor related behaviors of people living in relatively small communities. This was accomplished by using mass media alone in one town, Gilroy, and by using the same mass media in the other town, Watsonville, in combination with a program of face–to–face intensive instruction.

Despite some reservations and shortcomings, the results provide support for both approaches to behavior change, but also suggest the need for improved methods to achieve change in some risk areas and ways of making such improvements. Finding that a community–based field application of mediated and face–to–face instruction in beneficial health habits can affect knowledge and behavior, when these methods were used to teach specific behavioral skills and not merely to exhort, is encouraging. Ways were discovered to assist some individuals in small groups to make recommended changes in certain risk–related behaviors, e.g., smoking and diet, but did not achieve long–term change in others, e.g., weight control and exercise habits. Some highly cost– and effort–effective means of obtaining these effects were developed in some

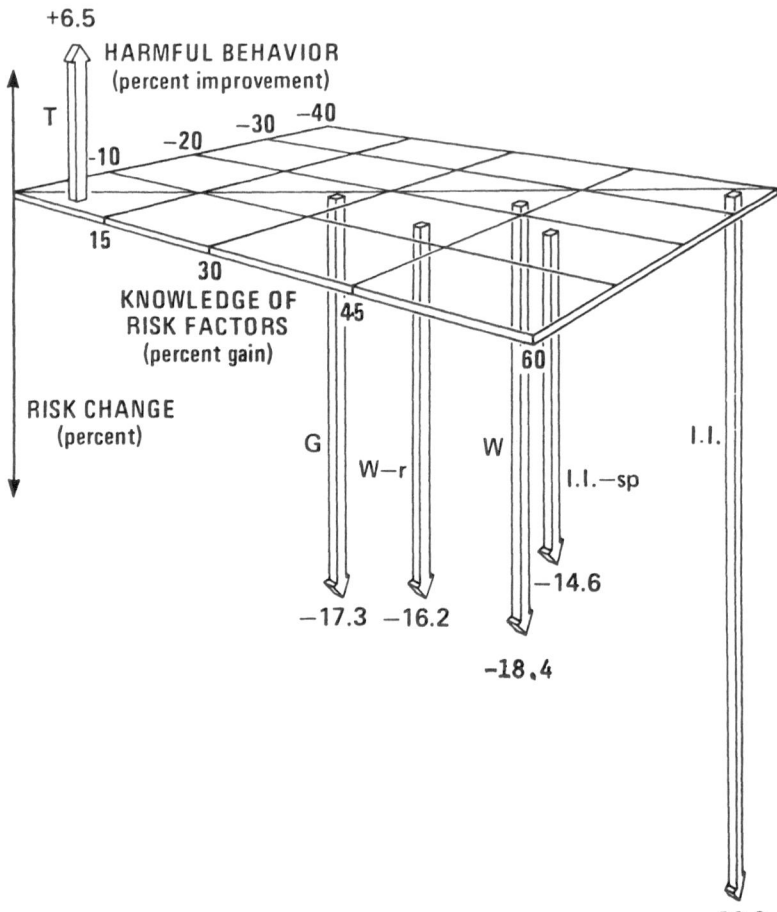

Fig. 6. Relationship between changes in knowledge, behavior, and risk at the end of the two years of health education in various study groups. The groups are defined in Table 3. Harmful behavior is a composite of dietary intake of saturated fat and cholesterol and of smoking; dietary and smoking behavior were given equal weight. Knowledge of risk factors is derived from the 25–item questionnaire. Cardiovascular risk is measured by a multiple logistic function of risk factors; figures on the vertical axis represent the percentage of change in risk (T = Tracy total participants; G = Gilroy total participants; W = Watsonville total participants; W–R = Watsonville reconstituted sample; W–I.I. = intensive instruction group at Watsonville; I.I.-spouses = spouses of intensive instructees in Watsonville).

instances, e.g., diet, and other effects, e.g., smoking reduction, were achieved only through relatively cost– and effort–intensive means.

It is important to note that beneficial changes in risk factors that might be considered to be of relatively minor degree individually can, when entered into the multiple logistic function of risk, add up to a sizable reduction in overall cardiovascular risk. The results provide evidence that behavior change for better health can indeed be accomplished through sustained community–based education, but the optimal strategy for conducting that education has only just begun to be defined.

IMPLICATIONS FOR FUTURE INTERVENTIONS

The Three Community Study together with continued research has suggested ways that should enhance the ability of individuals to make the kind of lasting changes in their behavior that will lead to meaningful risk reduction. Future interventions into whole communities should seek a behavior–oriented risk reduction program that employs a mix of techniques for delivering health education to large general populations in an economical way. Methods must be developed that would provide guidance and validation for more cost- and effort–effective ways than the face–to–face instruction and media combination used in the Three Community Study.

The relative success of mediated methods for promoting habits conducive to health opens an avenue toward cost–effectiveness which would not be utilized if health education were applied only through the more restricted avenues currently in use by established health professionals. It is nevertheless germane to inquire whether the present environments of medical offices and hospitals and clinics can improve their ability to deliver risk reduction through mediated methods of instruction. It seems reasonable that carefully planned treatment programs that rely (almost entirely) on the mediated instruction can result in significant changes in risk factors that are maintained over long periods of time.

In order to achieve maximum risk reduction, future interventions should use both mediated methods as well as group process, face–to–face communication, and the networks of interpersonal influence within communities. The campaign created to produce change should achieve a synergistic relationship among all of the intervention components. The power of the mass media, with its potential for social action and change, should be linked at the individual level through a group process. The judicious combination of the mass–media campaign with the utilization of existing community groups, enhanced by a process of feedback from ongoing interviewing and on the basis of information obtained from formative laboratory evaluation, will allow continuous modification of intervention tactics from both the field and the laboratory. This will yield even greater and more lasting changes in risk reduction than was the case for the Three Community Study.

ACKNOWLEDGMENTS

Dr. Nash was a postdoctoral fellow with the Stanford Heart Disease Prevention Program, Stanford University. Dr. Farquhar is Professor of Medicine, Stanford University, and Director, Stanford Heart Disease Prevention Program. Others participating in the Three Community Study included Nathan Maccoby, Peter D. Wood, Janet K. Alexander, Henry Breitrose, Byron W. Brown, Jr., William L. Haskell, Alfred L. McAlister, Anthony J. Meyer, and Michael P. Stern. This research was supported by grant HL-14174 to the Stanford Specialized Center for Research in Arteriosclerosis and contract NIH-71-2151-L to the Stanford Lipid Research Clinic from the National Heart, Lung, and Blood Institute.

REFERENCES

1. American Heart Association. Report of inter-society commission for heart disease resources: Primary prevention of the atherosclerotic diseases. *Circulation*, vol. 42, December 1970.

2. Bandura, A. *Principles of Behavior Modification*. New York: Holt, Rinehart and Winston, 1969.

3. Blackburn, H. Progress in the epidemiology and prevention of coronary heart disease, in P. Yu and J. Goodwin (eds.), *Progress in Cardiology*. Philadelphia: Lea and Febiger, 1974, pp. 1-36.

4. Campbell, D.T., and Stanley, J.C. *Experimental and Quasi-experimental Designs for Research*. Chicago: Rand McNally and Company, 1963.

5. Department of Health, Education and Welfare, Public Health Service: *Forward Plan for Health, FY 1978-82*. DHEW Pub. No. (OS) 76-50046, Washington, D.C.; Stock No. 017-000-00172-8, 1976.

6. Department of Health, Education and Welfare, Public health Service: *Forward Plan for Health, FY 1977-81*. DHEW Pub. No. (OS) 76-50024, Washington, D.C.; Stock No. 017-000-00153-1, 1975.

7. Farquhar, J.W., Maccoby, N., Wood, P.D., et al. Community education for cardiovascular health. *Lancet* 1:1192-1195, June 4, 1977.

8. Fox, S.M., and Haskell, W.L. Physical activity and the prevention of coronary heart disease. *Bulletin of the New York Academy of Medicine*, vol. 44, 1968, pp. 950-967.

9. Griffiths, W., and Knutson, A.L. *The Role of Mass Media in Public Health*. American Journal of Public Health, Vol. 50, No. 4, pp. 515-523, 1960.

10. Hingson, R. Obtaining optimal attendance at mass immunization programs. *Health Services Reports*, vol. 89, no. 1, pp. 53-64, 1974.

11. Jenkins, C.D. Recent evidence supporting psychologic and social risk factors for coronary disease: Parts I and II. *N. Engl. J. Med.* 294:987-994, 1033-1038, 1976.

12. Jenkins, C.D. Psychologic and social precursors of coronary disease. *N. Engl. J. Med.* 284:244-255, 307-317, 1971.

13. Maccoby, N., and Farquhar, J.W. Communication for health: Unselling heart disease. *Journal of Comm.* 23(3):114-126, 1975.

14. McAlister, A.L., Farquhar, J.W., Thoresen, C.E., and Maccoby, N. Behavioral science

applied to cardiovascular health: Progress and research needs in the modification of risk-taking habits in adult populations. *Health Education Monographs* 4(1):45-74, 1976.

15. Mendelsohn, H. Which shall it be: Mass education or mass persuasion for health. *Am. J. Public Health* 58:131-137, 1968.

16. Meyer, A.J., and Henderson, J.B. Multiple risk factor reduction in the prevention of cardiovascular disease. *Prevent. Med.* 3:225-236, 1974.

17. Robinson, J.P. Toward defining the functions of television, in E. Rubenstein et al. (eds.), *Television and Social Behavior,* vol. IV, DHEW, 1972.

18. Stamler, J. Epidemiology of coronary heart disease. *Medical Clinics of North America* 57:5-46, 1973.

19. Stern, M.P., Farquhar, J.W., Maccoby, N., and Russell, S.H. Results of a two-year health education campaign on dietary behavior: The Stanford three community study. *Circulation* 54(5):826-833, 1976.

20. Swinehart, J.W. Voluntary exposure to health communications. *Am. J. Public Health* 58(7):1265-1275, 1968.

21. Task Force on Arteriosclerosis, National Heart and Lung Institute: *Arteriosclerosis,* DHEW Pub. No. (NIH) 72-137, Washington, D.C.; Stock No. 1743-0005, Vol. 1, June 1971.

22. Truett, J., Cornfield, J. and Kannel, W. Multivariate analysis of the risk of coronary heart disease in Framingham. *Journal of Chronic Disease,* Vol. 20, p. 511, 1967.

23. *World Health Statistics Annual, 1967,* Vol. 1, Vital Statistics and Causes of Death, World Health Organization, 1970.

Index